DEFENSE, SECURITY AND STRATEGY SERIES

VETERANS' BENEFITS AND CARE

DEFENSE, SECURITY AND STRATEGY SERIES

Military Satellites: Issues, Goals and Challenges
Abel Chirila (Editor)
2009. ISBN: 978-1-60741-238-0

Evaluating Military Compensation
Jaime G. Duenas (Editor)
2009. ISBN: 978-1-60741-476-6

The Army's Future Combat System Program
Christian N. Feliciano (Editor)
2009. ISBN: 978-1-60741-262-5

Strategizing Resilience and Reducing Vulnerability
Peter R. J. Trim and Jack Caravelli (Editors)
2009. ISBN: 978-1-60741-693-7

Counterinsurgency and the Armed Forces
Laure Paquette
2009. ISBN: 978-1-60741-763-7

U.S. Nuclear Stockpile: Maintenance and Replacement of Warheads
Robin A. Kraemer (Editor)
2010. ISBN: 978-1-60741-483-4

Security in Iraq
James L. Jones, Jennifer K. Elsea, and Nina M. Serafino (Editors)
2010. ISBN: 978-1-60692-127-2

War in Afghanistan: Strategy, Military Operations and Congressional Issues
Easton H. Ussery (Editor)
2010. ISBN: 978-1-60741-579-4

Border Security and Who is Responsible for it
Nevio Graziano (Editor)
2010. ISBN: 978-1-60741-804-7

Misleading Information from the Battlefield
Gene P. Stewart (Editor)
2010. ISBN: 978-1-60741-110-9

National Defense, Security, and Strategy
Norman P. Geise (Editor)
2010. ISBN: 978-1-60692-347-4

National Security Initiatives
Vivian B. Hickey (Editor)
2010. ISBN: 978-1-60692-354-2

Veterans' Benefits and Care
Mathew H. Bradley (Editor)
2010. ISBN: 978-1-60692-500-3

DEFENSE, SECURITY AND STRATEGY SERIES

VETERANS' BENEFITS AND CARE

MATHEW H. BRADLEY
EDITOR

Nova Science Publishers, Inc.

New York

LIBRARY OF CONGRESS CATALOGING-IN-PUBLICATION DATA

Veterans' benefits and care / editor, Mathew H. Bradley.
p. cm.
Includes index.
ISBN 978-1-60692-500-3 (hardcover)
1. Veterans--Services for--United States. 2. Veterans--Legal status, laws, etc.--United States. 3. United States. Dept. of Veterans Affairs. 4. Veterans--Medical care--United States. 5. Disabled veterans--Medical care--United States. 6. Military pensions--United States. 7. Veterans--Education--United States. I. Bradley, Mathew H.
UB357.V385 2009
362.860973--dc22

2009038424

Published by Nova Science Publishers, Inc. † New York

CONTENTS

PREFACE

The Department of Veterans Affairs (VA) provides services and benefits to veterans who meet certain eligibility criteria. Benefits to veterans range from disability compensation and pensions to hospital and medical care. Furthermore, veterans' education benefits have evolved substantially over the last 60-plus years. This book reviews the two disability programs administered by the VA, one of which is called the Disability Compensation, and the other which is known as a Disability pension. The authors of this book discuss the eligibility criteria and the fundamentals of these VA-administered disability benefit programs and related issues. The evolution of veterans' education benefit programs are also examined and the types of education benefits made available under these programs are described. Furthermore, the VA administers several pension benefit programs for the surviving spouses and dependent children of veterans. This book describes these programs, including the eligibility criteria and current benefit levels. Other chapters in this book examine the provisions of the National Defense Authorization Act, reflecting the congressional concern about the quality and availability of medical, mental health and dental care services for service members returning from active duty in Iraq and Afghanistan. It is well-known that veterans have a number of risk factors that increase their chance of attempting suicide. This book discusses suicide prevention efforts by the VA.

This book consists of public documents which have been located, gathered, combined, reformatted, and enhanced with a subject index, selectively edited and bound to provide easy access.

Chapter 1 - The Department of Veterans Affairs (VA) provides benefits to veterans who meet certain eligibility rules. Benefits to veterans range from disability compensation and pensions to hospital and medical care. The VA provides these benefits through three major operating units: the Veterans Health Administration (VHA), the Veterans Benefits Administration (VBA), and the National Cemetery Administration (NCA). The VHA is primarily a direct service provider of primary care, specialized care, and related medical and social support services to veterans through the nation's largest integrated health-care system.

On February 4, 2008, the President submitted his FY2009 budget proposal to Congress. The Administration is requesting a total of $39.2 billion (excluding collections) for VHA. This is a 5.3% increase (or $2.0 billion) over the FY2008 enacted level. Including total available resources (including medical collections) the Administration's budget would provide $41.1 billion for VHA.

On March 7, 2008, the House (H.Con.Res. 312) and Senate (S.Con.Res. 70) reported its respective budget resolutions. After negotiations between the House and Senate, the House agreed to an amended version of S.Con.Res. 70 (Conference Report; H.Rept. 110-659). The conference agreement provides $48.2 billion for FY2009 for discretionary veterans' programs, including medical care, and provides $45.1 billion in mandatory funding for veterans programs.

On June 24, the House Appropriations Committee marked up the Military Construction and Veterans Affairs Appropriations bill (H.R. 6599; H.Rept. 110-775) for FY2009. The House Appropriations Committee recommended $40.8 billion (excluding collections) for VHA, a $1.6 billion increase over the Administration's FY2009 request and $3.6 billion over the FY2008 enacted amount.

On July 17, 2008, the Senate Appropriations Committee marked up its version of the FY2009 Military Construction and Veterans Affairs and Related Agencies Appropriations bill (S. 3301; S.Rept. 110-428). The Senate Appropriations Committee recommended $41.1 billion (excluding collections) for VHA for FY2009. This is a 4.8% increase over the FY2009 request, and $294 million above the House Appropriations Committee-recommended amount.

H.R. 6599 and S. 3301 *did not* include any bill language authorizing fee increases as requested by the Administration's budget proposal for the VHA for FY2009. The House and Senate Committees are directing the VA to increase Priority Group 8 enrollment in FY2009, and have provided additional funding to accomplish this. With escalating gasoline prices, the House and Senate Appropriations Committees have also included report language to increase the mileage reimbursement rate, and has provided additional funding in their respective bills for this purpose.

This chapter will track the FY2009 appropriations process, and will be updated as legislative activities warrant.

Chapter 2 - Congress, through the United States Department of Veterans Affairs (VA), provides a variety of benefits and services to veterans and to certain members of their families. These benefits range from health care and related services to burial benefits. The veteran's basic eligibility for these programs and services is usually determined by the local VA office. Veterans not satisfied with the VA's decision(s) may wish to have them reviewed and may appeal the decision(s). This chapter traces the various steps involved in the appeal process — starting with the original application for benefits and concluding with an appeal to the U.S. Supreme Court. A flow chart outlining all of the steps in the appeal process is provided.

Following the filing of the initial appeal, the local VA office will either allow or disallow the claim. If the veteran/claimant wishes to appeal, a written request for appeal must be filed and various time deadlines and other requirements must be met prior to the case being considered by the Board of Veterans' Appeals (BVA). The appeal before the BVA may be a hearing at the local VA office by a traveling Board member; a hearing at the BVA office in Washington, DC; or a videoconference hearing at the local VA office. Various filing requirements and time limits must be met by the veteran/claimant in his/her appeal. There are specific guidelines for a person representing a veteran before the BVA. Legislation enacted in the 109th Congress changed traditional guidelines to allow for legal representation for veterans throughout the administrative appeals process.

The veteran/claimant may appeal the decision of the BVA to the Court of Appeals for Veterans Claims (CAVC), which is an independent federal court and not part of the VA. The decision of the CAVC may be appealed by either the veteran/claimant or the VA to the U.S. Court of Appeals for the Federal Circuit (Federal Circuit), an Article III court that sits in Washington, DC and has exclusive jurisdiction to hear cases challenging CAVC rulings. Decisions of the Federal Circuit may be appealed to the U.S. Supreme Court, which has final jurisdiction.

The VA has various statutory obligations to assist the veteran in the preparation of his/her application for benefits and any subsequent appeal(s). Among these obligations are assistance in the preparation of the initial application; provision of various records; medical exams; and other related issues. Certain legal and factual presumptions are established by statute that may be favorable to the veteran's claim. These issues are examined in the appendix to this chapter.

Legislation introduced in the 110th Congress concerning the appeal process is summarized in the appendix. These bills are H.R. 67, H.R. 653, H.R. 797, H.R. 1435, H.R. 1444, H.R. 1490, H.R. 1538, H.R. 2257, H.R. 2855, H.R. 3047, H.R. 5089, S. 1283, S. 1363, and S. 2737. H.R. 1318 is also discussed. One of the bills, H.R. 797, has been enacted into law (P.L. 110-157).

Chapter 3 - Federal educational assistance programs have been authorized for veterans of the Armed Forces since 1944. The Servicemen's Readjustment Act of 1944 (P.L. 78-346), or the GI Bill of Rights, provided support, including education benefits, to veterans of World War II. Subsequently, other programs were implemented for similar purposes (e.g., the Korean GI Bill and the Vietnam Era GI Bill). These new programs were primarily, if not exclusively, funded by the federal government and were intended to support veterans returning from war. The implementation of the Post-Vietnam Era Veterans' Educational Assistance Program (VEAP) marked the first time that an educational benefit had been established during peacetime and for anall-volunteerforce; the first time that education benefits wereviewedasamilitary recruiting tool; and the first time that servicemembers were required to make a contribution toward their veterans' education benefits. Many of the principles of VEAP were carried over during the creation of its successor program, the Montgomery GI Bill (MGIB), which was implemented in 1985.

Veterans' education benefits have evolved substantially over the last 60-plus years. When first established, veterans' education benefits were completely subsidized by the federal government; payments were issued to educational institutions on behalf of the veteran; they could be used for avarietyof education and training programs; and separate subsistence payments were also provided. Currently, veterans' education benefits are partially subsidized; they are paid directly to the veteran; and they may be used to pay tuition, fees and expenses associated with a variety of education and training programs.

During the period since veterans' education benefits first were made available, college prices have increased substantially. In addition, the manner in which federal student financial aid is calculated and awarded has shifted several times during the evolution of the veterans' education benefits programs. At present, federal student assistance is calculated according to the federal need analysis system, which considers the receipt of veterans' education benefits when determining eligibility for some student aid programs. These policy and program changes have altered the role that veterans' education benefits play in supporting access to postsecondary education for veterans.

This chapter reviews the evolution of veterans' education benefit programs and describes the types of education benefits that have been made available under these programs. It also examines how changes in the estimated value of these benefits compares with changes in average college prices, and provides a discussion of the interaction between veterans' education benefits and federal student aid benefits made available under Title IV of the Higher Education Act of 1965 (HEA), as amended.

Chapter 4 - The military Survivor Benefit Plan (SBP) was created in 1972. Since its creation, it has been subjected to a number of substantial legislative changes. This chapter describes the basic provisions of the military Survivor Benefit Plan and all relevant changes or modifications that have occurred.

Specifically, the military Survivor Benefit Plan is described and explained in terms of its eligibility provisions, costs, benefits, and its integration with other federal programs (including social security and Veterans' Administration Dependency and Indemnity Compensation) for members and retirees of active duty military service and the Reserve Components (both the reserves and National Guard). In addition, tables and work sheets are provided to assist the reader in computing the costs and benefits available under this program.

Nearly every Congress since 1972 has, in some way, modified the provisions of the military Survivor Benefit Plan. These modifications have had a significant effect on current and prospective participants and beneficiaries. In nearly every instance, these changes have made the SBP more generous. Furthermore, these modifications involve complex issues and processes, and are, therefore, a source of numerous requests for information from constituents to their congressional representatives.

Chapter 5 - Congress provides various benefits to American veterans and their dependents through the United States Department of Veterans Affairs (VA). One of these benefits is *disability compensation*, which is a monthly cash benefit program for veterans currently impaired from past service-connected activities.

A claim for disability compensation is initially analyzed by the VA at the local level to determine: 1) whether the claimant is considered a "veteran" (eligible for benefits); 2) whether the veteran qualifies for disability compensation (entitled to benefits); 3) the extent of the impairment and the "rate" of the disability; and 4) the effective date for the compensation.

Three requirements to qualify for disability compensation are: 1) medical diagnosis of the current impairment; 2) evidence of an in-service occurrence or an aggravation of the disease or injury; and 3) medical proof of a connection between the in-service incident or aggravation of an injury or illness and the current disability. The requisite standard of proof and certain medical presumptions are set by statute. The VA is required to provide assistance to the veteran in his/her case preparation by providing records and medical examinations. Special rules have been established for certain specific situations involving combat veterans, prisoners of war, and veterans exposed to Agent Orange.

If the veteran is found eligible for disability compensation, the VA then uses the Schedule for Rating Disabilities (SRD) to set the amount of earnings impairment on a percentage basis; the higher the percentage, the greater the compensation will be. Certain complications arise with the use of the rating system. A veteran's rating may be increased or decreased over time — depending on his/her medical condition. Rating decisions may be appealed administratively.

Legislation passed in the First Session of the 110th Congress increased the 2008 monthly disability compensation payments. Other legislation has been introduced that would provide veterans a cost-of-living (COLA) for their VA benefits equal to the COLA for Social Security benefits. The 110th Congress has considered additional legislation that may affect service-connected disabilities. One bill would change the manner in which disabled veterans could qualify to receive Social Security Disability Insurance (SSDI) benefits. Several bills have been introduced to deal with the claims processing backlog at the VA and issues related to the receipt of disability benefits.

Chapter 6 - On February 18, 2007, the *Washington Post* published the first in a series of articles describing problems with outpatient medical care and other services provided at the Walter Reed Army Medical Center (WRAMC). The series noted, among other things, concerns about the processes used to evaluate disability in injured military servicemembers. Both the Department of Defense (DOD) and the Department of Veterans Affairs (VA) conduct disability evaluations and assign disability ratings to servicemembers or veterans under their respective authorities. An individual's disability rating, from either department, affects the scope of pay and benefits for which he or she is eligible, and the cost to the respective department of providing such benefits.

There are significant differences between the disability evaluations performed by DOD and VA, as well as civilian disability evaluations conducted by the Social Security Administration (SSA) and workers' compensation programs. Most notably, the DOD disability evaluation is focused on the effect of any disabling condition on the performance of the servicemember's duties in the military, while the other three systems evaluate the impact of a disability on gainful employment in the civilian economy.

Congress has followed recent news reports with interest, and several legislative initiatives are under consideration. For example, H.R. 1538, the Wounded Warrior Assistance Act of 2007, passed unanimously in the House on March 28, 2007. The bill includes numerous provisions to improve or streamline medical care and benefits processing for returning injured servicemembers. Title XVI of the National Defense Authorization Act for FY2008 (H.R. 4986, P.L. 110-181), contains Wounded Warrior provisions related to the care and transition of injured servicemembers.

This chapter is intended as a primer to describe disability evaluation in general, including evaluations used by DOD and VA, as well as civilian evaluations used by the SSA and by workers' compensation programs. Next, the DOD and VA disability rating processes are described, respectively, in greater detail. Finally, recent congressional and executive actions and recommendations regarding DOD and VA disability evaluations are described. This chapter emphasizes the disability evaluation systems at DOD and VA, with illustrative comparisons made to civilian systems when appropriate. It will be updated as warranted.

Chapter 7 - A broad range of benefits is offered to American veterans and to certain members of their families by the United States Department of Veterans Affairs (VA). Among these benefits are various types of financial benefits and assistance — which include disability compensation and pensions.

The VA administers two disability programs. These programs pay monthly cash benefits to disabled veterans. *Disability compensation* provides a monthly benefit if the veteran is disabled as a result of his/her military service. Disability compensation relates specifically to a disability which directly resulted from military service. A *disability pension* is paid to a wartime veteran if the veteran has limited income, is no longer able to work, or is age 65 or older. The pension is not related to a service-connected injury or medical condition. Award of the pension takes into consideration the material needs of the veteran (i.e., it is a "needs-based" pension).

There is no deadline or time limit for applying for disability benefits. A veteran cannot simultaneously receive both disability compensation and a disability pension. There are certain basic criteria which must be met in order to be eligible to receive either of these benefits.

This chapter examines the eligibility criteria and the fundamentals of the VA-administered disability benefit programs and related issues.

Chapter 8 - The Department of Veterans Affairs (VA) administers several pension benefit programs for veterans as well as their surviving spouses and dependent children. The most current pension programs available (for those meeting the eligibility criteria on or after January 1, 1979) are the Improved Disability Pension for certain low-income veterans and the Improved Death Pension for certain low-income surviving spouses or children of veterans. There is also a special pension for Medal of Honor recipients. This chapter describes these programs, including the eligibility criteria and current benefit levels. This chapter will be updated as needed to reflect legislative activity and changes to benefits or eligibility requirements.

Chapter 9 - The Civilian Health and Medical Program of the Department of Veterans Affairs (CHAMPVA) is primarily a fee-for-service program that provides reimbursement for most medical care for certain eligible dependents and survivors of veterans rated permanently and totally disabled from a service-connected condition. This chapter provides an overview of CHAMPVA and includes a series of questions and answers about the program. The report will be updated as legislative or programmatic changes warrant.

Chapter 10 - This chapter summarizes provisions in Division A, Titles XVI and XVII, of the National Defense Authorization Act for Fiscal Year 2008, P.L. 110-181, signed by the President on January 28, 2008. Titles XVI and XVII address matters related to the care and treatment of servicemembers and former servicemembers (i.e., veterans) who were wounded, or who contracted an illness, while serving on active duty. These individuals are widely referred to as "wounded warriors."

Provisions in the act reflect congressional concern about the quality and availability of medical, mental health, and dental care services for servicemembers returning from active duty in Iraq and Afghanistan, and the difficulties that some of theseindividuals haveexperiencedin their transition from military service to veteran status. The provisions vary in scope. Some of them alter specific aspects of existing services or benefits programs in either the Department of Defense (DOD) or the Department of Veterans Affairs (VA). Others call for comprehensive and long-term redesign of programs or systems in one or both of the departments. Congress and others have determined that certain programs and systems that involve both departments are particularly problematic in providing continuity and quality of care and services to wounded warriors. Among the problems addressed in the act are the efficient maintenance and transfer of servicemembers' health and benefits records between the departments, and the separate evaluations of disability by each department. Efforts to address these and other transition problems were already underway in both departments, partly in response to the recommendations of several DOD and independent commissions and task forces. The act codifies various mandates for these activities, including deadlines.

This chapter does not attempt to analyze provisions in the act, but provides brief outlines of the matters addressed.

Chapter 11 - Numerous news stories in the popular print and electronic media have documented suicides among servicemembers and veterans returningfrom Operation Iraqi

Freedom (OIF) and Operation Enduring Freedom (OEF). In the United States, there are more than 30,000 suicides annually. Suicides among veterans are included in this number, but it is not known in what proportion. There is no nationwide system for surveillance of suicide specifically among veterans. Recent data show that about 20% of suicide deaths nationwide could be among veterans. It is not known what proportion of these deaths are among OIF/OEF veterans.

Veterans have a number of risk factors that increase their chance of attempting suicide. These risk factors include combat exposure, post-traumatic stress disorder (PTSD) and other mental health problems, traumatic brain injury (TBI), poor social support structures, and access to lethal means.

Several bills addressing suicide in veterans have been introduced in the 110th Congress. On November 5, 2007, the Joshua Omvig Veterans Suicide Prevention Act (P.L. 110-110) was signed into law, requiring the Department of Veterans Affairs (VA) to establish a comprehensive program for suicide prevention among veterans. More recently, the Veterans Suicide Study Act (S. 2899) was introduced. This bill would require the VA to conduct a study, and report to Congress, regarding suicides among veterans since 1997.

The VA has carried out a number of suicide prevention initiatives, including establishing a national suicide prevention hotline for veterans, conducting awareness events at VA medical centers, and screening and assessing veterans for suicide risk.

This chapter discusses data sources and systems that can provide information about suicides in the general population and among veterans, and known risk and protective factors associated with suicide in each group. It also discusses suicide prevention efforts by the VA. It does not discuss Department of Defense (DOD) activities, or VA's treatment of risk factors for suicide, such as depression, PTSD, and substance abuse.

Chapter 12 - Budget authority — the amount of money a federal department or agency can spend or obligate to spend by law — for veterans' benefits and services has increased significantly since FY1 940. In FY1 940, the budget authority for veterans' benefits and services was $561.1 million, and in FY2007 the budget authority was $82. 0 billion, or *146 times* the FY1940 budget authority. In constant 2007 dollars (i.e., inflation-adjusted), the FY2007 budget authority is *9.9 times* the FY1 940 budget authority. The increases over time have reflected the impact of increases in the number of veterans as the result of wars and other conflicts, the aging of the veteran population, and changes in benefits and services provided for veterans. This chapter provides information on the historical budget authority of the Department of Veterans Affairs (formerly the Veterans Administration) for FY1 940 through FY2007. Budget authority is presented in both current dollars and constant 2007 dollars (i.e., inflation-adjusted).

Chapter 13 - The Department of Veterans Affairs (VA) faces challenges in bridging language and cultural barriers as it seeks to provide quality health care services to an increasingly diverse veteran population in terms of race, ethnicity, sex, and age. To meet the needs of veterans with limited English proficiency (LEP), VA issued an LEP Directive that provides guidance for medical centers in assessing language needs and, if needed, developing language access services designed to ensure effective communication between English-speaking providers and those with LEP. In addition, VA is also challenged to deliver health care services in ways that are culturally appropriate—that is, respectful of and responsive to the cultural values of a diverse veteran population. In light of these challenges, GAO was asked to discuss the (1) actions VA has taken to implement its LEP Directive and the status of veterans' utilization of language access services, and (2) efforts VA has made to provide culturally appropriate health care services.

GAO reviewed VA's policies and the LEP Directive, interviewed VA officials and reviewed efforts by 6 VA medical centers and 10 other VA facilities to implement VA's LEP Directive and to provide culturally appropriate health care services. GAO also reviewed documents from 17 other VA medical centers related to implementation of the LEP Directive.

To view the full product, including the scope and methodology, click on GAO-08-535. For more information, contact Randall B. Williamson, (202) 512-7114, williamsonr@ gao. gov.

Chapter 14 - The Post-9/11 Veterans Educational Assistance Act of 2008, enacted as Title V of P.L. 110-252 on June 30, 2008, provides enhanced educational benefits for veterans and servicemembers. It establishes the Post-9/11 Veterans Educational Assistance program, under which veterans and servicemembers who have served on active duty in the armed forces on or after September 11, 2001, may receive assistance towards the cost of tuition and fees, a monthly housing allowance, and a stipend for books and supplies. The Act grants authority for servicemembers who meet certain criteria to be permitted to transfer unused veterans education benefits to family members. It also increases maximum monthly benefits amounts under the Montgomery GI Bill-Active Duty program and the Reserve Educational Assistance Program.

Chapter 15 - The Department of Veterans Affairs (VA) provides services and benefits to veterans who meet certain eligibility criteria. VA carries out its programs nationwide through three administrations and the Board of Veterans Appeals (BVA). The Veterans Health Administration (VHA) is responsible for veterans' health care programs. The Veterans Benefits Administration (VBA) is responsible for providing compensation, pensions, and education assistance, among other things. The National Cemetery Administration's (NCA) responsibilities include maintaining national veterans cemeteries.

VHA operates the nation's largest integrated health care system. Unlike most other federal health programs, VHA is a direct service provider rather than a health insurer or payer for health care. VA health care services are generally available to all honorably discharged veterans of the U.S. Armed Forces who are enrolled in VA's health care system. VA has a priority enrollment system that places veterans in priority groups based on various criteria. Under the priority system, VA decides each year whether its appropriations are adequate to serve all enrolled veterans. If not, VA could stop enrolling those in the lowest-priority groups.

Since the terrorist attacks of September 11, 2001, U.S. Armed Forces have been deployed in two major theaters of operation. Operation Enduring Freedom (OEF) in Afghanistan and Operation Iraqi Freedom (OIF) constitute the largest sustained ground combat mission undertaken by the United States since the Vietnam War. Veterans from these conflicts and from previous wars are exerting tremendous stress on the VA health care system. With increased patient workload and rising health care costs, the 110th Congress is focused on such issues as how to contain costs and at the same time maintain high-quality health care services to veterans who need them. Among other things, Congress may address the best method of funding for veterans' health care, while continuing to focus on ensuring a "seamless transition" process for servicemembers moving from the military health system into the VA health care system, improving mental health care services for veterans with Post Traumatic Stress Disorder (PT SD), and improving rehabilitation and mental health services for those with Traumatic Brain Injuries (TBI).

In recent years, VA has made an effort to realign its capital assets, primarily its buildings, to better serve veterans' needs. VA established the Capital Asset Realignment for Enhanced Services (CARES) initiative to identify how well the geographic distribution of VA health care resources matches the projected needs of veterans. Given the tremendous interest in the implementation of the CARES initiative in the previous Congress, the 110th Congress will likely continue to monitor the CARES implementation. H.R. 327 was enacted into law (P.L. 110-110) on November 5. The House has passed several measures to improve and expand health care services to veterans: H.R. 327, H.R. 612, H.R. 1315, H.R. 1470, H.R. 2199, H.R. 2623, and H.R. 2874. The Senate VA Committee has reported the following measures: S. 1233, S. 2004, S. 2142, S. 2160, and S. 2162.

In: Veterans' Benefits and Care
Editor: Mathew H. Bradley

ISBN: 978-1-60692-500-3

Chapter 1

VETERANS MEDICAL CARE: FY2009 APPROPRIATIONS

Sidath Viranga Panangala

SUMMARY

The Department of Veterans Affairs (VA) provides benefits to veterans who meet certain eligibility rules. Benefits to veterans range from disability compensation and pensions to hospital and medical care. The VA provides these benefits through three major operating units: the Veterans Health Administration (VHA), the Veterans Benefits Administration (VBA), and the National Cemetery Administration (NCA). The VHA is primarily a direct service provider of primary care, specialized care, and related medical and social support services to veterans through the nation's largest integrated health-care system.

On February 4, 2008, the President submitted his FY2009 budget proposal to Congress. The Administration is requesting a total of $39.2 billion (excluding collections) for VHA. This is a 5.3% increase (or $2.0 billion) over the FY2008 enacted level. Including total available resources (including medical collections) the Administration's budget would provide $41.1 billion for VHA.

On March 7, 2008, the House (H.Con.Res. 312) and Senate (S.Con.Res. 70) reported its respective budget resolutions. After negotiations between the House and Senate, the House agreed to an amended version of S.Con.Res. 70 (Conference Report; H.Rept. 110-659). The conference agreement provides $48.2 billion for FY2009 for discretionary veterans' programs, including medical care, and provides $45.1 billion in mandatory funding for veterans programs.

On June 24, the House Appropriations Committee marked up the Military Construction and Veterans Affairs Appropriations bill (H.R. 6599; H.Rept. 110-775) for FY2009. The House Appropriations Committee recommended $40.8 billion (excluding collections) for VHA, a $1.6 billion increase over the Administration's FY2009 request and $3.6 billion over the FY2008 enacted amount.

On July 17, 2008, the Senate Appropriations Committee marked up its version of the FY2009 Military Construction and Veterans Affairs and Related Agencies Appropriations bill (S. 3301; S.Rept. 110-428). The Senate Appropriations Committee recommended $41.1 billion (excluding collections) for VHA for FY2009. This is a 4.8% increase over the FY2009 request, and $294 million above the House Appropriations Committee-recommended amount.

H.R. 6599 and S. 3301 *did not* include any bill language authorizing fee increases as requested by the Administration's budget proposal for the VHA for FY2009. The House and Senate Committees are directing the VA to increase Priority Group 8 enrollment in FY2009, and have provided additional funding to accomplish this. With escalating gasoline prices, the House and Senate Appropriations Committees have also included report language to increase the mileage reimbursement rate, and has provided additional funding in their respective bills for this purpose.

This chapter will track the FY2009 appropriations process.

MOST RECENT DEVELOPMENTS

On July 17, 2008, the Senate Appropriations Committee marked up its version of the FY2009 Military Construction and Veterans Affairs and Related Agencies Appropriations bill (S. 3301 and S.Rept. 110-428). The Senate Appropriations Committee recommended $41.1 billion (excluding collections) for the Veterans Health Administration (VHA) for FY2009 (see **Table 1**). This is a 4.8% increase over the FY2009 request. S. 3301 *did not* include any bill language authorizing fee increases as requested by the Administration's budget proposal for the VHA for FY2009.

On June 24, 2008, the House Committee on Appropriations, approved its version of the Military Construction and Veterans Affairs Appropriations bill, FY2009 (H.R. 6599 and H.Rept. 110-775). This bill recommends a total of $40.8 billion for VHA (see **Table 1**), a $1.6 billion increase over the Administration's FY2009 request and $3.6 billion over the FY2008 enacted amount. H.R. 6599 *did not* include any bill authorizing fee increases as requested by the Administration's budget proposal for the VHA for FY2009.

This chapter provides a brief background on the veterans health care system, followed by a discussion of the FY2009 VHA budget request, and House and Senate Appropriation Committee action. The report concludes with a discussion of major VHA budget issues.

BACKGROUND

The Department of Veterans Affairs (VA) provides a range of benefits and services to veterans who meet certain eligibility rules, including disability compensation and pensions, education, training and rehabilitation services, hospital and medical care, assistance to homeless veterans,[1] home loan guarantees, and death benefits that cover burial expenses.[2] The VA carries out its programs nationwide through three administrations and the board of veterans appeals (BVA). The Veterans Health Administration (VHA) is responsible for health-care services and medical research programs.[3] The Veterans Benefits Administration (VBA) is responsible, among other things, for providing compensations, pensions, and education assistance.[4] The National Cemetery Administration (NCA)[5] is responsible for maintaining national veterans cemeteries; providing grants to states for establishing, expanding, or improving state veterans cemeteries; and providing headstones and markers for the graves of eligible persons, among other things.

The VA's budget includes both mandatory and discretionary spending accounts. Mandatory funding supports disability compensation, pension benefits, vocational rehabilitation, and life insurance, among other benefits and services. Discretionary funding supports a broad array of benefits and services, including medical care. In FY2008, discretionary budget authority accounted for about 49% of the total VA budget authority of approximately $88 billion, with about 86% of this discretionary funding going toward supporting VA health-care programs.

THE VETERANS HEALTH CARE SYSTEM

The VHA operates the nation's largest integrated direct health-care delivery system.[6] The VA's health-care system is organized into 21 geographically defined Veterans Integrated Service Networks (VISNs). Although policies and guidelines are developed at VA headquarters to be applied throughout the VA health-care system, management authority for basic decision making and budgetary responsibilities are delegated to the VISNs.[7]

Table 1. VA and VHA Appropriations, FY2008-FY2009 ($ thousands)

	FY2008 request	FY2008 House	FY2008 Senate	FY2008 enacted	FY2009 request	FY2009 House Committee (H.Rept. 110-775)	FY2009 Senate Committee (S.Rept. 110-428)
Total Department of Veterans Affairs (VA)	$83,903,751	$87,696,839	$87,501,280	$87,595,142	$90,761,057	$93,685,057	$94,792,750
Total Veterans Health Administrati on (VHA)	$34,612,671	$37,122,000	$37,213,220	$37,201,220	$39,178,503	$40,783,270	$41,078,232
Total Discretionary	$39,416,501	$43,209,589	$43,014,030	$43,107,892	$44,764, 132	$47,688,132	$48,049,825
Total Mandatory	$44,487,250	$44,487,250	$44,487,250	$44,487,250	$45,996,925	$45,996,925	$46,742,925

Sources: S.Rept. 109-286; H.Rept. 109-464; H.Rept. 110-186; S.Rept. 110-85; Congressional Record, vol.153 (December 17, 2007), pp.H16249-H16431; H.Rept. 110-775; and S.Rept. 110-428.

Note: Does not include funding included in the Supplemental Appropriation Act, 2008 (P.L. 110-252).

Recently, VA's Inspector General (IG) for Health Care Inspections has stated that the current VISN management structure is ineffective. According to the IG's statement "VHA has an organizational bias in favor of local decision makers over national leaders which impedes the provision of one standard of excellent medical care for all eligible veterans. The lack of a standard organizational structure leads to differences in financial systems, medical data systems, and management and committee structures from VISN to VISN."[8]

Congressionally appropriated medical care funds are allocated to the VISNs based on the Veterans Equitable Resource Allocation (VERA) system, which generally bases funding on patient workload.[9] Prior to the implementation of the VERA system, resources were allocated to facilities primarily on the basis of their historical expenditures. Unlike other federally funded health insurance programs, such as Medicare and Medicaid, which finance medical care provided through the private sector, the VHA provides care directly to veterans.

In FY2008, VHA operated 153 medical centers, 135 nursing homes, 795 ambulatory care and community based outpatient clinics (CBOCs),[10] 6 independent outpatient clinics, and 232 Readjustment Counseling Centers (Vet Centers).[11] The VHA also pays for care provided to veterans by private-sector providers on a fee basis under certain circumstances. Inpatient and outpatient care is also provided in the private sector to eligible dependents of veterans under the Civilian Health and Medical Program of the Department of Veterans Affairs (CHAMPVA).[12] In addition, the VHA provides grants for construction of state-owned nursing homes and domiciliary facilities, and collaborates with the Department of Defense (DOD) in sharing health-care resources and services.

Table 2. Number of Veterans Enrolled in the VA Health Care System

Priority Groups	FY2006 Actual	FY2007 Actual	FY2008 Estimate	FY2009 Estimate
1	912,787	977,389	957,792	977,773
2	522,829	545,196	566,829	584,605
3	996,063	1,023,256	1,047,724	1,063,512
4	241,716	244,159	250,920	260,106
5	2,538,228	2,413,796	2,461,855	2,468,941
6	265,253	312,256	274,482	278,437
Subtotal Priority Groups 1-6	*5,476,876*	*5,516,052*	*5,559,302*	*5,633,374*
7	218,248	202,049	615,581	625,570
8	2,177,314	2,115,344	1,738,801	1,728,535
Subtotal Priority Groups 7-8	*2,395,562*	*2,317,393*	*2,354,382*	*2,354,105*
Total Enrollees	**7,872,438**	**7,833,445**	**7,913,684**	**7,987,479**

Source: U.S. Department of Veterans Affairs, *FY2009 Budget Submission, Medical Programs and Information Technology Programs*, Vol. 2 of 4.

Note: See **Appendix A** for the Priority Groups and their eligibility criteria.

Table 3. Number of Patients Receiving Care from VA

Priority Groups	FY2006 Actual	FY2007 actual	FY2008 Estimate	FY2009 Estimate
1	768,537	820,410	815,432	832,622
2	342,023	358,270	374,182	386,660
3	568,740	590,860	605,066	616,123
4	177,563	181,572	200,001	207,994
5	1,645,781	1,544,328	1,657,210	1,672,504
6	134,425	155,939	143,483	145,666
Subtotal Priority Groups 1-6	*3,637,069*	*3,651,379*	*3,795,374*	*3,861,569*
7	197,901	173,149	373,285	380,934
8	1,195,612	1,191,161	1,020,644	1,015,616
Subtotal Priority Groups 7-8	*1,393,513*	*1,364,310*	*1,393,929*	*1,396,550*
Subtotal Unique Veteran Patients[a]	*5,030,582*	*5,015,689*	*5,189,303*	*5,258,119*
Non-Veterans[b]	*435,488*	*463,240*	*492,117*	*513,232*
Total Unique Patients	**5,466,070**	**5,478,929**	**5,681,420**	**5,771,351**

Source: U.S. Department of Veterans Affairs, *FY2009 Budget Submission, Medical Programs and Information Technology Programs*, Vol. 2 of 4.

a. Unique veteran patients include Operation Iraqi Freedom (OIF) and Operation Enduring Freedom (OEF) veterans. These patients numbered: 155,272 in FY2006 and 205,628 in FY2007 and are estimated to be 293,345 in FY2008 and 333,275 in FY2009.

b. Non-veterans include CHAMPVA patients, reimbursable patients with VA- affiliated hospitals and clinics, care provided on a humanitarian basis, and employees receiving preventive occupational immunizations.

The Veteran Patient Population

During FY2008, the VHA had an estimated total enrolled veteran population of 7.9 million and provided medical care to about 5.2 million unique veteran patients (see **Tables 2** and **3**).[13] According to VHA estimates, the number of unique veteran patients is estimated to increase by approximately 69,000, from 5.189 million in FY2008 to 5.258 million in FY2009. As shown in **Table 3**, there would be a 1.6% increase in the total number of unique patients (both veterans and non-veterans), from 5.681 million in FY2008 to approximately 5.771 million in FY2009. This includes veterans from Operation Iraqi Freedom (OIF) and Operation Enduring Freedom (OEF). In FY2009, VHA estimates that it would treat 333,275 OIF and OEF veterans, an increase of 39,930 patients, or 13.6%, over the FY2008 level. In FY2009, VA would be treating over 513,000 non-veterans, an increase of over 21,000, or 4.3%, over the FY2008 level.[14]

The total number of outpatient visits, including visits to Vet Centers, reached 63 million during FY2007 and is projected to increase to approximately 65 million in FY2008 and 70.4 million in FY2009.[15] In FY2008, the VHA estimates that it will spend approximately 63.7% of its medical services obligations on outpatient care.[16]

ELIGIBILITY FOR VETERANS' HEALTH CARE

"Promise of Free Health Care"

To understand some of the issues discussed later in this chapter, it is important to understand eligibility for VA health care, the VA's enrollment process, and its enrollment priority groups. Unlike Medicare or Medicaid, VA health care is not an entitlement program. Contrary to numerous claims made concerning "promises" to military personnel and veterans with regard to "free health care for life," not every veteran is automatically entitled to medical care from the VA.[17] Prior to eligibility reform in 1996, provisions of law governing eligibility for VA care were complex and not uniform across all levels of care. All veterans were technically "eligible" for hospital care and nursing home care, but eligibility did not by itself ensure access to care.

The Veterans' Health Care Eligibility Reform Act of 1996, P.L. 104-262, established two eligibility categories and required the VHA to manage the provision of hospital care and medical services through an enrollment system based on a system of priorities.[18] P.L. 104-262 authorized the VA to provide all needed hospital care and medical services to veterans with service-connected disabilities, former prisoners of war, veterans exposed to toxic substances and environmental hazards such as Agent Orange, veterans whose attributable income and net worth are not greater than an established "means test," and veterans of World War I. These veterans are generally known as "higher priority" or "core" veterans (see **Appendix A**, discussed in more detail below).[19] The other category of veterans are those with no service-connected disabilities and with attributable incomes above an established means test (see **Appendix C**).

P.L. 104-262 also authorized the VA to establish a patient enrollment system to manage access to VA health care. As stated in the report language accompanying P.L. 104-262, "the Act would direct the Secretary, in providing for the care of 'core' veterans, to establish and operate a system of annual patient enrollment and require that veterans be enrolled in a manner giving relative degrees of preference in accordance with specified priorities. At the same time, it would vest discretion in the Secretary to determine the manner in which such enrollment system would operate."[20]

Furthermore, P.L. 104-262 was clear in its intent that the provision of health care to veterans was dependent upon the available resources. The committee report accompanying P.L. 104-262 states that the provision of hospital care and medical services would be provided to "the extent and in the amount provided in advance in appropriations Acts for these purposes. Such language is intended to clarify that these services would continue to depend upon discretionary appropriations."[21]

VHA Health-Care Enrollment

As stated previously, P.L. 104-262 required the establishment of a national enrollment system to manage the delivery of inpatient and outpatient medical care. The new eligibility standard was created by Congress to "ensure that medical judgment rather than legal criteria will determine when care will be provided and the level at which care will be furnished."[22]

For most veterans, entry into the veterans' health-care system begins by completing the application for enrollment. Some veterans are exempt from the enrollment requirement if they meet special eligibility requirements.[23] A veteran may apply for enrollment by completing the Application for Health Benefits (VA Form 10-10EZ) at any time during the year and submitting the form online or in person at any VA medical center or clinic, or mailing or faxing the completed form to the medical center or clinic of the veteran's choosing.[24] Once a veteran is enrolled in the VA health-care system, the veteran remains in the system and does not have to reapply for enrollment annually. However, those veterans who have been enrolled in Priority Group 5 (see **Appendix A**, discussed in more detail below) based on income must submit a new VA Form 10-10EZ annually with updated financial information demonstrating inability to defray the expenses of necessary care.[25]

Veteran's Status

Eligibility for VA health care is based primarily on "veteran's status" resulting from military service. Veteran's status is established by active-duty status in the military, naval, or air service and an honorable discharge or release from active military service. Generally, persons enlisting in one of the armed forces after September 7, 1980, and officers commissioned after October 16, 1981, must have completed two years of active duty or the full period of their initial service obligation to be eligible for VA health-care benefits. Servicemembers discharged at any time because of service-connected disabilities are not held to this requirement. Also, reservists that were called to active duty and who completed the term for which they were called, and who were granted an other than dishonorable discharge, are exempt from the 24 continuous months of active duty requirement. National Guard members who were called to active duty by federal executive order are also exempt from this two-year requirement if they (1) completed the term for which they were called, and (2) were granted an other than dishonorable discharge.

When not activated to full-time federal service, members of the reserve components and National Guard have limited eligibility for VA health-care services. Members of the reserve components may be granted service-connection for any injury they incurred or aggravated in the line of duty while attending inactive duty training assemblies, annual training, active duty for training, or while going directly to or returning directly from such duty. In addition, reserve component service members may be granted service-connection for a heart attack or stoke if such an event occurs during these same periods. The granting of service-connection makes them eligible to receive care from the VA for those conditions. National Guard members are not granted service-connection for any injury, heart attack, or stroke that occurs while performing duty ordered by a governor for state emergencies or activities.[26]

After veteran's status has been established, the VA next places applicants into one of two categories. The first group is composed of veterans with service- connected disabilities or with incomes below an established means test. These veterans are regarded by the VA as "high priority" veterans, and they are enrolled in Priority Groups 1-6 (see **Appendix A**). Veterans enrolled in Priority Groups 1-6 include

- veterans in need of care for a service-connected disability;[27]
- veterans who have a compensable service-connected condition;

- veterans whose discharge or release from active military, naval, or air service was for a compensable disability that was incurred or aggravated in the line of duty;
- veterans who are former prisoners of war (POWs);
- veterans awarded the Purple Heart;
- veterans who have been determined by VA to be catastrophically disabled;
- veterans of World War I;
- veterans who were exposed to hazardous agents (such as Agent Orange in Vietnam) while on active duty; and
- veterans who have an annual income and net worth below a VA-established means test threshold.

The VA looks at applicants' income and net worth to determine their specific priority category and whether they have to pay copayments for nonservice-connected care. In addition, veterans are asked to provide the VA with information on any health insurance coverage they have, including coverage through employment or through a spouse. The VA may bill these payers for treatment of conditions that are not a result of injuries or illnesses incurred or aggravated during military service. **Appendix B** provides information on what categories of veterans pay for which services.

The second group of veterans is composed of those who do not fall into one of the first six priority groups — primarily veterans with nonservice-connected medical conditions and with incomes and net worth above the VA-established means test threshold. These veterans are enrolled in Priority Group 7 or 8.[28] **Appendix C** provides information on income thresholds for VA health-care benefits.

Operation Enduring Freedom (OEF) and Operation Iraqi Freedom (OIF) Veterans

The National Defense Authorization Act (NDAA), FY2008 was signed by the President (P.L. 110-181) on January 28, 2008. This Act extended the period of enrollment for VA health care from two to five years for veterans who served in a theater of combat operations after November 11, 1998 (generally, OEF and OIF veterans who served in a combat theater).

According to the VA, currently enrolled combat veterans will have their enrollment eligibility period extended to five years from their most recent date of discharge. New servicemembers discharged from active duty on or after January 28, 2003, could enroll for a period of up to five years after their most recent discharge date from active duty. Veterans who served in a theater of combat, and who never enrolled, and were discharged from active duty between November 11, 1998 and January 27, 2003, may apply for this enhanced enrollment opportunity through January 27, 2011.

Generally, new OEF and OIF veterans are assigned to Priority Group 6, unless eligible for a higher Priority Group, and are not charged copays for medication and/or treatment of conditions that are potentially related to their combat service. Veterans who enroll in the VA health care system under this extended enrollment authority will continue to be enrolled even after the five-year eligibility period ends. At the end of the five-year period, veterans enrolled in Priority Group 6 may be re-enrolled in Priority Group 7 or 8, depending on their service-connected disability status and income level, and may be required to make copayments for nonservice-connected conditions. The above criteria apply to National Guard and Reserve personnel who were called to active duty by federal executive order and served in a theater of combat operations after November 11, 1998.

Priority Groups and Scheduling Appointments

The VHA is mandated to provide priority care for non-emergency outpatient medical care for *any* condition of a service-connected veteran rated 50% or more, or for a veteran's service- connected condition.[29] According to VHA policies, patients with emergency or urgent medical needs must be provided care, or must be scheduled to receive care as soon as practicable, independent of service-connected status and whether care is purchased or provided directly by the VA. Veterans who are service-connected 50% or more need to be scheduled to be seen within 30 days of the desired date for any condition.

Veterans who are rated less than 50% service-connected disabled, and who require care for a service-connected condition, need to be scheduled to be seen within 30 days of the desired date. When VHA staff are in doubt as to whether the request for care is for a service-connected condition, they are required to assume, on behalf of the veteran, that the veteran is entitled to priority access and schedule within 30 days of the desired date.[30]

Veterans in other priority groups are to be scheduled to be seen within 120 days of the desired date. According to VHA policies, all outpatient appointment requests must be acted on as soon as possible, but no later than seven calendar days from the date of the request. The VHA also requires that priority scheduling of any veteran must not affect the medical care of any other previously scheduled veteran. Furthermore, VHA guidelines state that veterans with service-connected conditions cannot be prioritized over other veterans with more acute health-care needs.[31]

FUNDING FOR THE VHA

The VHA is funded through multiple appropriations accounts that are supplemented by other sources of revenue. Although the appropriations account structure has been subject to change from year to year, the appropriation accounts used to support the VHA traditionally include medical care, medical and prosthetic research, and medical administration. In addition, Congress also appropriates funds for construction of medical facilities through a larger appropriations account for construction for all VA facilities. In FY2004, "to provide better oversight and [to] receive a more accurate accounting of funds," Congress changed the VHA's appropriations structure.[32] The Department of Veterans Affairs and Housing and Urban Development and Independent Agencies Appropriations Act, 2004 (P.L. 108-199, H.Rept. 108-401), funded VHA through four accounts: (1) medical services, (2) medical administration, (3) medical facilities, and (4) medical and prosthetic research. Provided below are brief descriptions of these accounts.

Medical Services

The medical services account covers expenses for furnishing inpatient and outpatient care and treatment of veterans and certain dependents, including care and treatment in non-VA facilities; outpatient care on a fee basis; medical supplies and equipment; salaries and expenses of employees hired under Title 38, United States Code; and aid to state veterans homes. In its FY2008 budget request to Congress, the VA requested the transfer of food service operations costs from the medical facilities appropriations to the medical services appropriations. The House and Senate Appropriations Committees have concurred with this request.[33]

In its FY2009 budget request to Congress, the Administration requested the consolidation of the medical services and medical administration account. While the House Appropriations Committee did not concur with this request, the Senate Appropriations Committee has consolidated the medical services and medical administration accounts (see discussion under Senate Committee Action below).

Medical Support and Compliance (Previously Medical Administration)

The medical support and compliance account provides funds for the expenses in the administration of hospitals, nursing homes, and domiciliaries, billing and coding activities, public health and environmental hazard program, quality and performance management, medical inspection, human research oversight, training programs and continuing education, security, volunteer operations, and human resources.

Medical Facilities

The medical facilities account covers, among other things, expenses for the maintenance and operation of VHA facilities; administrative expenses related to planning, design, project management, real property acquisition and deposition, construction, and renovation of any VHA facility; leases of facilities; and laundry services.

Medical and Prosthetic Research

This account provides funding for VA researchers to investigate a broad array of veteran-centric health topics, such as treatment of mental health conditions, rehabilitation of veterans with limb loss, traumatic brain injury and spinal cord injury, organ transplantation, and the organization of the health-care delivery system. VA researchers receive funding not only through this account but also from the DOD, the National Institutes of Health (NIH), and private sources.

As seen in **Figure 1**, the total level of funding for VHA increased between FY2006 and FY2008, and most of this increase has been due to the increase in spending on medical services. As a percentage of total VHA funding, spending on medical facilities, medical administration, and medical and prosthetic research has been fairly stable (see **Appendix D** for FY2005 and FY2006 VHA funding levels).

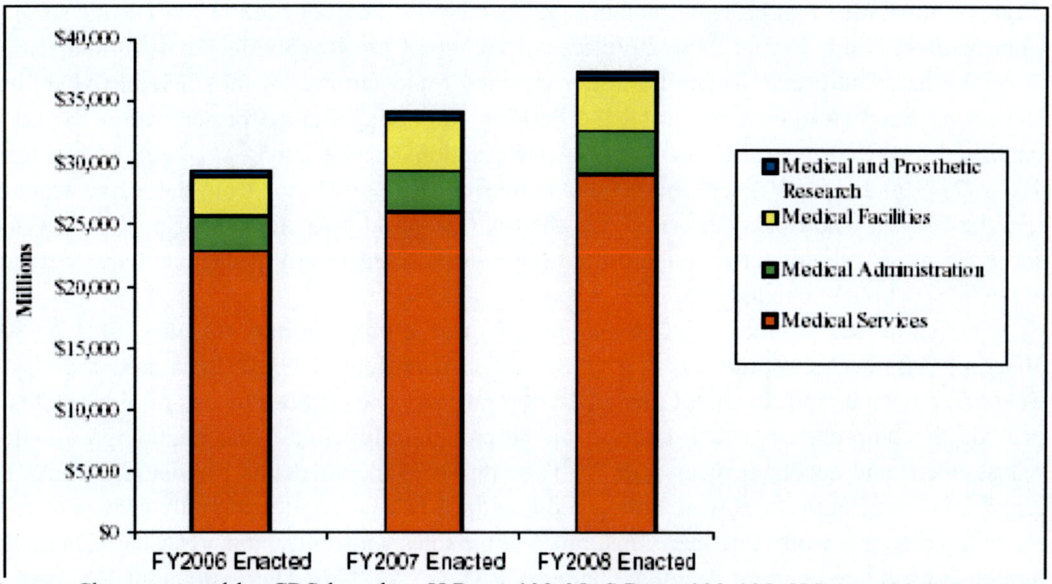

Source: Chart prepared by CRS based on H.Rept. 109-95; S.Rept. 109-105; H.Rept. 109-305; H.Rept. 109-359; H.Rept. 109-464; H.Rept. 109-494; S.Rept. 109-286; P.L. 110-5; H.Rept. 110-64; S.Rept. 110-37; H.Rept. 110-60; *Congressional Record*, vol. 153, (May 24, 2007), H5786-H5787; H.Rept. 110-186; S.Rept. 110-85; *Congressional Record*, vol. 153, (September 7, 2007), S1 1271-S1 1278; and *Congressional Record*, vol.153 (December 17, 2007), pp.H1 6249-H1 6431.

Figure 1. VHA Funding FY2006-FY2008

Medical Care Collections Fund (MCCF)

In addition to direct appropriations for the above accounts, the Committees on Appropriations include medical care cost recovery collections when considering the amount of resources needed to provide funding for the VHA. The Consolidated Omnibus Budget Reconciliation Act of 1985 (P.L. 99-272), enacted into law in 1986, gave the VHA the authority to bill some veterans and most health-care insurers for nonservice-connected care provided to veterans enrolled in the VA health-care system, to help defray the cost of delivering medical services to veterans.[34] This law also established means testing for veterans seeking care for nonservice-connected conditions. However, P.L. 99-272 did not provide the VA with specific authority to retain the third-party payments it collected and VA was required to deposit these third-party collections in the General Fund of the U.S. Treasury.

The Balanced Budget Act of 1997 (P.L. 105-33) gave the VHA the authority to retain these funds in the Medical Care Collections Fund (MCCF). Instead of returning the funds to the Treasury, the VA can use them for medical services for veterans without fiscal year limitations.[35] To increase the VA's third-party collections, P.L. 105-33 also gave the VA the authority to change its basis of billing insurers from "reasonable costs" to "reasonable charges."[36] This change in billing was intended to enhance VA collections to the extent that reasonable charges result in higher payments than reasonable costs.[37] In FY2004, the Administration's budget requested consolidating several medical existing collections accounts into one MCCF. The conferees of the Consolidated Appropriations Act of 2004 (H.Rept. 108-401) recommended that collections that would otherwise be deposited in the Health Services Improvement Fund (former name), Veterans Extended Care Revolving Fund (former name), Special Therapeutic and Rehabilitation Activities Fund (former name), Medical Facilities Revolving Fund (former name), and the Parking Revolving Fund (former name) should be deposited in MCCF.[38] The Consolidated Appropriations Act of 2005; (P.L. 108-447, H.Rept. 108-792) provided the VA with permanent authority to deposit funds from these five accounts into the MCCF. The funds deposited into the MCCF would be available for medical services for veterans. These collected funds do not have to be spent in any particular fiscal year and are available until expended.

The conferees of the FY2006 Military Construction, Military Quality of Life and Veterans Affairs Appropriations Act (P.L. 109-114, H.Rept. 109-305) required the VA to establish a revenue improvement demonstration project. The purpose of this pilot project is to provide a "comprehensive restructuring of the complete revenue cycle including cash-flow management and accounts receivable."[39] The conferees included this provision because the Appropriations Committees were concerned that the VHA was collecting only 41% percent of the billed amounts from third-party insurance companies. Currently, the VHA has established a pilot Consolidated Patient Account Center (CPAC) in VISN 6. There are eight VA medical centers under the CPAC management initiative. In a report issued in June 2008, the Government Accountability Office (GAO) stated that VA had ineffective controls over medical center billings.[40]

As shown in **Table 4**, MCCF collections increased by 45%, from $1.5 billion in FY2003 to $2.2 billion in FY2007. During this same period, first-party collections increased by 33.6%, from $685 million to $915 million. In FY2007, first-party collections represented approximately 41% of total MCCF collections.

FY2008 Budget Summary[41]

On February 5, 2007, the President submitted his FY2008 budget proposal to Congress. The total amount requested by the Administration for the VHA for FY2008 was $34.6 billion, a 1.93% increase in funding compared with the FY2007 enacted amount. The total amount of funding that would have been available for the VHA under the President's budget proposal for FY2008, including collections, was approximately $37.0 billion (see **Table 5** and **Appendix E**). For FY2008, the Administration requested $27.2 billion for medical services, a $1.2 billion, or 4.8%, increase in funding over the FY2007 enacted amount. The Administration's budget proposal also requested $3.4 billion for medical administration, $3.6 billion for medical facilities, and $411 million for medical and prosthetic research (see **Table 5** and **Appendix E**). As in FY2003, FY2004, FY2005, FY2006, and FY2007, the Administration' FY2008 budget request included several cost-sharing proposals.

House Action

On June 6, 2007, the House Appropriations Committee recommended $37.1 billion for the VHA for FY2008, a 9.3% increase over the FY2007 enacted amount of $34.0 billion and 7.3% above the President's request. The Military Construction and Veterans Affairs appropriations bill for FY2008 (H.R. 2642, H.Rept. 110-186) was reported out of committee on June 11.

Table 4. Medical Care Collections, FY2003-FY2007
($ in thousands)

	FY2003 Actual	FY2004 Actual	FY2005 Actual	FY2006 Actual	FY2007 Actual
First-party pharmacy copayments[a]	$576,554	$623,215	$648,204	$723,027	$760,616
First-party copayments for inpatient and outpatient care	104,994	113,878	118,626	135,575	150,964
First-party long-term care copayments[b]	3,461	5,077	5,411	4,347	3,699
Third-party insurance collections	804,141	960,176	1,055,597	1,095,810	1,261,346
Enhanced use leasing revenue[c]	234	459	26,861	3,379	1,692
Compensated work therapy collections[d]	38,834	40,488	36,516	40,081	43,296
Parking fees[e]	3,296	3,349	3,443	3,083	3,136
Compensation and pension living expenses[f]	376	634	2,431	2,075	1,904
MCCF Total	**$1,531,890**	**$1,747,276**	**$1,897,089**	**$2,007,377**	**$2,226,653**

Sources: Table prepared by CRS based on data provided by the VA, and U.S. Department of Veterans Affairs, *FY2009 Budget Submission, Medical Programs and Information Technology Programs*, Vol. 2 of 4, pp. 1C-11.

Notes: The following accounts were not consolidated into the MCCF until FY2004: enhanced use leasing revenue, compensated work therapy collections, parking fees, and compensation and pension living expenses. Collection figures for these accounts for FY2003 are provided for comparison purposes.

a. In FY2002, Congress created the Health Services Improvement Fund (HSIF) to collect increases in pharmacy copayments (from $2 to $7 for a 30-day supply of outpatient medication) that went into effect on February 4, 2002. The Consolidated Appropriations Resolution, 2003 (P.L. 108-7) granted the VA the authority to consolidate the HSIF with the MCCF and granted permanent authority to recover copayments for outpatient medications.

b. Authority to collect long-term care copayments was established by the Millennium Health Care and Benefits Act (P.L. 106-117). Certain veteran patients receiving extended care services from VA providers or outside contractors are charged copayments.

c. Under the enhanced-use lease authority, the VA may lease land or buildings to the private sector for up to 75 years. In return the VA receives fair consideration in cash and/or in-kind. Funds received as monetary considerations may be used to provide care for veterans.

d. The compensated work therapy program is a comprehensive rehabilitation program that prepares veterans for competitive employment and independent living. As part of their work therapy, veterans produce items for sale or undertake subcontracts to provide certain products and/or services, such as providing temporary staffing to a private firm. Funds collected from the sale of these products and/or services are deposited into the MCCF.

e. The Parking program provides funds for construction and acquisition of parking garages at VA medical facilities. The VA collects fees for use of these parking facilities.

f. Under the compensation and pension living expenses program, veterans who do not have either a spouse or child would have their monthly pension reduced to $90 after the third month a veteran is admitted for nursing home care. The difference between the veteran's pension and the $90 is used for the operation of the VA medical facility.

On June 15, 2007, the House passed H.R. 2642.[42] As amended, H.R. 2642 provided $29.0 billion for medical services. The MILCON-VA appropriations bill, as amended, also provided: $3.5 billion for the medical administration account, $68.6 million above the FY2008 request and $82.6 million above the FY2007 enacted amount; $4.1 billion for medical facilities, a 14% increase over the President's request; and $480 million for medical and prosthetic research, a 17% increase over the President's request of $411 million (see **Table 5**).

Senate Action

On June 14, 2007, the Senate Appropriations Committee approved its version of the MILCON-VA appropriations bill. The bill was reported to the Senate on June 18 (S. 1645, S. Rept.1 10-85). S. 1645, as reported, provided a total of $37.2 billion for the VHA.

On September 6, 2007, the Senate passed H.R. 2642 with an amendment in the nature of a substitute to reflect the Senate Appropriations Committee-approved measure (S. 1645, S. Rept.1 10-85). As amended by the Senate, H.R. 2642 provided $29.1 billion for medical services — a $3.2 billion (12.3%) increase over the FY2007 enacted amount and $1.9 billion over the FY2008 budget request — and $3.5 billion would have been available for medical administration, $75 million above the FY2008 Administration's request. H.R. 2642, as passed by the Senate, provided $4.1 billion for medical facilities — a 14.0% increase over the FY2008 request and 1.7% less than the FY2007 enacted amount — and $500 million for medical and prosthetic research — a 12% increase over the FY2007 enacted amount, a 22.0% increase over the FY2008 request, and 4.2% above the House-passed amount (see **Table 5**).

Consolidated Appropriations Act for FY2008

At the end of 2007, Congress passed the Consolidated Appropriations Act for FY2008 (H.R. 2764), an omnibus measure that combined the 11 outstanding appropriations bills for FY2008.[43] H.R. 2764 was passed by the House on December 17, 2007; the Senate passed the measure the next day, December 18, with an amendment (McConnell Amendment — adding funding for the Iraq war). The House agreed to the McConnell Amendment on December 19. The bill was signed into law (P.L. 110-161) on December 26. Division I of H.R. 2764 included the Military Construction and Veterans Affairs and Related Agencies Appropriations Act, 2008 (MILCON-VA Appropriations Act).

The MILCON-VA Appropriation Act provided $37.2 billion for VHA for FY2008, which is $2.6 billion above the Administration's request for FY2008 (see **Table 5**). Of this amount $2.6 billion (the amount above the Administration's request) was designated as contingent emergency funding, and was to be available for obligation only after the President submitted a budget request to Congress. On January 17, 2008, the President submitted a budget request to Congress, requesting this additional amount and designating it as an emergency requirement.

FY2009 VHA BUDGET

On February 4, 2008, the President submitted his FY2009 budget proposal to Congress. The Administration is requesting a total of $39.2 billion (excluding collections) for VHA. This is a 5.3% increase, or a $2.0 billion increase, over the FY2008 enacted level. Including total available resources (including medical collections) the Administration's budget would provide $ 41.1 billion for VHA. The President's FY2009 budget submission also proposes to abolish the medical administration account and consolidate these activities in the medical services account. Under this account structure the Administration is requesting $34.1 billion for the medical services account which is approximately $5 billion above the FY2008 enacted amount (**Table 5**). The VHA is estimating an overall medical inflation rate of 4.63% for FY2009. The major cost drivers for VHA medical care are increases in costs of goods and services beyond the control of the VHA, as well as increases in utilization of services by existing patients, and increases in intensity of care (more complex care).

The President's budget proposal also requests $4.7 billion for the medical facilities account, an increase of $561 million over the FY2008 enacted level. The Administration's budget proposal for FY2009 requests $442 million for the medical and prosthetic research account, a 7.9% decrease ($38 million) below the FY2008 enacted level. According to the Senate Committee on Veterans' Affairs, the President's proposal would result in the loss of 49 full time positions and 294 research projects.[44]

As in FY2003, FY2004, FY2005, FY2006, FY2007, and FY2008. the Administration included several cost-sharing proposals. These legislative proposals are discussed in detail in the key budget issues section at the end of this chapter.

FY2009 Congressional Budget Resolution[45]

On March 7, 2008, the House (H.Con.Res. 312) and Senate (S.Con.Res. 70) reported their respective budget resolutions.[46] The House budget resolution provided $48.2 billion in funding for discretionary veterans programs and $45.1 billion in mandatory spending for FY2009. The House budget resolution also rejected health care enrollment fees and prescription drug copayment increases as proposed by the President. Similar to the House amounts, the Senate budget resolution provided $48.2 billion for discretionary veterans programs including health care, and $45.1 billion for mandatory programs. The House passed its budget resolution on March 13 and the Senate passed its version the following day. After negotiations between the House and Senate, the House agreed to an amended version of S.Con.Res. 70 (Conference Report; H.Rept. 110-659). The Senate adopted H.Rept. 110-659 on June 4 and the House adopted the conference agreement the next day. The conference agreement provides $48.2 billion for FY2009 for discretionary veterans' programs, including medical care. This amount is $4.9 billion more than the FY2008 enacted level, and $3.3 billion more than the President's budget proposal for FY2009. The conference agreement also provides $45.1 billion in mandatory funding for veterans programs.

House Committee Action

On June 12, 2008, the House Committee on Appropriations, Subcommittee on Military Construction, Veterans Affairs, and Related Agencies, marked up a draft Military Construction and Veterans Affairs Appropriations bill. On June 24, the House Appropriations Committee marked up the Military Construction and Veterans Affairs Appropriations bill (H.R. 6599; H.Rept. 110-775), for FY2009 (MILCONVA Appropriations bill). The House Appropriations Committee recommended \$40.8 billion for VHA, a \$1.6 billion increase over the Administration's FY2009 request, and \$3.6 billion over the FY2008 enacted amount. This amount includes \$3 1billion for the medical services account. The committee did not concur with the President's proposed account structure of consolidating the medical administration account with the medical services account. The House Appropriations Committee-recommended amount for the medical services account is 6% above the FY2008 enacted amount (**Table 5**). The Committee has included bill language stipulating that VA must spend not less than \$3.8 billion on specialty mental health care, including Post-traumatic Stress Disorder (PTSD).

The Committee also recommended \$4.4 billion for the medical support and compliance account (previously known as the medical administration account). This amount is 25% above the FY2008 enacted amount. H.R. 6599 also provides approximately \$5 billion for the medical facilities account, a \$368 million increase over the Administration's request, and \$929 million above the FY2008 enacted level. This increase includes funding for non-recurring maintenance. The Committee is directing the VHA to use these funds to address life/safety and suicide prevention deficiencies in mental health wards. Lastly, the House MILCON-VA appropriations bill provides \$500 million for the medical and prosthetic research account, a 13.1 % increase over the FY2009 request, and a 4.2 % increase over the FY2008 enacted amount (**Table 5**).

Construction Projects

The MILCON-VA appropriations bill (H.R. 6599) recommends \$923 million for the construction major account, a 58% increase over the FY2009 request and a 13 % decrease from the FY2008 enacted level. H.R. 6599 also provides \$991.5 million for the construction minor projects account, an increase of 200% over the FY2009 request and 57% above the FY2008 enacted amount. In total (excluding grants for construction of state veterans cemeteries), the Committee has recommended \$2.1 billion for VA construction projects, including construction projects identified under the Capital Asset Realignment for Enhanced Services (CARES) initiative, and grants for construction of state extended care facilities. This level of funding is a 108% increase in funding over the FY2009 request, and 11.5% over the FY2008 enacted amount (**Table 6**).

Senate Committee Action

On July 17, 2008, the Senate Appropriations Committee marked up its version of the FY2009 Military Construction and Veterans Affairs and Related Agencies Appropriations bill (S. 3301, S.Rept. 110-428). The Senate Appropriations Committee recommended \$41.1

Table 5. VHA Appropriations by Account, FY2007-FY2009
($ in thousands)

Program	FY2007 Enacted	FY2008 Request	FY2008 House	FY2008 Senate	FY2008 Enacted	FY2009 Request	FY2009 House Committee (H.Rept. 110-775)	FY2009 Senate Committee (S.Rept. 110-428)
Medical Services	$25,518,254	$27,167,671	$29,031,400	$29,104,220	$27,167,671	$34,075,503	$30,854,270	$35,590,432
Emergency appropriations — U.S. Troop Readiness, Veterans' Care, Katrinia Recovery (P.L. 110-28)	$400,778[a]	—	—	—	—	—	—	—
Contingent emergency (P.L. 110-161)	—	—	—	—	$1,936,549	—	—	—
Subtotal Medical Services	***$25,919,032***	***$27,167,671***	***$29,031,400***	***$29,104,220***	***$29,104,220***	***$34,075,503***	***$30,854,270***	***$35,590,432***
Medical Support and Compliance (Previously Medical Administration)	$3,177,968	$3,442,000	$3,510,600	$3,517,000	$3,442,000	—	$4,400,000	—
Emergency appropriations — U.S. Troop Readiness, Veterans' Care, Katrinia Recovery (P.L. 110-28)	$250,000	—	—	—	—	—	—	—
Contingent emergency (P.L. 110-161)	—	—	—	—	$75,000	—	—	—
Subtotal Medical Support and Compliance (Previously Medical Administration)	***$3,427,968***	***$3,442, 000***	***$3,510,600***	***$3,517,000***	***$3,517,000***	—	***$4,400,000***	—
Medical Facilities	$3,569,533	$3,592,000	$4,100,000	$4,092,000	$3,592,000	$4,661,000	$5,029,000	$4,961,000
Emergency appropriations — U.S. Troop Readiness, Veterans' Care, Katrinia Recovery (P.L. 110-28)	$595,000	—	—	—	—	—	—	—
Contingent emergency (P.L. 110-161)	—	—	—	—	$508,000	—	—	—
Subtotal Medical Facilities	***$4,164,533***	***$3,592,000***	***$4,100,000***	***$4,092,000***	***$4,100,000***	***$4,661,000***	***$5,029,000***	$4,961,000
Medical and Prosthetic Research	$413,980	$411,000	$480,000	$500,000	$411,000	$442,000	$500,000	$526,800
Emergency appropriations — U.S. Troop Readiness, Veterans' Care, Katrinia Recovery (P.L. 110-28)	$32,500	—	—	—	—	—	—	—

Table 5. (Continued)

Program	FY2007 Enacted	FY2008 Request	FY2008 House	FY2008 Senate	FY2008 Enacted	FY2009 Request	FY2009 House Committee (H.Rept. 110-775)	FY2009 Senate Committee (S.Rept. 110-428)
Contingent emergency (P.L. 110-161)	—	—	—	—	$69,000	—	—	—
Subtotal Medical and Prosthetic Research	***$446,480***	***$411,000***	***$480,000***	***$500,000***	***$480,000***	***$442,000***	***$500,000***	***$526,800***
Total VHA appropriations (without collections)	**$33,958,013**	**$34,612,671**	**$37,122,000**	**$37,213,220**	**$37,201,220**	**$39,178,503**	**$40,783,270**	**$41,078,232**
Medical care cost collections (MCCF)	$2,329,000	$2,414,000	$2,414,000	$2,414,000	$2,414,000	$1,879,000	$2,544,000	$2,544,000
Total VHA appropriations (with collections)	**$36,287,013**	**$37,026,671**	**$39,536,000**	**$39,627,220**	**$39,615,220**	**$41,057,503**	**$43,327,270**	**$43,622,232**

Sources: Table prepared by the Congressional Research Service based on H.Rept. 109-464; H.Rept. 109-494; S.Rept. 109-286; P.L. 110-5; H.Rept. 110-64; S.Rept. 110-37; H.Rept. 110-60; *Congressional Record*, vol. 1 53,(May 24, 2007), H5786-H5787; H.Rept. 110-186; S.Rept. 110-85; *Congressional Record*, vol. 153, (September 7, 2007), S1 1271-S1 1278; *Congressional Record*, vol. 153 (December 17, 2007),H1 6249-H1 6431; H.Rept. 110-775; and S.Rept. 110-428.

Note: FY2008 enacted does not include funding included in the Supplemental Appropriation Act, 2008 (P.L. 110-252).

a. P.L. 110-161 (H.R. 2764) transferred $66 million from the FY2007 medical services account to the construction major, projects account for FY2007.

Table 6. Appropriations for VA Construction Projects, FY2008-FY2009 ($ in thousands)

	FY2008 Request	FY2008 House	FY2008 Senate	FY2008 enacted	FY2009 Request	FY2009 House Committee (H. Rept. 110-775)	FY2009 Senate Committee (S.Rept. 110-428)
Construction, major projects[a]	$727,400	$1,410,800	$727,400	$727,400	$581,582	$923,382	$1,217,747
Contingent emergency (P.L. 110-161)	—	—	—	341,700	—	—	—
Subtotal construction, major projects	***727,400***	***1,410,800***	***727,400***	***1,069,100***	***581,582***	***923,382***	***1,217,747***
Construction, minor projects[b]	233,396	615,000	751,398	233,396	329,418	991,492	729,418
Contingent emergency (P.L.110-161)	—	—	—	397,139	—	—	—
Subtotal construction, minor projects	***233,396***	***615,000***	***751,398***	***630,535***	***329,418***	***991,492***	***729,418***
Grants for construction of state extended care facilities[c]	85,000	165,000	250,000	85,000	85,000	165,000	250,000
Contingent emergency (P.L.110-161)	—	—	—	80,000	—	—	—
Subtotal Grants for construction of state extended care facilities	***85,000***	***165,000***	***250,000***	***165,000***	***85,000***	***165,000***	***250,000***
Total	**$1,045,796**	**$2,190,800**	**$1,728,798**	**$1,864,635**	**$996,000**	**$2,079,874**	**$2,197,165**

Sources: Table prepared by CRS based on H.Rept. 110-186; S.Rept. 110-85; *Congressional Record*, vol. 153, (September 7, 2007), S11271-S11278; *Congressional Record*, vol.153 (December 17, 2007), H16249-H16431; H.Rept. 110-775; and S.Rept. 110-428.

Note: This table excludes grants for construction of state veterans cemeteries.

a. This account provides funds for constructing, altering, extending, and improving any VA facility, including planning, assessments of needs, architectural and engineering services, CARES projects, and site acquisition, where the estimated cost of a project is *$10 million or more* or where funds for a project were made available in a previous major project appropriation. Emphasis is placed on correction of safety code deficiencies in existing VA medical facilities.

b. This account provides funds for constructing, altering, extending and improving any VA facility, including planning, architectural and engineering services, CARES projects, and site acquisition, where the estimated cost of a project is *less than $10 million*. VA medical center projects that need minor improvements costing $500,000 or more are funded from this account.

c. This account provides grants to states to acquire or construct state nursing home and domiciliary facilities, and to remodel, modify, or alter existing hospitals, nursing homes, and domiciliary facilities in state homes. A grant may not exceed 65% of the total cost of the project. P.L. 102-585 granted permanent authority for this program, and P.L. 104-262 added Adult Day Health Care as another level of care that may be provided by state homes. This is a no-year account.

billion (excluding collections) for VHA for FY2009 (see **Table 5**). This is a 4.8% increase over the FY2009 request, and $294 million above the House Appropriations Committee-recommended amount. The Senate Appropriations Committee concurred with the President's proposal to merge the medical services account with the medical administration account. The Committee has stated that the "current account structure has created bureaucratic confusion at the medical center level often slowing effective delivery of health care."[47] The Committee recommends merging the medical services account with the medical administration account in order to provide more spending flexibility to medical center directors.

Under the proposed new account structure the Committee is recommending $35.6 billion for the medical services account, a 4.4% ($1.5 billion) increase over the FY2009 request. S. 3301, as marked up by the Committee, also provides $5.0 billion for medical facilities. This is a 21% increase compared to the FY2008 enacted amount, 6.4% above the FY2009 request, and $68 million below the House Committee-recommended amount (see **Table 5**).

The Senate marked up MILCON-VA appropriations bill also provides $527 million for the medical and prosthetic research account. This is a 19.2% increase over the FY2009 request and 9.8% above the FY2008 enacted amount.

Construction Projects

The Committee recommended bill (S. 3301) provides $1.2 billion for the construction major projects account, a 109% increase over the FY2009 request and 32% above the House Appropriations Committee- recommended amount. S. 3301 also provides $729 million for the construction minor projects account, a 26% decrease from the House Committee recommended amount (see **Table 6**). In total, S. 3301 provides $2.2 billion for VA construction projects (excluding grants for state veterans cemeteries), including projects identified under the CARES initiative.

Major Areas of Committee Interest

Priority Group 8 Veterans

The Veterans Health Care Eligibility Reform Act of 1996 (P.L. 104-262) included language that stipulated that medical care to veterans will be furnished to the extent appropriations were made available by Congress on an annual basis. Based on this statutory authority, the Secretary of Veterans Affairs announced on January 17, 2003 that VA would temporarily suspend enrolling Priority Group 8 veterans.[48] Those who were in VA's health care system prior to January 17, 2003 were not to be affected by this suspension.

The House Appropriations Committee, in its report to accompany H.R. 6599 (H.Rept. 110-775) states that the VA "should do everything possible to increase access to medical care for all our veterans, but not in a manner that will negatively impact the medical care [provided to] currently enrolled patients."[49] The Committee is directing the VA to increase Priority Group 8 enrollment by 10%, and has provided $568 million above the Administration's request for this purpose.

Likewise the Senate Appropriations Committee has included $350 million within the medical services account so that the VA could "raise the income threshold to an amount commensurate with the increased level of funding" in order to enroll more Priority Group 8 veterans.[50]

Beneficiary Travel Milage Reimbursement

In general, the beneficiary travel program reimburses certain veterans for the cost of travel to VA medical facilities when seeking health care. P.L. 76-432, passed by Congress on March 14, 1940, mandated VA to pay either the actual travel expenses, or an allowance based upon the mileage traveled by any veteran traveling to and from a VA facility or other place for the purpose of examination, treatment, or care. P.L. 85-857, signed into law on September 2, 1958, authorized VA to pay necessary travel expenses to any veteran traveling to or from a VA facility or other place in connection with vocational rehabilitation counseling or for the purpose of examination, treatment, or care. However, this law changed VA's travel reimbursement into a discretionary authority by stating that VA "may pay" expenses of travel.

Due to rapidly increasing costs of the beneficiary travel program, on March 12, 1987, VA published final regulations that sharply curtailed eligibility for the beneficiary travel program.[51] Under these regulations beneficiary travel payments to eligible veterans were paid when specialized modes of transportation, such as ambulance or wheelchair van, were medically required. In addition, payment was authorized for travel in conjunction with compensation and pension examinations, as well as travel beyond a 100-mile radius from the nearest VA medical care facility. It also authorized the VA to provide transportation costs, when necessary, to transfer any veteran from one health care facility (either a VA or contract care facility) to another in order to continue care paid for by the VA. The following transportation costs were not authorized under these regulations:

- Cost of travel by privately owned vehicle in any amount in excess of the cost of such travel by public transportation unless public transportation was not reasonably accessible or was medically inadvisable.
- Cost of travel in excess of the actual expense incurred by any person as certified by that person in writing.
- Cost of routine travel in conjunction with admission for domiciliary care, or travel for family members of veterans receiving mental health services from the VA except for such travel performed beyond a 100-mile radius from the nearest VA medical care facility.

Travel expenses of all other veterans were not authorized unless the veterans were able to present clear and convincing evidence to show the inability to pay the cost of transportation; or except when medically-indicated ambulance transportation was claimed and an administrative determination was made regarding the veteran's ability to bear the cost of such transportation.[52]

The Veterans' Benefits and Services Act of 1988 (P.L. 100-322, section 108), in large part restored VA travel reimbursement benefits. It required that if VA provides any beneficiary travel reimbursement under Section 111 of Title 38 U.S.C. in any given fiscal year, then payments must be provided in that year in the case of travel for health care services for all the categories of beneficiaries specified in the statute. In order to limit the overall cost of this program, the law imposed a $3 one-way deductible applicable to all travel, except for veterans otherwise eligible for beneficiary travel reimbursement who are traveling by special modes of transportation such as ambulance, air ambulance, wheelchair van, or to receive a compensation and pension examination. In order to limit the overall impact on veterans whose clinical needs dictate frequent travel for VA medical care, an $18- per-calendar-month cap on the deductible was imposed for those veterans who are pre-approved as needing to travel on a frequent basis.

Veterans may qualify for travel reimbursement if (1) they have a service-connected disability rated 30% or more; (2) they are traveling for treatment of a service-connected disability; (3) they receive a VA pension; (4) their income does not exceed the maximum annual VA pension rate; or (5) traveling for a scheduled compensation or pension examination; (6) they are participating in an authorized Vocational Rehabilitation Program.

The FY2008 Appropriations Act (P.L. 110-161) provided funding for VA to increase the beneficiary travel mileage reimbursement rate from 11 cents per mile to 28.5 cents per mile. The increase went into effect on February 1, 2008. While increasing the payment, VA, as mandated by law, also increased proportionately the deductible amounts applied to certain mileage reimbursements. The new deductibles are $7.77 for a one way trip, $15.54 for a round trip, with a maximum of $46.62 per calendar month. However, these deductibles can be waived if they cause a financial hardship to the veteran.

VA regulation with respect to waiving deductibles

Under current regulations 38 CFR 17.144 (b) when it is determined that charging a deductible would cause a severe financial hardship to the veteran, the VA could waive the deductible requirement. Currently, VA determines severe financial hardship as (1) annual income for the year immediately preceding the application for benefits does not exceed the maximum annual rate of pension which would be payable if the person were eligible for pension; or (2) the person is able to demonstrate that due to circumstances such as loss of employment, or incurrence of a disability, income in the year of application will not exceed the maximum annual rate of pension which would be payable if the person were eligible for pension.

With gasoline prices at record high levels, the House and Senate Appropriations Committees have included report language to further increase the mileage reimbursement rate. The House Appropriations Committee has provided an additional $100 million to increase the beneficiary travel reimbursement mileage rate to 41.5 cents per mile from the current rate of 28.5 cents per mile. The Senate Appropriations Committee has included an additional $138 million above the Administration's request to raise the mileage reimbursement rate to 50.5 cents per mile, which raises VA's reimbursement rate to conform with the General Services Administration's (GSA) rate at which federal employees are reimbursed when using private automobiles for official business.

KEY BUDGET ISSUES

In its FY2009 budget request, the Administration has put forward several legislative proposals. These proposals are similar to previous ones included in the Administration's budget requests for FY2003, FY2004, FY2005, FY2006, FY2007, and FY2008 and rejected by Congress each year.[53] Similar to the FY2008 budget proposals, revenue from the proposals in the FY2009 budget request would not be deposited in the Medical Care Collections Fund (MCCF), but would be classified as mandatory receipts to the Treasury. None of these proposals have received any consideration by the House and Senate Appropriation Committees.

The President's FY2009 budget request includes three major policy proposals:

- Assess a tiered annual enrollment fee for all Priority 7 and 8 veterans based on the family income of the veteran.
- Increase pharmaceutical copayments from $8 to $15 (for each 30- day prescription) for all enrolled veterans in Priority Groups 7 and 8.
- Bill veterans receiving treatment for nonservice-connected conditions for the entire copayment amount.

A detailed description of these budget proposals follows.

Assess an Annual Enrollment Fee

The Administration is proposing a tiered annual enrollment fee, which is structured to charge $250 for Priority 7 and 8 veterans with family incomes from $50,000 to $74,999; $500 for those with family incomes from $75,000 to $99,999; and $750 for those with family incomes equal to or greater than $100,000. The VA has estimated that this proposal would contribute more than $129 million to the Treasury annually, beginning in FY2010, and will increase revenue by $1.1 billion over 10 years.

Increase Pharmacy Co-payments

The Administration proposes increasing the pharmacy copayments from $8 to $15 for all enrolled Priority Group 7 and Priority Group 8 veterans whenever they obtain medication from the VA on an outpatient basis for the treatment of a nonservice-connected condition. The Administration put forward this proposal in its FY2004, FY2005, FY2006, FY2007, and FY2008 budget requests as well, but did not receive any approval from Congress. At present, veterans in Priority Groups 2-8 pay $8 for a 30-day supply of medication, including over-the-counter medications.[54]

The Omnibus Budget Reconciliation Act of 1990 (P.L. 101-508) authorized the VA to charge most veterans $2 for each 30-day supply of medication furnished on an outpatient basis for treatment of a nonservice-connected condition. The Veterans Millennium Health Care and Benefits Act of 1999 (P.L. 106-117) authorized the VA to increase the medication copayment amount and establish annual caps on the total amount paid, to eliminate financial hardship for veterans enrolled in Priority Groups 2-6.[55] When veterans reach the annual cap, they continue to receive medications without making a copayment.

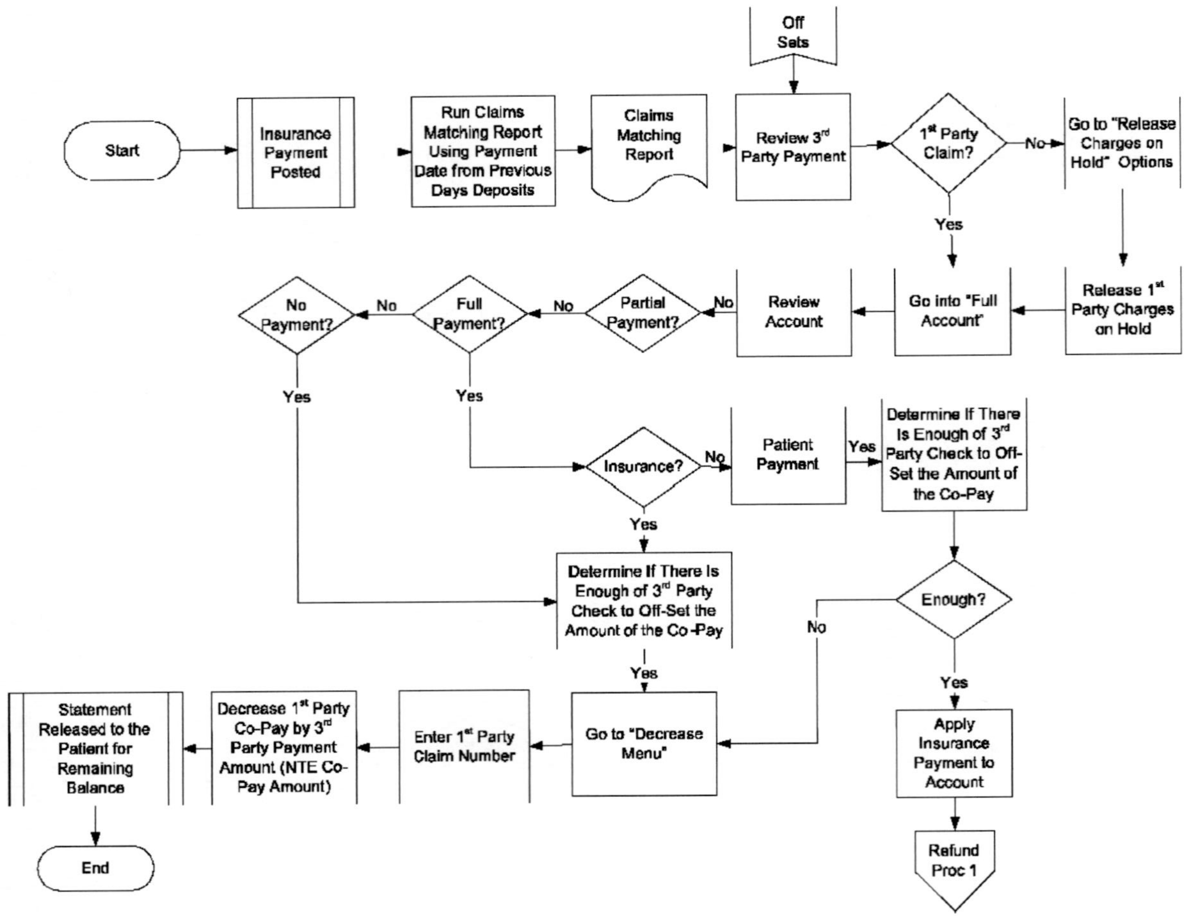

Source: Department of Veterans Affairs.

Figure 2. Present Copayment Process

On November 15, 2005, the VHA issued a directive stating that effective January 1, 2006, the medication co-payment will be increased to $8 for each 30-day supply of medication furnished on an outpatient basis for treatment of a nonserviceconnected condition, and that the annual cap for veterans enrolled in Priority Groups 2-6 will be $960.[56] There is no cap for veterans in Priority Groups 7 and 8 (see **Appendixes B** and **C**). The VA estimates that if the current proposal to raise the copayment were enacted, it would contribute $355 million to the Treasury in FY2009 and will increase revenue by $3.7 billion over 10 years.

Impact of Fee Proposals

According to the VA, in FY2009, as many as 444,000 veterans would choose not to enroll in the VA health care system and 146,000 unique veteran patients would not seek VA health care if enrollment fees are imposed and pharmacy copays are increased.

Third-Party Offset of First-Party Debt

The Administration is requesting that Congress amend the VA's statutory authority by eliminating the practice of reducing first-party copayment debts with third-party health insurance collections. The VA asserts that this proposal would align the VA with the DOD health-care system for military retirees and with the private sector.

With the enactment of P.L. 99-272 in 1986, Congress authorized the VA to collect payments from third-party health insurers for the treatment of veterans with nonservice-connected disabilities; it also established copayments from veterans for this care.[57] Under current law, the VA is authorized to collect from third-party health insurers to offset the cost of medical care furnished to a veteran for the treatment of a nonservice-connected condition.[58] If the VA treats an insured veteran for a nonservice-connected disability, and the veteran is also determined by the VA to have copayment responsibilities, the VA will apply the payment collected from the insurer to satisfy the veteran's copayment debt related to that treatment.

Under the current copayment billing process, in cases where the cost of a veteran's medical care for a nonservice-connected condition appears to qualify for billing under reimbursable insurance and copayment, the VA medical facilities sends the bill to the insurance provider. The veteran's copayment obligation is placed on hold for 90 days pending payment from the third-party payer. If no payment is received from the third-party payer within 90 days, a bill is sent to the veteran for the full copayment amount. However, when insurers reimburse the VA after the 90-day period, the VA must absorb the cost of additional staff time for processing a refund if the veteran has already paid the bill. On all insurance policies, the entire amount of the claim payment is applied first to the copayment. The veteran is then billed only for the portion of the copayment not covered by the insurance reimbursement and the portion of the copayment for services not covered by the veteran's insurance plan (see **Figure 2**).

Under the Administration's proposal, veterans receiving medical care services for treatment of nonservice-connected disabilities will receive a bill for their entire copayment, and the copayment will not be reduced by collection recoveries from third-party health plans. This proposal would apply to all veterans who make copayments.

According to VA estimates, this proposal will increase revenue by $44 million in FY2009 and $415 million over 10 years. The House and Senate Appropriations Committees have not addressed this issue because it is an issue in the purview of the authorizing committees.

APPENDIX A. PRIORITY GROUPS AND THEIR ELIGIBILITY CRITERIA

Priority Group 1 Veterans with service-connected disabilities rated 50% or more disabling
Priority Group 2 Veterans with service-connected disabilities rated 30% or 40% disabling
Priority Group 3 Veterans who are former POWs Veterans awarded the Purple Heart Veterans whose discharge was for a disability that was incurred or aggravated in the line of duty Veterans with service-connected disabilities rated 10% or 20% disabling Veterans awarded special eligibility classification under Title 38, U.S. C., Section 1151, "benefits for individuals disabled by treatment or vocational rehabilitation"
Priority Group 4 Veterans who are receiving aid and attendance or housebound benefits Veterans who have been determined by the VA to be catastrophically disabled
Priority Group 5 Nonservice-connected disabled veterans and noncompensable service-connected veterans rated 0% disabled whose annual income and net worth are below the established VA Means Test thresholds Veterans receiving VA pension benefits Veterans eligible for Medicaid benefits
Priority Group 6 Compensable 0% service-connected disabled veterans World War I veterans Mexican Border War veterans Veterans solely seeking care for disorders associated with — exposure to herbicides while serving in Vietnam; or — ionizing radiation during atmospheric testing or during the occupation of Hiroshima and Nagasaki; or — for disorders associated with service in the Gulf War; or — for any illness associated with service in combat in a war after the Gulf War or during a period of hostility after November 11, 1998.
Priority Group 7 Veterans who agree to pay specified copayments who have income and/or net worth *above* the VA Means Test threshold and income *below* the HUD geographic index — Subpriority a: Noncompensable 0% service-connected disabled veterans who were enrolled in the VA Health Care System on a specified date and who have remained enrolled since that date — Subpriority c: Nonservice-connected disabled veterans who were enrolled in the VA Health Care System on a specified date and who have remained enrolled since that date. — Subpriority e: Noncompensable 0% service-connected disabled veterans not included in Subpriority a above — Subpriority g: Nonservice-connected disabled veterans not included in Subpriority c above
Priority Group 8 Veterans who agree to pay specified copayments with income and/or net worth *above* the VA Means Test threshold and the HUD geographic index — Subpriority a: Noncompensable 0% service-connected disabled veterans enrolled as of January 16, 2003 and who have remained enrolled since that date — Subpriority c: Nonservice-connected disabled veterans enrolled as of January 16, 2003 and who have remained enrolled since that date — Subpriority e: Noncompensable 0% service-connected disabled veterans applying for enrollment after January 16, 2003

Source: Department of Veterans Affairs.

Note: Service-connected disability means with respect to disability, that such disability was incurred or aggravated in the line of duty in the active military, naval, or air service.

APPENDIX B. VETERANS' PAYMENTS FOR HEALTH-CARE SERVICES, BY PRIORITY GROUP

	Copayments				Insurance Billing	Humanitarian Emergency Billing
	Inpatient		Out-patient	Medication[a]		
	Geographic Means Test Copayment	VA Means Test				
Priority Group 1	No	No	No	No	Yes, but only if care was for nonservice-connected condition	No
Priority Groups 2, 3,[b] 4[c]	No	No	No	Yes, but only for veterans with less than 50% service connected disability and medication is for nonservice-connected condition. Former POWs are exempt from allmedications copayments	Yes, but only if care was for nonservice-connected condition	No
Priority Group 5	No	No	No	Yes	Yes, but only if care was for nonservice-connected condition	No
Priority Group 6 (WWI, and 0% service- connected compensable)	No	No	No	Yes	Yes, but only if care was for nonservice-connected condition	No
Priority Group 6 (Veterans receiving care for exposure or experience)[d]	No	No[d]	No[d]	No[d]	Yes, but only if care was for nonservice-connected condition	No
Priority Group 7a	Yes	No	Yes	Yes, but only if care was for nonservice-connected condition	Yes, but only if care was for nonservice-connected condition	No
Priority Group 7c	Yes	No	Yes	Yes, but only if care was for nonservice-connected condition	Yes, but only if care was for nonservice-connected condition	No
Priority Group 8a	No	Yes	Yes	Yes, but only if care was for nonservice-connected condition	Yes, but only if care was for nonservice-connected condition	No
Priority Group 8c	No	Yes	Yes	Yes, but only if care was for nonservice-connected condition	Yes, but only if care was for nonservice-connected condition	No

Source: Table prepared by CRS based on information from the Department of Veterans Affairs.

Notes: Priority Group 7a and 7c veterans have income above the VA Means Test threshold but below the Geographic Means Test threshold and are responsible for 20% of the inpatient copayment and 20% of the inpatient per diem copayment. The geographic means test copayment reduction does not apply to outpatient and medication copayment, and veterans will be assessed the full applicable copayment charges. Note that reduced inpatient copayments can apply to veterans in Priority Groups 4 and 6 based on the income of the veteran.

Priority Group 8a and 8c veterans have income above the VA Means Test threshold and above the Geographic Means Test threshold. Veterans enrolled in this priority group are responsible for the full inpatient copayment and the inpatient per diem copayment for care of their nonservice-connected conditions. Veterans in this priority group are also responsible for outpatient and medication copayments for care of their nonservice-connected conditions.

a. An annual medication copayment cap has been established for veterans enrolled in Priority Groups 2-6. Medication will continue to be dispensed after copayment cap is met. An annual copayment cap has not been established for veterans enrolled in Priority Groups 7 or 8.

b. Veterans in receipt of a Purple Heart are in Priority Group 3. This change occurred with the enactment of the Veterans Millennium Health Care and Benefits Act (P.L. 106-117) on Nov. 30, 1999.

c. Priority Group 7 veterans who are determined to be catastrophically disabled and who are placed in Priority Group 4 for treatment are still subject to the copayment requirements as a Priority Group 7 veteran.

d. Priority Group 6 — veterans claiming exposure to Agent Orange; veterans claiming exposure to environmental contaminants; veterans exposed to Ionizing Radiation; combat veterans within two years of discharge from the military; veterans who participated in Project 112/SHAD; veterans claiming military sexual trauma; and veterans with head and neck cancer who received nasopharyngeal radium treatment while in the military are subject to copayments when their treatment or medication is not related to their exposure or experience. The initial registry examination and follow-up visits to receive results of the examination are not billed to the health insurance carrier and are not subject to copayments. However, care provided that is not related to exposure, if it is nonservice-connected, will be billed to the insurance carrier and copayments can apply.

APPENDIX C. FINANCIAL INCOME THRESHOLDS FOR VA HEALTH-CARE BENEFITS, CALENDER YEAR 2008

Veterans with —	Free VA prescriptions and travel benefits for veterans with incomes of —	Free VA inpatient and outpatient care for veterans with incomes of —
No dependents	$11,181 or less	$28,429 or less
1 dependent	$14,643 or less	$34,117 or less
2 dependents	$16,552 or less	$36,026 or less
3 dependents	$18,461 or less	$37,935 or less
4 dependents	$20,370 or less	$39,844 or less
For each additional dependent, add:	$1,909	$1,909

Source: Department of Veterans Affairs.

Appendix D. VHA Appropriations for FY2005 and FY2006
($ in thousands)

Program	FY2005 Request	FY2005 House	FY2005 Senate	FY2005 Enacted	FY2006 Request	FY2006 House	FY2006 Senate	FY2006 Enacted
Medical services	—	$19,498,600	$19,498,600[a]	$19,316,995	$19,995,141	$20,995,141	$21,331,011	$21,322,141
Supplemental appropriations (P.L. 108-324)	$38,283	—	—	38,283	—	—	—	—
Supplemental appropriations	975,000[b]	975,000[c]	1,500,000[d]	1,500,000[e]	—	—	—	—
Emergency appropriations	—	—	—	—	1,977,000[f]	—	1,977,000[g]	1,225,000[h]
Emergency appropriations- Gulf Coast Hurricanes (P.L. 109-148)	—	—	—	—	198,265	—	—	198,265
Emergency appropriations-Avian Flu Pandemic (P.L. 109-148)	—	—	—	—	27,000	—	—	27,000
Subtotal medical services	***1,013,283***	***20,473,600***	***20,998,600***	***20,855,278***	***22,197,406***	***20,995,141***	***23,308,011***	***22,772,406***
Medical administration	—	4,705,000	4,705,000	4,667,360	4,517,874	4,134,874	2,858,442	2,858,442
Supplemental appropriations (P.L. 108-324)	1,940	—	—	1,940	—	—	—	—
Subtotal medical administration	***1,940***	***4,705,000***	***4,705,000***	***4,669,300***	***4,517,874***	***4,134,874***	***2,858,442***	***2,858,442***
Medical facilities	—	3,745,000	3,745,000	3,715,040	3,297,669	3,297,669	3,297,669	3,297,669
Supplemental appropriations (P.L. 108-324)	46,909	—	—	46,909	—	—	—	—
Subtotal medical facilities	***46,909***	***3,745,000***	***3,745,000***	***3,761,949***	***3,297,669***	***3,297,669***	***3,297,669***	***3,297,669***
Medical and prosthetic research	384,770	384,770	405,593	402,348	393,000	393,000	412,000	412,000
Information technology	—	—	—	—	—	—	1,456,821	—
Medical care[i]	26,748,600	—	—	—	—	—	—	—
Total VHA appropriations (without collections)	**28,195,502**	**28,308,370**	**28,854,193**	**29,688,875**	**30,405,949**	**28,820,684**	**31,332,943**	**29,340,517**
Medical care cost collection (MCCF)[j]	2,002,000	2,002,000	2,002,000	1,985,984	2,170,000	2,170,000	2,170,000	2,170,000
Total: VHA (appropriations and collections)	**$30,197,502**	**$31,310,370**	**$30,856,193**	**$31,674,859**	**$32,575,949**	**$30,990,684**	**$33,502,943**	**$31,510,517**

Source: Table prepared by the Congressional Research Service based on H.Rept. 108-674; S.Rept. 108-353; H.Rept. 109-95; S.Rept. 109-105; H.Rept. 109-305; H.Rept. 109-359; and House Appropriations Committee data.

Notes: Appropriation amounts for FY2005 adjusted to account for the 0.8% across-the-board reduction in most discretionary accounts as called for in Division J, Section 122 (a)(1) of P.L. 108-447. Supplemental appropriations for FY2005 are not subject to the 0.8% across-the-board reductions. Appropriation amounts for FY2006 *are not* subject to any cross-theboard reductions as stipulated in Division B, Title III, Section 3801(c)(2) of P.L. 109-148.

a. This amount includes $1.2 billion designated as an emergency requirement.

b. On June 30, 2005, the Administration requested an additional $975 million for medical services for FY2005.

c. On June 30, 2005, the House passed H.R. 3130.

d. On June 29, 2005, the Senate passed an amendment to H.R. 2361, the Department of the Interior, Environment, and Related Agencies Appropriations bill, 2006 to add $1.5 billion in emergency funds for medical services.

e. On August 2, 2005, the FY2006 Department of the Interior, Environment, and Related Agencies appropriations bill (H.R. 2361, P.L. 109-54) was signed into law.

f. On July 14, 2005, the Administration requested an additional $1.977 billion for medical services for FY2006.

g. On July 21, 2005, the Senate Committee on Appropriations reported H.R. 2528 favorably out of committee (S.Rept. 109-105) and designated this amount as an emergency appropriation.

h. On November 18, 2005, the House and Senate adopted the conference report (H.Rept. 109-305) to accompany H.R. 2528 and designated this amount as an emergency appropriation.

i. This amount includes funding for medical services, medical administration, and medical facilities.

j. Medical Care Cost Collection Fund (MCCF) receipts are restored to the VHA as an indefinite budget authority equal to the revenue collected, estimated to be $1.985 billion in FY2005, $2.17 billion in FY2006, and $2.33 billion in FY2007.

APPENDIX E. VHA APPROPRIATIONS FOR FY2007 AND FY2008 ($ in thousands)

Program	FY2007 request	FY2007 House	FY2007 Senate	FY2007 enacted	FY2008 request	FY2008 House	FY2008 Senate	FY2008 enacted
Medical services	$25,512,000	$25,412,000	$28,689,000	$25,518,254	$27,167,671	$29,031,400	$29,104,220	$27,167,671
Emergency appropriations — U.S. Troop								
Readiness, Veterans' Care, Katrina Recovery, and Iraq Accountability (P.L. 110-28)	—	414,982	454,131	400,778[a]	—	—	—	—
Contingent emergency (P.L. 110-161)	—	—	—	—	—	—	—	1,936,549
Subtotal medical services	***25,512,000***	***25,826,982***	***29,143,131***	***25,919,032***	***27,167,671***	***29,031,400***	***29,104,220***	***29,104,220***
Medical administration	3,177,000	3,277,000	—	3,177,968	3,442,000	3,510,600	3,517,000	3,442,000
Emergency appropriations (P.L. 110-28)	—	256,300	250,000	250,000	—	—	—	—
Contingent emergency (P.L. 110-161)								75,000

Table (Continued)

Program	FY2007 request	FY2007 House	FY2007 Senate	FY2007 enacted	FY2008 request	FY2008 House	FY2008 Senate	FY2008 enacted
Subtotal medical administration	***3,177,000***	***3,533,300***	***250,000***	***3,427,968***	***3,442,000***	***3,510,600***	***3,517,000***	***3,517,000***
Medical facilities	3,569,000	3,594,000	3,569,000	3,569,533	3,592,000	4,100,000	4,092,000	3,592,000
Emergency appropriations (P.L. 110-28)	—	595,000	595,000	595,000	—	—	—	—
Contingent emergency (P.L. 110-161)	—	—	—	—	—	—	—	508,000
Subtotal medical facilities	***3,569,000***	***4,189,000***	***4,164,000***	***4,164,533***	***3,592,000***	***4,100,000***	***4,092,000***	***4,100,000***
Medical and prosthetic research	399,000	412,000	412,000	413,980	411,000	480,000	500,000	411,000
Emergency appropriations (P.L. 110-28)	—	35,000	30,000	32,500	—	—	—	—
Contingent emergency (P.L. 110-161)	—	—	—	—	—	—	—	69,000
Subtotal medical and prosthetic research	***399,000***	***447,000***	***442,000***	***446,480***	***411,000***	***480,000***	***500,000***	***480,000***
Total VHA appropriations (without collections)	**32,657,000**	**33,996,282**	**33,999,131**	**33,958,013**	**34,612,671**	**37,122,000**	**37,213,220**	**37,201,220**
Medical care cost collection (MCCF)	2,329,000	2,329,000	2,329,000	2,329,000	2,414,000	2,414,000	2,414,000	2,414,000
Total: VHA (appropriations and collections)	**$34,986,000**	**$36,325,282**	**$36,328,131**	**$36,287,013**	**$37,026,671**	**$39,536,000**	**$39,627,220**	**$39,615,220**

Sources: Table prepared by the Congressional Research Service based on H.Rept. 109-95; S.Rept. 109-105; H.Rept. 109-305; H.Rept. 109-359; H.Rept. 109-464; H.Rept. 109-494; S.Rept. 109-286; P.L. 110-5; H.Rept. 110-64; S.Rept. 110-37; H.Rept. 110-60; *Congressional Record*, vol. 153, (May 24, 2007), H5786-H5787; H.Rept. 110-186; S.Rept. 110-85; *Congressional Record*, vol. 153, (September 7, 2007), S11271-S11278; and *Congressional Record*, vol. 153 (December 17, 2007), H16249-H16431.

Note: FY2008 enacted does not include funding included in the Supplemental Appropriation Act, 2008 (P.L. 110-252).

a. P.L. 110-161 (H.R. 2764) transferred $66 million from the FY2007 medical services account to the construction major, projects account for FY20

End Notes

[1] For detailed information on homeless veterans programs, see CRS Report RL34024, *Veterans and Homelessness*, by Libby Perl.

[2] For a detailed description on eligibility for veterans disability benefits programs, see CRS Report RL33113 *Veterans Affairs: Basic Eligibility for Disability Benefit Programs*, by Douglas Reid Weimer.

[3] For a detailed description of veterans' health-care issues, see CRS Report RL33993, *Veterans' Health Care Issues*, by Sidath Viranga Panangala.

[4] For a detailed description of veterans' benefits issues, see CRS Report RL33985, *Veterans' Benefits: Issues in the 110th Congress*, by Carol D. Davis (Coordinator).

[5] Established by the National Cemeteries Act of 1973 (P.L. 93-43).

[6] Established on January 3, 1946, as the Department of Medicine and Surgery by P.L. 79- 293, succeeded in 1989 by the Veterans Health Services and Research Administration, renamed the Veterans Health Administration in 1991.

[7] Jian Gao, Ying Wang and Joseph Engelhardt, "Logistic Analysis of Veterans' Eligibility- Status Change," *Health Services Management Research*, vol. 18, (August 2005), p. 175.

[8] U.S. Congress, House Committee on Appropriations, Subcommittee on Military Construction, Veterans Affairs, and Related Agencies Appropriations, *Military Construction, Veterans Affairs, and Related Agencies Appropriations for FY2009*, hearings, 110th Congress, 2nd sess., February 2008, p. 295.

[9] About 90% of the VHA appropriation is allocated through VERA. Networks also receive appropriated funds not allocated through VERA for such things as prosthetics, homeless programs, readjustment counseling, and clinical training programs. VA facilities could also retain collections from insurance reimbursements and copayments, and use these funds for the care of veterans.

[10] Data on the number of CBOCs differ from source to source. Some count outpatient clinics located at VA hospitals while others count only freestanding CBOCs. The number represented in this chapter excludes clinics located in VA hospitals. On June 26, 2008, VA announced that it would be establishing 44 new CBOCs in FY2008 and FY2009. The new CBOCs are to be located in: Marshall County, and Wiregrass, AL; Matanuska-Susitna Borough area, AK; Ozark, and White County, AR; East Bay-Alameda County area, CA; Summerfield, FL; Baldwin County, Coweta County, Glynn County, and Liberty County, GA; Miami County, and Morgan County, IN; Wapello County, IA; Lake Charles, Leesville, Natchitoches, St. Mary Parish, and Washington Parish, LA; Lewiston-Auburn area, ME; Douglas County, and Northwest Metro, MN; Franklin County, MO; Rio Rancho, NM; Robeson County, and Rutherford County, NC; Grand Forks County, ND; Gallia County, OH; Altus, Craig County, Enid, and Jay, OK; Giles County, Maury County, and McMinn County, TN; Katy, Lake Jackson, Richmond, Tomball, and El Paso County, TX; Augusta County, Emporia, and Wytheville, VA; and Greenbrier County, WV.

[11] On July 9, 2008, VA announced that it would be establishing 39 new Vet Centers. The new Vet Centers are to be located in the following counties: Madison, AL; Maricopa, AZ; Kern, Los Angeles, Orange, Riverside, Sacramento, San Bernardino, and San Diego, CA; Fairfield, CT; Broward, Palm Beach, Pasco, Pinellas, Polk, and Volusia, FL; Cobb, GA; Cook, and DuPage, IL; Anne Arundel, Baltimore, and Prince George's, MD; Macomb and, Oakland, MI; Hennepin, MN; Greene,MO; Onslow, NC; Ocean, NJ; Clark, NV; Comanche, OK; Bucks, and Montgomery, PA; Bexar, Dallas, Harris, and Tarrant, TX; Virginia Beach, VA; King, WA; and Brown, WI. VA plans to have the 39 sites fully operational by the end of December 2009.

[12] For further information on CHAMPVA, see CRS Report RS22483, *Health Care for Dependents and Survivors of Veterans*, by Sidath Viranga Panangala and Susan Janeczko.

[13] "Enrolles" are veterans who have enrolled in the VA health care system. "Unique patients" are those receiving medical care who are counted only once. In any given year, some enrollees do not seek any medical care, either because they do not become sick or because they rely on other health care systems, such as private health insurance, for care.

[14] Non-veterans include CHAMPVA patients, reimbursable patients with VA affiliated hospitals and clinics, care provided on a humanitarian basis, and employees receiving preventive occupational immunizations.

[15] This number excludes outpatient care provided on a contract basis and outpatient visits to readjustment counseling centers. U.S. Department of Veterans Affairs, *FY2009 Budget Submission, Medical Programs and Information Technology Programs*, Vol. 2 of 4.

[16] Ibid., p.1C-20.

[17] For a detailed discussion of "promised benefits," see CRS Report 98-1006, *Military Health Care: The Issue of "Promised" Benefits*, by David F. Burrelli.

[18] U.S. Congress, House Committee on Veterans Affairs, *Veterans' Health Care Eligibility Reform Act of 1996*, report to accompany H.R. 3118, 104th Cong. 2nd sess., H.Rept. 104-690 p. 2.

[19] Ibid., p.5.

[20] Ibid., p.6.

[21] Ibid., p.5.

[22] Ibid., p.4.

[23] Veterans do not need to apply for enrollment in the VA's health-care system if they fall into one of the following categories: veterans with a service-connected disability rated 50% or more (percentages of disability is based upon the severity of the disability; those with a rating of 50% or more are placed in Priority Group 1); less than one year has passed since the veteran was discharged from military service for a disability that the military determined was incurred or aggravated in the line of duty, but the VA has not yet rated; or the veteran is seeking care from the VA only for a service-connected disability (even if the rating is only 10%).

[24] VA Form 10-1 0EZ is available at [https://www. 101 0ez.med.va.gov/sec/vha/1 01 0ez/ #Process].

[25] 38 C.F.R. § 17.36 (d)(3)(iv) (2007).

[26] 38.U.S.C. §101(24); 38 C.F.R. §3.6(c).

[27] The term "service-connected" means, with respect to disability, that such disability was incurred or aggravated in the line of duty in the active military, naval, or air service. The VA determines whether veterans have service-connected disabilities and, for those with such disabilities, assigns ratings from 0 to 100% based on the severity of the disability. Percentages are assigned in increments of 10%.

[28] The VA considers a veteran's previous year's total household income (both earned and unearned income, as well as his/her spouse's and dependent children's income). Earned income is usually wages received from working. Unearned income includes interest earned, dividends received, money from retirement funds, Social Security payments, annuities, and earnings from other assets. The number of persons in the veterans family will be factored into the calculation to determine the applicable income threshold. 38 C.F.R. § 1 7.36(b)(7) (2006).

[29] VHA Directive 2006-05 5, October 11, 2006.

[30] Ibid.

[31] Ibid.

[32] U.S. Congress, Conference Committees, *Consolidated Appropriations Act, 2004,* conference report to accompany H.R. 2673, 1 08th Cong., 1st sess., H.Rept. 108-401, p. 1036.

[33] The cost of food service operations support hospital food service workers, provisions, and supplies related to the direct care of patients.

[34] Veterans' Health-Care and Compensation Rate Amendments of 1985;100 Stat. 372, 373, 383.

[35] For a detailed history of funding for VHA from FY1995 to FY2004, see CRS Report RL32732, *Veterans' Medical Care Funding FY1995-FY2004*, by Sidath Viranga Panangala.

[36] Under "reasonable costs," the VA billed insurers based on its average cost to provide a particular episode of care. Under "reasonable charges," the VA bills insurers based on market pricing for health-care services.

[37] U.S. Government Accountability Office (GAO), *VA Health Care: Third-Party Charges Based on Sound Methodology; Implementation Challenges Remain*, GAO/HEHS-99- 124, June 1999.

[38] For a detailed description of these former accounts, see CRS Report RL32548, *Veterans' Medical Care Appropriations and Funding Process*, by Sidath Viranga Panangala.

[39] U.S. Congress, Conference Committees, *Military Construction, Military Quality of Life and Veterans Affairs Appropriations Act, 2006*, conference report to accompany H.R. 2528, 109th Congress, 1st session, H.Rept. 109-305, p. 43.

[40] For details on whether medical centers under the CPAC initiative had more effective controls over third-party billings and collections, see U.S. Government Accountability Office, *VA Health Care: Ineffective Controls over Medical Center Billings and Collections Limit Revenue from Third- Party Insurance Companies,* GAO-08-675, June 2008.

[41] For a detailed description of VA Medical Care Appropriations for FY2008, see CRS Report RL34063, *Veterans' Medical Care: FY2008 Appropriations*, by Sidath Viranga Panangala.

[42] H.R. 2642 as passed by the House on June 15, 2007, was not enacted into law. Provisions in this bill were amended and later incorporated into the Consolidated Appropriations Act, 2008 (H.R. 2764, P.L. 110-161). H.R. 2642 subsequently became the vehicle for the Supplemental Appropriations Act, 2008 (P.L. 110-252).

[43] The only appropriations bill that passed as a stand alone measure was the Department of Defense Appropriations Act, 2008 (H.Rept. 110-434), which was signed into law on November 13, 2007 (P.L. 110-116).

[44] Senate Committee on Veterans Affairs (majority), *Views and Estimates Letter for FY2009,* to the Senate Committee on the Budget, February 22, 2008.

[45] For a detailed analysis of the FY2009 budget resolution see CRS Report RL344 19, *The Budget for Fiscal Year 2009,* by D. Andrew Austin.

[46] H.Rept. 110-543 and S. Prt. 110-039.

[47] U.S. Congress, Senate Committee on Appropriations, *Military Construction, and Veterans Affairs, and Related Agencies Appropriations Bill, 2009*, report to accompany S. 3301, 110th Cong., 2nd sess., S.Rept. 110-428, p.40.

[48] Department of Veterans Affairs, "Enrollment — Provision of Hospital and Outpatient Care to Veterans Subpriorities of Priority Categories 7 and 8 and Annual Enrollment Level Decision; Final Rule," *68 Federal Register* 2670, January 17, 2003.

[49] U.S. Congress, House Committee on Appropriations, *Military Construction, Veterans Affairs, and Related Agencies Appropriations Bill, 2009*, report to accompany H.R. 6599, 110th Cong., 2nd sess., H.Rept. 110-775, p.39.

[50] U.S. Congress, Senate Committee on Appropriations, *Military Construction, and Veterans Affairs, and Related Agencies Appropriations Bill, 2009*, report to accompany S. 3301, 110th Cong., 2nd sess., S.Rept. 110-428, p.50.

[51] Veterans Administration, "Transportation of Claimants and Beneficiaries," final regulations, 52 FR 7575-01, March 12, 1987. These regulations became effective on April 13, 1987.

[52] Ibid.

[53] In FY2003, the VA proposed a $1,500 deductible for all Priority Group 7 veterans for nonservice-connected disabilities. For proposals included in FY2004, FY2005, FY2006, FY2007,and FY2008, see CRS Report RL32548, *Veterans' Medical Care Appropriations and Funding Process*, by Sidath Viranga Panangala; CRS Report RL32975, *Veterans' Medical Care: FY2006 Appropriations*, by Sidath Viranga Panangala; CRS Report RL33409, *Veterans' Medical Care: FY2007 Appropriations*, by Sidath Viranga Panangala; and CRS Report RL34063, *Veterans' Medical Care: FY2008 Appropriations*, by Sidath Viranga Panangala.

[54] The following veterans are exempt from paying copayments: veterans receiving a pension for a nonservice-connected disability from the VA; veterans with incomes below $11,181 (if no dependents) and $14,643 (with one dependent plus $1,909 for each additional dependent); veterans receiving care for conditions such as Agent Orange or Military Sexual Trauma, and combat veterans within five years of discharge; and veterans who are former POWs.

[55] This law allowed the VA to increase the copayment amount for each 30-day or less supply of medication provided on an outpatient basis (other than medication administered during treatment) for treatment of a nonservice-connected condition. Accordingly, the VA increased the copayment amount from $2 to $7. The medication copayment charge for each subsequent calendar year after 2002 is established by using the prescription drug component of the Medical Consumer Price Index. When an increase occurs, the copayment increases in whole dollar amounts. The amount of the annual cap increases $120 for each $1 increase in the copayment amount.

[56] VHA Directive 2005-05 2, *Implementation of Medication Copayment Changes*, November 15, 2005.

[57] Consolidated Omnibus Budget Reconciliation Act of 1985, 100 Stat. 372, 373, 383.

[58] 38 U.S.C. § 1729; 38 U.S.C. § 1710; and 38 U.S.C. 1722A.

In: Veterans' Benefits and Care
Editor: Mathew H. Bradley

ISBN: 978-1-60692-500-3

Chapter 2

VETERANS AFFAIRS: THE APPEAL PROCESS FOR VETERANS' CLAIMS

Douglas Reid Weimer

SUMMARY

Congress, through the United States Department of Veterans Affairs (VA), provides a variety of benefits and services to veterans and to certain members of their families. These benefits range from health care and related services to burial benefits. The veteran's basic eligibility for these programs and services is usually determined by the local VA office. Veterans not satisfied with the VA's decision(s) may wish to have them reviewed and may appeal the decision(s). This chapter traces the various steps involved in the appeal process — starting with the original application for benefits and concluding with an appeal to the U.S. Supreme Court. A flow chart outlining all of the steps in the appeal process is provided.

Following the filing of the initial appeal, the local VA office will either allow or disallow the claim. If the veteran/claimant wishes to appeal, a written request for appeal must be filed and various time deadlines and other requirements must be met prior to the case being considered by the Board of Veterans' Appeals (BVA). The appeal before the BVA may be a hearing at the local VA office by a traveling Board member; a hearing at the BVA office in Washington, DC; or a videoconference hearing at the local VA office. Various filing requirements and time limits must be met by the veteran/claimant in his/her appeal. There are specific guidelines for a person representing a veteran before the BVA. Legislation enacted in the 109th Congress changed traditional guidelines to allow for legal representation for veterans throughout the administrative appeals process.

The veteran/claimant may appeal the decision of the BVA to the Court of Appeals for Veterans Claims (CAVC), which is an independent federal court and not part of the VA. The decision of the CAVC may be appealed by either the veteran/claimant or the VA to the U.S. Court of Appeals for the Federal Circuit (Federal Circuit), an Article III court that sits in Washington, DC and has exclusive jurisdiction to hear cases challenging CAVC rulings.

Decisions of the Federal Circuit may be appealed to the U.S. Supreme Court, which has final jurisdiction.

The VA has various statutory obligations to assist the veteran in the preparation of his/her application for benefits and any subsequent appeal(s). Among these obligations are assistance in the preparation of the initial application; provision of various records; medical exams; and other related issues. Certain legal and factual presumptions are established by statute that may be favorable to the veteran's claim. These issues are examined in the appendix to this chapter.

Legislation introduced in the 110th Congress concerning the appeal process is summarized in the appendix. These bills are H.R. 67, H.R. 653, H.R. 797, H.R. 1435, H.R. 1444, H.R. 1490, H.R. 1538, H.R. 2257, H.R. 2855, H.R. 3047, H.R. 5089, S. 1283, S. 1363, and S. 2737. H.R. 1318 is also discussed. One of the bills, H.R. 797, has been enacted into law (P.L. 110-157).

INTRODUCTION

Veterans' Benefits

Congress, through the United States Department of Veterans Affairs (VA), provides a broad variety of benefits and services to veterans and certain members of their families.[1] Among the benefits that the VA extends to veterans are various types of health care and related services, such as nursing homes, clinics, and medical centers; various types of financial benefits, including disability compensation and pensions; education, vocational training, and related career assistance; home financing; life insurance; burial benefits; and benefits for certain family survivors.[2]

The veteran's basic eligibility for these various services and programs is usually determined by the local VA office.[3] Various criteria must be met in order for the veteran to be eligible for VA benefits and the local VA office scrutinizes the veteran's claim before determining eligibility.[4]

Appeals from the Local VA Office Decisions

Veterans not satisfied with the decisions made by the local VA office on their claims or benefits may wish to have the decisions reviewed on appeal.[5] The VA has stated that the two most common types of appeals are 1) the denial of benefits for a disability that the veteran believes is service-connected; and 2) the veteran believes that his/her disability is more severe than the VA has rated it.[6] The first issue involves *disability compensation,* which is a monthly cash benefit for veterans currently impaired from past service-connected activities.[7] The second issue involves the VA's *rating of the severity of the veteran's disability* — which is directly related to the amount of monthly disability compensation (a cash payment) the veteran receives.[8] While these two issues seem to be the most prevalent types of appeals, nearly any decision made by the local VA office concerning veterans' benefits may be appealed.[9]

An appeal of the local VA office's decision may be made to 1) the local VA office (which made the original decision) and/or 2) the Board of Veterans' Appeals (BVA), which is discussed below. The findings of the BVA may be appealed to the U.S. Court of Veterans Claims. Subsequent appeals may be made to the U.S. Court of Appeals for the Federal Circuit and ultimately to the U.S. Supreme Court.

THE APPEAL PROCESS

Flow Chart of the Various Steps in the Appeal Process

The appeal process consists of several steps. The following flow chart provides a simplified outline of the steps that must be taken by the veteran in his/her appeal. Each step is discussed in detail in the text following the chart.

Filing the *Original* Claim for Benefits at the VA

In order to apply for VA benefits, the veteran must file a claim at the local VA office or VA medical facility.[10] A claim for benefits may also be filed on-line.[11] The claim must specifically state the requested benefit(s).[12] Assistance to the veteran during the application process may be provided by representatives from Veterans Service Organizations (VSOs)[13] and/or by other persons or agents.[14] The VSOs have staff located at most local VA offices.

In addition to assistance that may be provided by the VSOs or other agents, the VA is obligated by statute and regulation to provide certain assistance to the claimant during the original claim procedure and during any subsequent appeal(s). Such assistance many involve locating and producing records and providing medical examinations. Certain presumptions relating to medical conditions are also mandated by statute. These obligations and presumptions are summarized in the Appendix to this chapter.[15]

Following receipt of the veteran's claim for benefits, the local VA office will review the claim and make a decision about the claim(s).[16] The local VA office will either allow or deny the claim.[17] Where relevant, the local VA office may also rate (on a percentage basis) the veteran's degree of service-connected disability.[18] The local VA office's determination will be mailed to the veteran.[19] If the veteran is not satisfied with the local VA office decision, the veteran may appeal.

The Appeal: The First Steps

An appeal[20] is a request for a review of a local VA determination[21] on a claim for benefits.[22] Anyone who has filed a claim for benefits with the VA and has received a determination from a local VA office is eligible to appeal a complete or a partial denial of a claim.[23] The veteran may also appeal the level of benefit granted.[24]

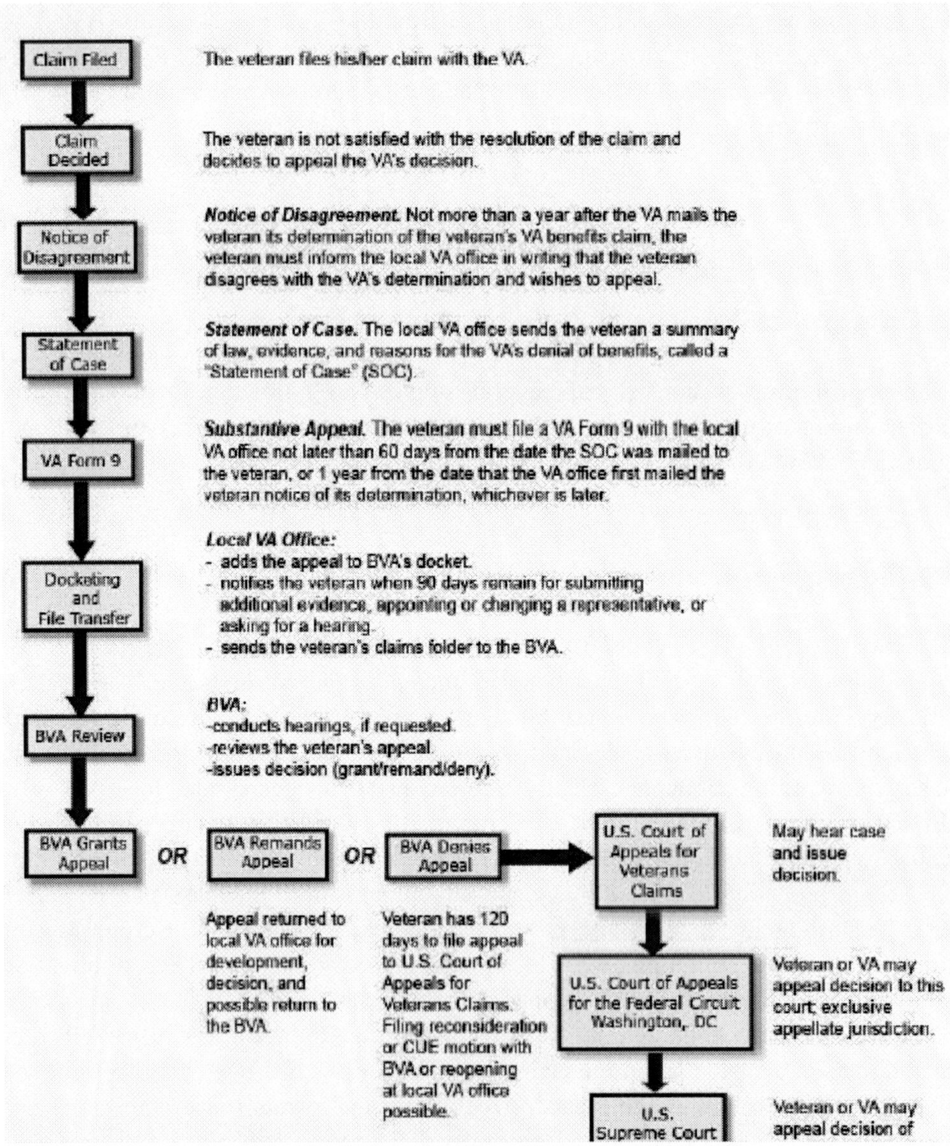

Source: Adapted from charts at *How Do I Appeal?* at 2 and *Understanding* at 32.
Note: These filing time limits apply in most cases. However, they do not apply to "simultaneously contested claims," when more than one person is trying to receive benefits that only one person is entitled to, such as life insurance proceeds. See *Understanding* at 11.

Figure 1. Appeal Process

Time Limit

The veteran seeking a review of the local VA office decision (called "the appellant") has one year from the date on which the local VA office mails the appellant its initial determination of the claim to appeal. After one year, the local VA office determination is considered final and cannot be appealed unless there is proof of clear and unmistakable error on the part of the VA.[25]

The Notice of Disagreement (NOD)[26]

There is no special form needed to initiate the appeal process. The appellant need only submit a written statement disagreeing with the local VA office's claim determination and stating the veteran's wish to appeal the claim determination. This statement is called the Notice of Disagreement (NOD).[27]

Appeal to the Local VA Office

The NOD is filed with the same local VA office that made the decision being appealed,[28] as this is the location of the appellant's claims file or claims folder,[29] unless the appellant has moved. After the NOD is filed, the appellant may request that his/her claims file be reviewed by a Decision Review Officer (DRO) from the local VA office. The DROs provide a second review of the entire file and may also hold a personal hearing on the claim.[30]

The Statement of the Case

At this point, the local VA office will either allow or not allow the claim. If the claim is disallowed, the local VA office will prepare and send to the appellant a Statement of Case (SOC) and a blank VA Form 9 to be used for continuation of the appeal. The SOC summarizes the submitted evidence and the relevant laws and regulations and provides the local VA office's reasons for making its determination and disallowing the claim.[31]

VA Form 9 and the Substantive Appeal[32]

To continue an appeal, the appellant must fill out and return the VA Form 9 — the Substantive Appeal — to the local VA office. Form 9 is available on-line.[33] The appellant must state the requested benefit, any mistakes in the SOC, and indicate whether a personal hearing is requested.[34] The Form 9 becomes part of the claims folder and is the basis for adding the appeal to the Board of Veterans Appeals docket. Specific provisions exist for the withdrawal of the appeal.[35]

Supplemental Statement of Case[36]

If the appellant submits new evidence or information, the local VA office will prepare a Supplemental Statement of Case (SSOC). The SSOC is similar to the SOC and includes the newly submitted information.[37] The appellant has 60 days from the date the SSOC was mailed to submit, in writing, any matter in dispute on the SSOC

Time Limitation[38]

The local VA office must receive the VA Form 9 within 60 days from the date that the VA mailed the SOC (or SSOC) or within one year of the date that the original decision denying the claim, whichever date is later.[39]

Withdrawal of Issue(s)

If the appellant does not wish the Board of Veterans Appeals to examine an issue that is contained in the SOC or the SSOC, the appellant may state on Form 9 that the appellant is withdrawing the issue(s) on the appeal.[40]

Issues Related to the Appeal Process

Filing Extensions[41]

An appellant may request an extension of the 60-day filing period for filing a Substantive Appeal or the 60-day period to respond to a Supplemental Statement of the Case.[42] The appellant makes this request in writing to the local VA office handling the appeal. The appellant needs to explain to the VA local office why extra time is needed to file.

Representation for the Appeal[43]

The appellant may represent him/herself at the appeal. However, the VA has reported that about 90 percent of appeals heard before the Board of Veterans Appeals (BVA) have some representation.[44]

There are three different categories of representatives that the appellant may engage. The first includes representatives of the VSO or from the state or local veterans' office. Usually, the representatives from the VSOs and the government veterans' offices do not charge for their services.[45] Second, the VA recognizes certain "agents" who are able to represent appellants and who are certified by the VA.[46] Third, the appellant may engage a lawyer for representation.[47]

The appellant must complete a **VA Form 21-22** to authorize representation by a VSO or a related entity on the appeal.[48] The appellant must complete a **VA Form 22a** to authorize representation by a lawyer[49] or a recognized agent for his/her appeal.[50] An appellant is limited to one representative recognized by the BVA.[51]

Attorney Representation: Recent Legislation

The Veterans Benefits, Health Care, and Information Technology Act of 2006,[52] enacted in the 109th Congress, modified attorney participation in the appeal process. The act also requires the Secretary of the VA to provide additional qualifications and standards for agents and attorneys who represent veterans before the VA, including standards that deal with (1) training and character and (2) fee criteria and limitations. The Secretary is authorized to charge and collect fees from the agents or attorneys to be used for administrative expenses for veterans' benefits programs. The following grounds for suspension of agents or attorneys are provided in the act: presenting frivolous claims, prior suspensions, charging excessive or unreasonable fees, or failure to comply with the Secretary's regulations.

The legislation significantly broadens opportunities for legal representation during administrative appeals. Previously, an attorney could not represent a veteran for a fee until the BVA made a final decision.[53] This had the effect of excluding an attorney from the process until all of the administrative appeals had been exhausted. The act now permits an attorney to enter the appeal process at a much earlier date — after the veteran has received a decision on his or her claim from the VA and decides to appeal this initial decision administratively through the filing of a NOD.[54] An attorney may now provide representation for a fee after the NOD is filed. The act requires the Secretary to provide Congress with an evaluation of the effect of the new system of representation. The Secretary is also authorized to review fee agreements, and the Secretary may order a reduction in an agreed upon fee if the Secretary finds the fee excessive or unreasonable. The Secretary's decision may be reviewed by the BVA, which is authorized to make the final review of the issue.[55]

Broadening attorney participation in the veterans' appeal process has been somewhat controversial. Opposition has focused on attorneys' fees and the possibility of additional delays in the appeal process. On March 5, 2007, Representative Ron Lewis introduced H.R. 1318,[56] which, if enacted, would repeal the authority for certain agent or attorney representation in veterans' benefit cases before the VA. In effect, the bill would return to the process that existed prior to the enactment of the 2006 law and would permit representation only after the BVA renders a final decision in the case. The bill has been referred to the House Committee on Veterans' Affairs and referred to the Subcommittee on Disability Assistance and Memorial Affairs.

Information for the Appeal

Should new evidence or medical proof supporting the appellant's claim arise during the appeal process, the evidence should be submitted to the VA. If the appellant's claims file is at the local VA office and the new evidence is sent there, the VA local office will send the appellant an SSOC if it does not allow the claim after reviewing the new evidence. The new evidence will be added to the claims file and considered during the appeal process.[57]

Location of the VA Form 9

After the Form 9 is filed, it becomes part of the claims file and serves as the basis for the appeal to the BVA. The Form 9, as part of the claims file, will be sent by the local VA office to the BVA and will be reviewed later by the BVA when the BVA considers the appeal and reviews the entire claims file.

THE BOARD OF VETERANS' APPEALS (BVA)

Organization[58]

Known as the "Gateway to VA Appeals,"[59] the Board of Veterans' Appeals (BVA) is a part of the VA based in Washington, DC.[60] The BVA reviews benefit claims appeals and issues decisions on those appeals. The BVA is composed of "Members of the Board" who are attorneys experienced in veterans' law, appointed by the Secretary of Veterans Affairs and approved by the President of the United States. Staff attorneys, who are designated as Counsel or Associate Counsel, assist Members of the Board in preparing decisions.[61] The function that they provide is similar to a law clerk who assists a judge in his/her legal capacities.[62]

The BVA's Docket

The BVA Docket and Docket Number

The local VA office will forward the appellant's claims file to the BVA's docket. The law requires that the BVA decide cases on a "first come, first served" basis.[63] Each appellant's case is added to the docket when the VA receives the substantive appeal — VA Form 9 — and the claims file from the local VA.[64]

On occasion, the BVA may, on a motion by the appellant, advance the order of a claim on its docket.[65] The appellant must demonstrate compelling need, exceptional circumstances, or proof of hardship.[66] The BVA seldom grants a request for "advancement on the docket," as the BVA feels that most appeals involve some form of hardship and the BVA wishes to treat all appellants fairly.[67]

Waiting Time

Once a case/claim has been entered on the BVA's docket, it is uncertain how long it may take for the BVA to reach a decision on the case. The VA has stated, that as of the fall of 1999, it took an average of two years from the time a NOD was filed, until a final decision was issued.[68] However, 2005 congressional testimony by the Undersecretary for Benefits of the VA appears to indicate that the decision time has been substantially reduced.[69]

PERSONAL HEARINGS

There are two types of personal hearings: a *local VA office hearing*[70] and a *BVA hearing*.

As previously discussed,[71] a local office hearing is held at the local VA office between the appellant and a *hearing officer* from the local VA office staff. Such a hearing is arranged between the appellant and the local VA office. The local VA office may find in favor of the appellant. The appellant may subsequently appeal the local office hearing through the BVA.

The appellant may present his/her case in person to a member of the BVA. There are three types of BVA hearings: a hearing by a Board member at a the local VA office (Regional Office), called a Travel Board hearing;[72] a hearing at the BVA office in Washington, DC; or a videoconference hearing at the local VA office, if it is equipped for videoconferencing. The VA does not provide travel expenses to the appellant.[73]

Request for a BVA Hearing

The typical way to request a BVA hearing is for the appellant to indicate on VA Form 9 the type of hearing that the appellant wishes. The appellant may also write to the BVA to request a hearing, indicating whether a hearing is requested at the local level or in Washington, DC.

Scheduling the BVA Hearing

The schedule of the hearing depends upon the type of hearing requested. The BVA has reported that the Travel Board hearings are usually held as soon as they can be scheduled on the hearing officer's calendar,[74] but that they may be difficult to arrange because of the schedules of the BVA Board members and the accumulation of a sufficient number of appeals to warrant a scheduled visit from a BVA member.[75] Videoconferenced hearings are less complicated to arrange and can be scheduled more quickly than Travel Board hearings, according to the BVA.[76]

Hearings that are held at the BVA offices in Washington DC are usually scheduled close to the time when the BVA will consider the case. In 2000, the BVA reported that the BVA will schedule a case about three months before the case is reviewed.[77]

The Ninety Day Rule

The local VA office will notify the appellant by letter when it transfers the claims file to the BVA in Washington, DC. The letter will inform the claimant that the claimant has ninety days from the date of the letter or until the BVA decides the case, whichever comes first, to add additional evidence to the file, request a hearing (if none was selected), and/or select or change representation.[78]

In order for the BVA to accept any of these materials after the expiration of the ninety day period, the appellant must submit a motion — a written request — asking the BVA to accept the item, even though it is late. The motion needs to include an explanation of why the item is late and demonstrate why the BVA should accept the item into the claims file.

The Appeal at the BVA

The local VA office will forward the appellant's file to the BVA. The appellant will be notified in writing when the file is officially transferred and received by the BVA.[79] The decision time in the appeal process varies from case to case. After the file is received by the BVA, the appellant's case will then be assigned to a Board member for review. When the docket number for the appeal has been reached, the file will be examined by a Board member and a staff attorney. They will check the file for completeness, review all of the evidence and arguments, the transcript of the local VA hearing, the statement of the appellant's representative (if the appellant has a representative), and any additional information that may be with the claims file.[80] The Board member may request the staff attorney to undertake additional research on the case and prepare recommendations for the review of the Board member. If the appellant requested a BVA hearing, the Board member assigned to the case will conduct the hearing before reaching a decision.

Before reaching a decision, the Board member will examine all of the material in the appellant's file, along with the recommendations prepared by the staff attorney. The Board member will then issue a decision on the appeal.[81]

Notification of the Board's Decision

The BVA will issue its decision in writing. The decision may contain legal documents and legal discussions as well as medical discussions. The decision will be mailed to the appellant's home address.[82]

The decision will allow, deny, or remand the claim. If the claim is allowed or denied, the BVA's decision is final. A remand is not a final decision and allows further work on the claim.[83]

If the appeal is denied, the BVA will send a copy of the "Notice of Appellate Rights" that describes additional actions that the appellant may choose to pursue.

The Remand

At times the BVA may review an appeal and determine that the case is not ready for a final decision. The BVA will send the case back to the local VA office with directions as to what should be done. The action of returning the case to the local VA office for additional work is called a remand. It is sometimes described as "additional development."[84]

After the case has been returned to the local VA office, it will perform the additional work on the file. The local VA office will review the case and issue a new determination. If the local VA office does not allow the claim, it will return the case to the BVA for a final decision. The case keeps its original place on the BVA's docket, so it is usually reviewed relatively soon after it is returned to the BVA.[85]

Certain cases are remanded because of new rulings by the U.S. Court of Appeals for Veterans Claims or changes in the law. The local VA office will then review them within the context of the new legislation or the court ruling.[86]

Additional Appeal Options

Should the appellant wish to appeal the BVA's decision, the appellant may appeal to the United States Court of Appeals for Veterans Claims (CAVC), an independent court and not part of the VA.[87] An appellant may also wish to pursue further motions with the BVA.

Notice of Appeal

Usually, the appellant must file the Notice of Appeal with the CAVC within 120 days from the date the BVA's decision is mailed. (The mailing date is stamped on the front of the BVA's decision.)

If the appellant filed a motion to reconsider with the BVA within the 120-day time period and that motion was denied, the appellant has a new 120-day period to file the Notice of Appeal with the CAVC.[88] The new 120-day period begins on the date the BVA mails the appellant a letter notifying the appellant that it has denied the motion to reconsider.

Motion for Reconsideration

If the appellant is able to demonstrate that the BVA made an obvious error of fact or of law in its decision, the appellant may file a written "motion to reconsider" of the appeal.[89] The appellant may have the VSO representative advise him/her whether to file the motion and the VSO representative may also provide assistance in its preparation. The motion to reconsider is sent directly to the BVA and not to the local VA office.

The appellant will need to demonstrate that the BVA made a mistake in law or in fact and that the BVA's decision would have been different if the mistake had not been made.[90]

Reopening the Case

If the appellant has "new and material" evidence relating to his/her claim, the appellant can request that the case be reopened.[91] In order to be considered "new and material," the evidence submitted needs to include information related to the case that was not included in the claims folder when the Board reviewed and decided the case.

To reopen a case, the appellant must submit the new evidence directly to the local VA office and not to the BVA.[92]

CUE Motion

A BVA decision may be reversed or revised if the appellant is able to show that the decision contained "clear and unmistakable error" (CUE).[93] The written request for the BVA to review its decision for CUE is called a motion. CUE motions are filed directly with the BVA and not with the local VA office.

The motion for CUE review must meet various requirements and if the motion is denied, the appellant cannot request another CUE review. The VA has reported that not many CUE motions are successful. In order to succeed, the conclusion must be reached that the BVA would have decided the case differently, but for the error. A difference in opinion is not sufficient.[94]

The appellant may file a motion to review a BVA decision for CUE at any time. However, if the motion for CUE is filed after filing a timely Notice of Appeal with the CAVC (120 days),[95] the BVA will not be able to rule on the CUE motion.[96]

Death of the Appellant Before a Decision Issued

The death of the appellant usually ends the appeal.[97] If the appellant dies, the BVA normally dismisses the appeal without issuing a decision. Any rights of a deceased appellant's survivors are not affected by this action. The survivors may file a claim at the VA regional office (RO) for any benefits to which they may be entitled.[98]

Subsequent Judicial Appeals

The *U.S. Court of Appeals for the Federal Circuit* (Federal Circuit) has exclusive jurisdiction to hear cases involving challenges to VA decisions in an appeal of a CAVC decision and in a direct challenge to VA regulation and VA policies of general applicability.[99] A decision of the CAVC may be appealed to the Federal Circuit by the persons who appealed to the CAVC or by the VA. An appeal to the Federal Circuit must be filed within 60 days of the final CAVC decision. After the Federal Circuit issues a final decision, either the claimant or the VA may petition the U.S. Supreme Court for certiorari (to hear the case) within ninety days of the Federal Circuit's final action.[100] The Supreme Court is the court of last resort and the Supreme Court's decision is final.

APPENDIX. DUTIES AND OBLIGATIONS OF THE VA TO THE CLAIMANT/APPELLANT

The Obligations of the VA to the Claimant/Appellant[101]

The VA[102] has various legal obligations to a claimant/appellant relating to the completeness of the application for benefits (or a subsequent appeal), the provision of medical and service records, and other issues related to the application/appeals process.

Application and Notice of Incomplete Application

The VA is required to provide to any person claiming or applying for any benefit, the "instructions and forms necessary to apply for that benefit."[103] These materials are to be provided "free of all expense" to the claimant.[104]

If the claimant's application for a VA benefit is incomplete, the VA is required to notify the claimant of the information that is necessary to complete the application.[105]

Required Information and Evidence; and Time Limitation[106]

After the VA receives a complete or a nearly complete application for benefits, the VA is required to notify the claimant of any information or medical or lay evidence that is needed to substantiate the claim.[107] As part of this notification requirement, the VA is required to indicate which information and evidence is to be provided by the claimant and which information the VA will attempt to obtain on the claimant's behalf to substantiate and complete the claim.

The claimant is required to submit the above-mentioned evidence to substantiate the claim *within one year of the date of the VA 's notification*. If no further evidence is obtained, no benefits will be paid or furnished on this claim.[108]

Duty to Assist Claimants: Records

The VA is required to make "reasonable efforts" to assist a claimant in obtaining evidence necessary to substantiate the claim for benefits.[109] However, certain exceptions exist to this requirement. The VA is not required to provide assistance to the claimant if "no reasonable possibility" exists that such assistance would aid in substantiating the claim.[110] The VA may defer providing assistance pending the claimant's submission of essential information that is missing from the claimant's application.[111]

Assistance in Obtaining Records

The VA is required to make "reasonable efforts" to obtain relevant records (including private records) that the claimant adequately identifies to the VA and authorizes the VA to obtain.[112] Federal regulations outline the procedures for obtaining records not in the custody of a federal department or agency[113] and obtaining records in the custody of a federal department or agency.[114] If after making reasonable efforts, the VA is unable to locate the records, the VA will notify the claimant that the VA is unable to obtain the records pursuant to this claim.[115] The notification is required to identify the records being sought, explain the efforts made to obtain the records, and describe any further action to be taken by the VA regarding this claim.[116] It is required that the VA's efforts to obtain records from the federal department or agency will continue until the records are obtained, unless it is reasonably certain that such records do not exist or that further efforts to obtain the records would be futile.[117]

Records for Compensation Claims

If the case involves a claim for disability compensation, additional assistance in obtaining records is required to be provided.[118] Assistance is to be provided in locating the claimant's service medical records and other relevant records relating to the claimant's active military, naval, or air service that are held or maintained by a governmental entity;[119] records of relevant medical treatment or examination at VA health-care facilities;[120] and any other relevant records held by any federal department or agency that the claimant identifies and authorizes the VA to obtain.[121]

Medical Examinations for Compensation Claims

If the case involves a claim for disability compensation, the VA is required to provide a medical examination or obtain a medical opinion when such an examination or opinion is necessary to make a decision on the claim.[122] The VA is required to treat an examination or opinion as being necessary to make a decision on a claim if the evidence on the record, taking in consideration all information and lay or medical evidence 1) contains competent evidence that the claimant has a current disability or persistent or recurrent symptoms of disability[123] or 2) indicates that the disability or symptoms may be associated with the claimant's active military, naval, or air service;[124] but does not contain sufficient medical evidence for the VA to make a decision on the claim.[125]

Disallowed Claims

The statute specifically provides that the VA is not required to reopen a claim that has been disallowed except when new and material evidence is presented or secured.[126]

Other Assistance not Precluded

The statute is not to be construed as precluding the VA from providing such other assistance to a claimant in substantiating a claim as the VA considers appropriate.[127]

Decisions and Notices of Decisions

When the VA makes a decision affecting the provision of benefits to a claimant, the VA is required, on a timely basis, to provide the claimant (and the claimant's representative) notice of the decision.[128] The notice must include an explanation of the procedure for obtaining a review of the decision.[129] If the VA denies a benefit, the notice is required to include a statement of the reason for the decision and a summary of the evidence considered by the VA.[130]

VA's Obligation to Assist in the Development of Claims

Federal regulations require the VA to assist the claimant "in developing the facts pertinent to the claim" and to render a decision that grants every benefit that can be supported in law while protecting the interests of the government.[131] Therefore, the VA has the duty to consider all legal theories upon which the claim could be granted,[132] regardless of whether the claimant argues or focuses on every possible legal theory.

Reopening Disallowed Claims

If any new or material evidence is presented or secured relating to a claim that has been disallowed, the VA is required to reopen the claim and review the former disposition of the claim.[133]

Revision of Decisions on Grounds of Clear and Unmistakable Error

A VA decision is subject to revision on the grounds of clear and unmistakable error, as previously discussed.[134] If there is evidence to establish the error, the prior decision is reversed or revised.[135] For the purposes of authorizing benefits, a rating, or other adjudicative decision that constitutes a reversal or revision of a prior decision on the grounds of clear and unmistakable error, has the effect as if the decision had been made on the date of the prior decision.[136] A review to determine whether a clear and unmistakable error exists in a case may be initiated by the VA or upon the request of the claimant.[137] A request for a revision of a VA decision based on clear and unmistakable error may be made at any time after the decision is made.[138] Such a request for a revision shall be submitted to the VA and shall be decided in the same manner as any other claim.[139]

Benefit of the Doubt Standard

The VA is required to consider all information and the legal and medical evidence of record in a case before the VA with respect to benefits under the laws administered by the VA.[140] When there is an approximate balance of positive and negative evidence regarding any issue material to the determination, the VA "shall give the benefit of the doubt to the claimant."[141] Regulations provide that when reasonable doubt arises, such doubt will be resolved in favor of the claimant.[142] For instance, in order to satisfy this element, the submitted medical evidence generally needs to show that it is as likely as not that there is a connection between the in-service injury, occurrence, or illness and the current disability. Thus, the VA can deny the claim only if the preponderance of the evidence is against the claim.

Certain Presumptions

In its analysis of certain claims, the VA is required by statute and/or regulation to make certain presumptions.

Presumption of Medical Soundness

In evaluating a veteran's claim, the VA generally presumes that the veteran entered the service in sound medical condition.[143] This may assist the veteran in proving a claim by making it difficult for the VA to claim that the condition or disease existed prior to service. However, if the medical impairment was noted at the time of entry into service, the veteran may have to prove that the condition was exacerbated in-service. If the VA is able to prove by "clear and unmistakable evidence" that the disease or injury was in existence prior to service, and that it was not worsened during service, the veteran's claim will be denied.

Special Rules for Certain In-Service Occurrences

Special rules exist under which the VA is required to consider a service-connected problem by presumption. For example, certain diseases associated with exposure to Agent Orange will be presumed to be service-related in the case of Vietnam veterans.[144]

A similar regulation holds that veterans who were held prisoners of war, or who served in combat, can be presumed to have suffered traumatic, stressful events during their military service.[145] Similarly, combat veterans have special rules applicable to them in proving an in-service injury or other incident.[146] Usually, if a combat veteran states that he/she suffered a disease, injury, or other event during the combat, the VA will usually accept that statement as fact. This is the case even if there are no service records to substantiate the claim.

LEGISLATION INTRODUCED IN THE 110TH CONGRESS

Legislation has been introduced in the 110th Congress, which, if enacted, may affect the appeal process. The summary below covers the following bills: H.R. 67, H.R. 653, H.R. 797, H.R. 1435, H.R. 1444, H.R. 1490, H.R. 1538, H.R. 2257, H.R. 2855, H.R. 3047, H.R. 5089, S. 1283, S. 1363, and S. 2737.

H.R. 67

H.R. 67 (sponsored by Representative Mike McIntyre),[147] the proposed Veterans Outreach Improvement Act of 2007, would establish procedures for coordinating activities of the VA and various related entities, including the Veterans Health Administration, the Veterans Benefits Administration, and the National Cemetery Administration. The Secretary would be required to review these procedures annually.

The bill would provide assistance to the states to help carry out veterans benefits and related programs. The Secretary could provide assistance to county veteran service programs, enter into agreements and arrangements with state veterans agencies, and make grants to state veterans agencies to assist in outreach activities and the submittal of benefits claims.

Outreach activities would be funded through a separate appropriation account. A sum of $25 million would be authorized for each fiscal year from 2007-2009.

The bill defines "outreach" within the context of the legislation as taking steps in a way to provide "information, services and benefits counseling to veterans" and their survivors who may be eligible for such benefits.[148]

H.R. 653

H.R. 653 (sponsored by Representative Thomas M. Reynolds)[149] would have the Secretary of Veterans Affairs accept that an injury or disease is service-connected (if there is no clear and convincing proof to the contrary), based upon the sworn affidavit of a veteran who served in combat on or before July 27, 1953 (prior to or during the Korean War).

H.R. 797

H.R. 797 (sponsored by Representative Tammy Baldwin), which was enacted into law,[150] expands disability compensation for veterans who are visually impaired in both eyes by a standard definition of blindness used by other federal agencies.

H.R. 1435

H.R. 1435, the proposed Department of Veterans Affairs Claims Backlog Reduction Act of 2007 (sponsored by Representative Joe Baca),[151] if enacted, would direct the Secretary to conduct a pilot program to reduce the backlog of pending benefits claims.

The bill would make various findings on claims backlogs and the quality of County Veterans Service Officers (CVSOs). The bill would establish a three-year pilot program to reduce the backlog of veterans' claims in the following states: California, Florida, Ohio, South Carolina, and Texas.[152] Claims identified as requiring further development would be referred to a CVSO, based upon the Officer's geographical proximity to the claimant. The bill outlines the procedures for the development of the claim by the CVSO and the claimant.[153] Under the program, the CVSO would serve as the claimant's advocate in developing and transmitting the claim. The CVSO could also cooperate with a veterans service organization to develop the claim. During the development of the claim, the CVSO would have access to client information, including information held by the VA.

Following the completion of the pilot program, the Secretary would report to Congress regarding backlog reduction, statistics, and other related information.

H.R. 1444

H.R. 1444 (sponsored by Representative John J. Hall),[154] if enacted, would direct the Secretary to make interim payments in cases remanded (referred back) to the VA by the BVA or the CAVC if the VA fails to decide the matter within 180 days of remand. If the Secretary does not make a decision within 180 days of the remand, then until the matter is finally decided, the Secretary would be required to pay an interim benefit of $500 per month. When a claim is finally decided, and if benefits are awarded, the interim payments would be considered advance benefit payments. If the final decision is not to award benefits, the interim benefits would not be considered an overpayment.

Under the bill, the Secretary would also be required to submit to Congress a report on measures that the Secretary intends to expedite the process of remanded claims for veterans benefits.

H.R. 1490

If enacted, H.R. 1490 (sponsored by Representative Joe Donnelly)[155] would provide for a presumption of service-connectedness in certain claims for benefits, upon the claimant proving service in a conflict and the nature of the claim, unless the Secretary determines that there is positive evidence to the contrary. The bill would require the Secretary to award benefits, at a "median level" as determined by the Secretary, immediately upon processing the claim until such time as the appropriate level of benefits is determined.[156]

The bill would also provide for the redeployment of VA claims workers freed up by the presumption of service-connectedness to assist veterans with their claims.[157] Such staff would be redeployed to veterans centers or other locations that the Secretary determines are appropriate.

H.R. 1538

H.R. 1538 (sponsored by Representative Ike Skelton)[158] deals primarily with improving the management of medical care, personnel actions, and quality of life issues for members of the Armed Forces. However, certain provisions could impact the appeal process. The bill addresses disability evaluations, a study by DOD and the VA concerning their individual evaluation systems, and the possibility of combining the two systems. The bill would also streamline record keeping and the transfer of records from DOD to the VA. Some of the bill's provisions are similar to those of S. 1283, discussed below.

H.R. 2257

H.R. 2257 (sponsored by Representative Peter Welch)[159] would require the Secretary of the VA to increase the number of benefits claims representatives. The bill would require that no fewer than two claims representative be located at each "vet center."[160]

H.R. 2855

In addition to providing new types of assistance, H.R. 2855 (sponsored by Representative Ciro D. Rodriguez),[161] the proposed Wounded Heroes Bill of Rights Act, would establish a Wounded Heroes Independent Review Board ("Board") to review certain cases involving a member of the Armed Forces or a veteran who was severely injured on or after September 11, 2001, while on active duty.[162]

Upon the request of a "Wounded Hero," the Board would expeditiously review the decision or determination of the VA or other federal department or agency relating to the eligibility for or the scope of benefits, including health care or vocational rehabilitation benefits. Following a review, the Board would render a written advisory opinion relating to such eligibility or provision of such care or benefits.

An advisory opinion rendered by the Board would be "considered as evidence" by the BVA and the CAVC in any case with respect to the "Wounded Hero" before the BVA or the CAVC, upon the submission of the opinion by the "Wounded Hero."[163] An advisory opinion rendered by the Board could not be reviewed by any other official or by any court, whether by an action in the nature of mandamus or otherwise.[164]

H.R. 3047

H.R. 3047 (sponsored by Representative Doug Lamborn),[165] the proposed Veterans Claims Processing Innovation Act of 2007, would provide changes to improve the processing of claims for benefits administered by the VA.

Among the changes proposed by the bill is the implementation of a work credit system for the BVA.[166] Under this system, a regional office of the BVA would receive work credit for a claim assigned to the regional office when the appellate period for the claim has expired or the BVA has issued a final decision with respect to the claim.[167]

The bill would also implement the electronic processing of claims for benefits administered by the Secretary of Veterans Affairs (Secretary).[168] The Secretary would be required to develop and maintain a system for processing claims for disability compensation using artificial intelligence. The system would use medical and military service data to generate recommendations with respect to disability ratings.[169]

Section 4 of the bill would provide for the treatment of the beneficiary of a deceased veteran's accrued benefits as the claimant for the purpose of incomplete claims at the time of the death of the veteran.[170] Thus, if a veteran claimant dies before completing the submission of a claim for any benefit administered by the Secretary, the person who would have received any accrued benefits due to the veteran would be treated as the claimant for the purpose of completing the submission of the claim.[171]

Section 5 of the bill would require an evaluation by a private contractor of training and performance assessment programs for VA employees.[172]

H.R. 5089

H.R. 5089, (sponsored by Representative John Barrow),[173] would propose to reform the veterans' disability determination process by requiring the Secretary of Veterans Affairs to pay disability compensation to certain veterans based on the concurring diagnosis of two physicians.

S. 1283

S. 1283, (sponsored by Senator Mark Pryor)[174] deals primarily with improving the management of medical care, personnel actions, and quality of life issues for members of the Armed Forces. However, certain provisions could impact the appeal process. Among these issues are evaluation of the disability evaluation system, a study by DOD and the VA concerning their individual evaluation systems, and the possibility of combining the two systems. Some of the bill's provisions are similar to those of H.R. 1538, discussed above.

S. 1363

S. 1363 (sponsored by Senator Hillary Rodham Clinton),[175] the proposed Bridging the Gap for Wounded Warriors Act, would improve health care for severely injured members and former members of the armed forces. The bill would create a Department of Defense-Department of Veterans Affairs Office of Transition ("Office").[176] Among the functions of this office would be to "develop uniform standards, to be applicable across the military departments and to the Department of Veterans Affairs, for the rating of disabilities incurred or aggravated by members of the Armed Forces during service in the Armed Forces."[177] The bill would also provide for the reform of the disability ratings systems of the Department of Defense and the Department of Veterans Affairs.[178]

S. 2737

S. 2737 (sponsored by Senator Daniel K. Akaka),[179] the proposed "Veterans' Rating Schedule Review Act" would amend title 38 of the United States Code to grant jurisdiction to the U.S. Court of Appeals for Veterans Claims to review compliance of ratings for disabilities under the schedule of 38 U.S.C. § 1151 with the statutory requirements applicable to entitlement to disability compensation.

End Notes

[1] See generally *Federal Benefits for Veterans and Dependents*, published by the Department of Veterans Affairs (2008 edition), available online at [http://www1 .va.gov/opa/vadocs/ fedben.pdf]. See CRS Report RL33113, *Veterans Affairs: Basic Eligibility for Disability Programs*, by Douglas Reid Weimer. This chapter deals with the fundamental requirements for disability benefit programs. See CRS Report RL33323, *Veterans Affairs: Benefits for Service-Connected Disabilities*, by Douglas Reid Weimer. This chapter discusses various aspects of disability compensation, a monthly cash benefit program for veterans currently impaired from past service-connected activities.

[2] See CRS Report RL33323.

[3] The *local VA office* is defined by the VA as "any local office of the Department of Veterans Affairs where claims for VA benefits are received and determined." This is usually a VA Regional Office or an administrative office at a VA medical center. The legal term for such an office is the "agency of original jurisdiction." A VA *Regional Office* is one of 58 VA regional offices located throughout the United States and its territories, and it is at these offices where most claims for VA benefits are filed and determined. *Thus, all Regional Offices are considered to be "local offices," but the concept of "local office" may also include administrative offices located at VA medical centers.* Therefore, all Regional Offices are "local offices," but not all "local offices" are Regional Offices. See *Board of Veterans' Appeals, Understanding the Appeal Process*, published by the Department of Veterans Affairs; VA Pamphlet 01-00-1 (January 2000) at 38-39 (cited to afterward as "Understanding"). See [http://www.va.gov/vbs/bva/y2000.pdf] for the publication online. Go to the website and click on "Understanding the Appeal Process."

[4] See CRS Report RL33323.

[5] *How Do I Appeal?*, published by the Board of Veterans Appeals, Department of Veterans Affairs; VA Pamphlet 1-02-02A (April 2002) at 1 (cited to afterward as *"How Do I Appeal?"*). See [http://www.va.gov/vbs/bva/pamphlet.htm]. Go to the website and click on "How Do I Appeal?" for an online copy of the pamphlet.

[6] *Id.*

[7] See CRS Report RL33323.

[8] *Id.* at 7-10. For instance, the local VA office may determine that the veteran is 10% disabled, while the veteran believes that he/she is 40% disabled.

[9] See *How Do I Appeal?* at 1. For example, a veteran may appeal a denial of education benefits made by the local VA office.

[10] The *local VA office* is defined by the VA as "any local office of the Department of Veterans Affairs where claims for VA benefits are received and determined." This is usually a VA Regional Office or an administrative office at a VA medical center. The legal term for such an office is the "agency of original jurisdiction." A VA *Regional Office* is one of 58 VA regional offices located throughout the United States and its territories, and it is at these offices where most claims for VA benefits are filed and determined. *Thus, all Regional Offices are considered to be "local offices," but the concept of "local office" may also include administrative offices located at VA medical centers.* Therefore, all Regional Offices are "local offices," but not all "local offices" are Regional Offices. See *Board of Veterans' Appeals, Understanding the Appeal Process*, published by the Department of Veterans Affairs; VA Pamphlet 01-00-1 (January 2000) at 38-39 (cited to afterward as "Understanding"). See [http://www.va.gov/vbs/bva/pamphlet.htm] for the publication online. Go to the website and click on "Understanding the Appeal Process."

[11] See *How Do I Appeal* at 3. File the claim at [http://www.vba.va.gov]. Go to the website, then go to "Apply Online" and click on "Compensation and Pension." This is the Veterans ON-line APPlication (VONAPP) website.

[12] Such benefits might relate to medical care, disability compensation, or educational benefits.

[13] Such organizations are the American Legion, the Disabled American Veterans, and other veterans' groups.

[14] See *How Do I Appeal?* at 3.

[15] See discussion at Appendix.

[16] See CRS Report RL33323.

[17] *Id.*

[18] *Id.* at 7-10.

[19] See *How Do I Appeal?* at 3.

[20] See 38 C.F.R. § 20.200. What Constitutes An Appeal. "An appeal consists of a timely filed Notice of Disagreement in writing and, after a Statement of the Case has been furnished, a timely filed Substantive Appeal."

[21] See *Understanding* at 6. Most local determinations are made by the local VA office. However, some determinations made by VA medical facilities, such as eligibility for medical treatment, may also be appealed.

[22] 38 U.S.C. § 511(a) outlines the authority of the Secretary of the VA to make decisions regarding benefits for veterans.

[23] Again, see *Understanding* at 6. Most local determinations are made by the local VA office. However, some determinations made by VA medical facilities, such as eligibility for medical treatment, may also be appealed.

[24] For example, a veteran may be determined to be 20% disabled and the veteran may believe that he/she is 40% disabled and appeal.

[25] See *Understanding* at 6-7.

[26] See 38 C.F.R. § 20.201.

[27] See *Understanding* at 39.

[28] 38 C.F.R. § 20.300.

[29] For the purpose of this chapter, the appellant's records will be referred to as "claims file."

[30] See *How Do I Appeal?* at 4.

[31] See *Understanding* at 8-9.

[32] 38 C.F.R. § 20.202.

[33] See [http://www.vba.va.gov]. Go to the website, then go to "Board of Veterans' Appeals," then go to "VA Forms," then type in VA9.

[34] A personal hearing must be requested. Without such a request, the BVA will review the claims file and the VA Form 9 and make a decision without meeting or speaking with the appellant and his/her representative.

[35] 38 C.F.R. § 20.204.

[36] 38 C.F.R. § 20.302(b), (c).

[37] See *Understanding* at 40-41.

[38] 38 C.F.R. § 20.302.

[39] Id. See *How Do I Appeal?* at 6.

[40] See *Understanding* at 10.

[41] 38 C.F.R. § 20.303.

[42] 38 U.S.C § 5105(d)(3); 38 C.F.R. § 20.303.

[43] See in general, 38 C.F.R. § 20.600. Legislation pending in the 110th Congress, discussed below, may change the representation available to appellants.

[44] See *Understanding* at 12.

[45] See *Understanding* at 12.

[46] 38 U.S.C. § 5904; 38 C.F.R. § 20.604.

[47] 38 C.F.R. § 20.603.

[48] 38 C.F.R. § 20.602.

[49] 38 C.F.R. § 20.603.
[50] 38 C.F.R. § 20.604.
[51] See *Understanding* at 12.
[52] P.L. 109-461, Title I.
[53] See Figure I. Appeal Process at 3.
[54] *Id.*
[55] 38 U.S.C. § 7104.
[56] 110th Cong., 1st Sess. (2007).
[57] See *Understanding* at 13-14.
[58] For a general overview of the BVA, see the website at [http://www.va.gov/vbs/bva].
[59] See note 57.
[60] 38 U.S.C. § 7101(a); 38 U.S.C. § 7104.
[61] See *Understanding* at 6.
[62] *Id.*
[63] 38 U.S.C. § 7107(a); 38 C.F.R. § 20.900.
[64] See *Understanding* at 15. Each case is assigned a docket number when it is added to the list of cases. The first two numbers are the year in which the case was filed and the remaining numbers indicate the order in which the case was added to that year's list/docket. For example, 05-00111, would indicate the 111th claim filed in 2005.
[65] 38 U.S.C. § 7107(a)92); 38 C.F.R. § 20.900.
[66] For example, terminal illness, bankruptcy, pending eviction, and other hardships.
[67] See *Understanding* at 16.
[68] *Id.*
[69] Testimony of Daniel L. Cooper, Undersecretary of Benefits, Department of Veterans Affairs before the Senate Veterans Affairs Committee (May 26, 2005). See [http://www.va.gov/OCA/testimony
[70] This is sometimes called a Regional Office hearing, an RO hearing, or a hearing officer hearing.
[71] See "Appeal to the Local VA Office" on page 6.
[72] See note 3.
[73] See *Understanding* at 18.
[74] *Id.* at 19.
[75] *Id.*
[76] *Id.*
[77] *Id.*
[78] 38 C.F.R. § 20.1304.
[79] See *Understanding* at 21. Appellants may check the status of their file after its transfer to by BVA by telephone at 202-565-5436.
[80] *Id.* at 22.
[81] *Id.* at 23.
[82] *Id.*
[83] See *How Do I Appeal* at 11.
[84] See *Understanding* at 24.
[85] *Id.*
[86] *Id.*
[87] See the CAVC' s website: [http://www.vetapp.uscourts.gov/].
[88] See *Understanding* at 25-26 for the appropriate addresses to file the Notice of Appeal and a copy of the Notice of Appeal.
[89] 38 U.S.C. § 7103; 38 C.F.R. § 20.1000; 38 C.F.R. § 20.1001.
[90] See *Understanding* at 27.
[91] 38 U.S.C. § 5108; 38 U.S.C. § 7104(b); 38 C.F.R. § 3.156; 38 C.F.R. § 20.1105.
[92] See *Understanding* at 27.
[93] 38 U.S.C. § 7111; 38 C.F.R. § 20, subpart O.
[94] *Id.*
[95] See "Nature of Appeal" at 11.
[96] See *Understanding* at 28.
[97] 38 U.S.C. § 7 104(a); 38 C.F.R. § 20.1302.
[98] See *Understanding* at 29.
[99] 38 U.S.C. § 7292. See CRS Report RS22561, *Veterans Affairs: The U.S. Court of Appeals for Veterans Claims — Judicial Review of VA Decision Making,* by Douglas Reid Weimer.
[100] 38 U.S.C. § 7292(c).
[101] See CRS Report RL33323.
[102] The statutory language provides that "the Secretary" is required to provide various assistance to the claimant. For the purposes of this summary and for consistency, the term "VA" is used instead.

[103] 38 U.S.C. § 5102(a); 38 C.F.R. § 3.150(a).
[104] 38 U.S.C. § 5102(a).
[105] 38 U.S.C. § 5102(b); 38 C.F.R. § 3.159(b)(2).
[106] These provisions are not applicable for any application or claim for government insurance benefits. 38 U.S.C. § 5103(b)(2).
[107] 38 U.S.C. § 5103(a); 38 C.F.R. § 3.159(b).
[108] 38 U.S.C. § 5103(a); 38 C.F.R. § 3.159(b)(1),
[109] 38 U.S.C. § 5103A(a)(1); 38 C.F.R. § 3.159(c)(1).
[110] 38 U.S.C. § 5103A(a)(2); 38 C.F.R. § 3.160(d).
[111] 38 U.S.C. § 5103A(a)(3).
[112] 38 U.S.C. § 5103A(b)(1); 38 C.F.R. § 3.160©).
[113] 38 C.F.R. § 3.159A(c)(1).
[114] 38 C.F.R. § 3.159A(c)(2).
[115] 38 U.S.C. § 5103A(b)(2); 38 C.F.R. § 3.160(e).
[116] *Id.*
[117] 38 U.S.C. § 5103A(b)(3).
[118] 38 U.S.C. § 5103A(c); 38 C.F.R. § 3.159(c)(3).
[119] 38 U.S.C. § 5103A(c)(1).
[120] 38 U.S.C. § 5103A(c)(2).
[121] 38 U.S.C. § 5103A(c)(3).
[122] 38 U.S.C. § 5103A(c)(4); 38 C.F.R. § 3.159(c)(4).
[123] 38 U.S.C. § 5103A(d)(2)(A).
[124] 38 U.S.C. § 5103A(d)(2)(B).
[125] 38 U.S.C. § 5103A(d)(2)(C).
[126] 38 U.S.C. § 5103A(f).
[127] 38 U.S.C. § 5103A(g).
[128] 38 U.S.C. § 5 104(a); 38 C.F.R. § 3.103(b).
[129] *Id.*
[130] 38 U.S.C. § 5104(b).
[131] 38 C.F.R. § 3.103(a).
[132] The VA would be required to consider all possible legal theories (e.g., secondary service connection, presumptive service connection, etc.) upon which the claim could be granted.
[133] 38 U.S.C. § 5108.
[134] 38 U.S.C. § 5109A(a). See discussion at 12.
[135] *Id.*
[136] 38 U.S.C. § 5109A(b).
[137] 38 U.S.C. § 5109A(c).
[138] 38 U.S.C. § 5109A(d).
[139] 38 U.S.C. § 5109A(e).
[140] 38 U.S.C. § 5107(b).
[141] *Id.* See 38 C.F.R. § 3.102.
[142] 38 C.F.R. § 3.102.
[143] 38 U.S.C. § 1111.
[144] 38 C.F.R. § 3.307(a)(6)(iii).
[145] 38 C.F.R. § 3.304(f).
[146] 38 U.S.C. § 1154(b); 38 C.F.R. § 3.304(d),(f).
[147] H.R. 67, 110th Cong., 1st Sess. (2007). The bill was introduced on January 4, 2007, passed the House on May 23, 2007, and was referred to the Senate Committee on Veterans' Affairs on May 24, 2007.
[148] *Id.* If enacted, to be codified at 38 U.S.C. § 564.
[149] H.R. 653, 110th Cong., 1st Sess. (2007). The bill was introduced on January 24, 2007, and was referred to the House Subcommittee on Disability Assistance and Memorial Affairs on March 2, 2007.
[150] H.R. 797, 110th Cong., 1st Sess. (2007), introduced on February 5, 2007; enacted as P.L. 110-157, 110th Cong., 1st Sess. (December 12, 2007).
[151] H.R. 1435, 110th Cong., 1st Sess. (2007). The bill was introduced on March 9, 2007, and referred to the House Committee on Veterans' Affairs on that date. The House Subcommittee on Disability Assistance and Memorial Affairs held hearings on April 17, 2007.
[152] *Id.* § 4.
[153] *Id.* § 4(d).
[154] H.R. 1444, 110th Cong., 1st Sess. (2007). The bill was introduced on March 9, 2007, and referred to the House Committee on Veterans' Affairs on that date. The House Subcommittee on Disability Assistance and Memorial Affairs held hearings on April 17, 2007.

[155] H.R. 1490, 110th Cong., 1st Sess. (2007). The bill was introduced on March 13, 2007, and referred to the House Committee on Veterans' Affairs on that date. The House Subcommittee on Disability Assistance and Memorial Affairs held hearings on April 17, 2007.

[156] *Id.* § 1.

[157] *Id.* § 2.

[158] H.R. 1538, 110th Cong., 1st Sess. (2007). The bill was introduced on March 15, 2007, passed the House on March 28, 2007, and passed the Senate with an amendment by Unanimous Consent on July 25, 2007. A message on Senate action was sent to the House on July 26, 2007. On September 5, 2007, the Senate ordered the measure printed as passed.

[159] H.R. 2257, 110th Cong., 1st Sess. (2007). The bill was introduced on May 9, 2007, and was referred to the House Subcommittee on Disability Assistance and Memorial Affairs on May 11, 2007.

[160] These "centers" provide readjustment counseling and related mental health services to veterans (38 U.S.C. § 1712A(i)(1)).

[161] H.R. 2855, 110th Cong., 1st Sess (2007). The bill was introduced on June 25, 2007, and referred to the House Subcommittee on Military Personnel, House Subcommittee on Health, and House Ways and Means on that date.

[162] H.R. 2855, § 311.

[163] *Id.* § 315(c).

[164] *Id.* § 315(d).

[165] H.R. 3047, 110th Cong., 1st Sess (2007). The bill was introduced on July 16, 2007, and referred to the House Committee on Veterans' Affairs. On July 23, 2007, it was referred to the House Subcommittee on Disability Assistance and Memorial Affairs. Subcommittee hearings were held on November 8, 2007.

[166] H.R. 3047, § 2

[167] *Id.* § 2(b). Presumably, this system could monitor and evaluate the workload and productivity of the regional offices of the BVA.

[168] *Id.* § 3.

[169] *Id.* § 3(a).

[170] *Id.* § 4.

[171] *Id.* § 4(a).

[172] *Id.* § 5(a).

[173] H.R. 5089, 110th Cong., 2d Sess (2008). The bill was introduced on January 22, 2008, and was referred to the House Committee on Veterans' Affairs on that same date.

[174] S. 1283, 100th Cong., 1st Sess (2007). The bill was introduced on May 3, 2007, and was referred to the Senate Committee on Armed Services on that date.

[175] S. 1363, 110th Cong., 1st Sess. The bill was introduced on May 10, 2007, and referred to the Senate Committee on Armed Services on that date.

[176] S. 1363, § 3.

[177] *Id.* § 3(c)(5).

[178] *Id.* § 4.

[179] S. 2737, 110th Cong., 2d Sess. (2008). The bill was introduced on March 10, 2008, and was referred to the Senate Committee on Veterans' Affairs on that date.

In: Veterans' Benefits and Care
Editor: Mathew H. Bradley

ISBN: 978-1-60692-500-3

Chapter 3

A Brief History of Veterans' Education Benefits and Their Value

David P. Smole and Shannon S. Loane

Summary

Federal educational assistance programs have been authorized for veterans of the Armed Forces since 1944. The Servicemen's Readjustment Act of 1944 (P.L. 78-346), or the GI Bill of Rights, provided support, including education benefits, to veterans of World War II. Subsequently, other programs were implemented for similar purposes (e.g., the Korean GI Bill and the Vietnam Era GI Bill). These new programs were primarily, if not exclusively, funded by the federal government and were intended to support veterans returning from war. The implementation of the Post-Vietnam Era Veterans' Educational Assistance Program (VEAP) marked the first time that an educational benefit had been established during peacetime and for anall-volunteerforce; the first time that education benefits wereviewedasamilitary recruiting tool; and the first time that servicemembers were required to make a contribution toward their veterans' education benefits. Many of the principles of VEAP were carried over during the creation of its successor program, the Montgomery GI Bill (MGIB), which was implemented in 1985.

Veterans' education benefits have evolved substantially over the last 60-plus years. When first established, veterans' education benefits were completely subsidized by the federal government; payments were issued to educational institutions on behalf of the veteran; they could be used for avarietyof education and training programs; and separate subsistence payments were also provided. Currently, veterans' education benefits are partially subsidized; they are paid directly to the veteran; and they may be used to pay tuition, fees and expenses associated with a variety of education and training programs.

During the period since veterans' education benefits first were made available, college prices have increased substantially. In addition, the manner in which federal student financial aid is calculated and awarded has shifted several times during the evolution of the veterans' education benefits programs. At present, federal student assistance is calculated according to the federal need analysis system, which considers the receipt of veterans' education benefits when determining eligibility for some student aid programs. These policy and program changes have altered the role that veterans' education benefits play in supporting access to postsecondary education for veterans.

This chapter reviews the evolution of veterans' education benefit programs and describes the types of education benefits that have been made available under these programs. It also examines how changes in the estimated value of these benefits compares with changes in average college prices, and provides a discussion of the interaction between veterans' education benefits and federal student aid benefits made available under Title IV of the Higher Education Act of 1965 (HEA), as amended. This chapter will be updated consistent with programmatic changes.

INTRODUCTION[1]

Since 1944, Congress has demonstrated an interest in providing education benefits to veterans of the Armed Forces. The Servicemen's Readjustment Act of 1944 (P.L. 78-346), or the GI Bill of Rights, provided support, including education benefits, to veterans of World War II. Following the expiration of the original GI Bill, other programs, including the Korean GI Bill, Vietnam Era GI Bill, the Post-Vietnam Era Veterans' Educational Assistance Program (VEAP), and the current GI Bill, known as the Montgomery GI Bill (MGIB), were implemented to make education benefits available to veterans of the Armed Forces. These programs were primarily, if not exclusively, funded by the federal government and were intended to provide assistance to veterans following the completion of their military service.

Veterans' education benefits have evolved substantially over the last 60-plus years. In the past, veterans' education benefits were completely subsidized by the federal government; they could be used for a variety of education and training programs; separate subsistence payments were provided; and payments were issued to educational institutions on behalf of the veteran. Currently, MGIB veterans' education benefits are partially subsidized; may be used to pay tuition, fees and expenses associated with a variety of education and training programs; and are paid directly to the student.

During the period since 1944, when veterans' education benefits first were made available, there have been numerous changes to the veterans' education programs and the benefit amounts made available. Also, during this period, other forms of federal financial assistance have been made to students, including students who are veterans, through the enactment of an array of federal student financial aid programs. At the same time, however, college prices and costs associated with obtaining a postsecondary education have continued to increase.[2]

The relationship between veterans' education benefits and federal student aid, and the manner by which federal student aid is calculated and awarded, have changed several times as veterans' education benefits programs have evolved. At present, federal student aid awards are calculated according to the federal need analysis system, which takes an individual's receipt of veterans' education benefits into account during the process of determining eligibility for certain federal student aid programs. The rules governing the interaction between the federal student aid programs and veterans' education benefits programs affect how much aggregate aid is made available to veterans to support their access to postsecondary education.

This chapter reviews the evolution of veterans' education benefit programs and describes the types of education benefits that have been made available under these programs.[3] The report is organized into three major sections. The first section provides an historical overview of education benefits for military veterans, beginning with the Servicemen's Readjustment Act of 1944 (GI Bill of Rights). The second section is an analysis of the estimated value of veterans' education benefits relative to average college prices. This section focuses on the estimated value of veterans' education benefits and college prices at four-year public and private institutions, and two-year public institutions. The final section briefly examines the interaction between veterans' education benefits and federal student aid benefits authorized under the Higher Education Act of 1965 (HEA), as amended.

VETERANS' EDUCATION BENEFIT PROGRAMS

This section provides a brief history of the education benefits programs that have been made available to veterans, beginning with the GI Bill of Rights. A summary of selected characteristics of the various programs is presented in **Table 1** at the end of this section.

GI Bill of Rights

The original GI Bill, the Servicemen's Readjustment Act of 1944, was intended to help veterans readjust to civilian life, avoid high levels of unemployment, and afford returning veterans an opportunity to receive the education and training that they missed while serving in the military. Under the GI Bill, the Veterans Administration, now the Department of Veterans Affairs (VA), paid up to $500 a year directly to an educational institution for tuition, books, fees, and other training costs.[4] The VA also paid as much as $50 a month (increased to $65 in 1946, and $75 in 1948) as a subsistence allowance to single veterans, and greater monthly amounts to veterans with one or more dependents. This program ended on July 25, 1956.

Korean GI Bill

The Veterans' Readjustment Assistance Act of 1952, the Korean GI Bill (P.L. 82-550), was authorized to help veterans returning from the Korean War to adjust to civilian life. The benefit provided up to $110 a month to single veterans for educational expenses and education-related expenses, and higher amounts for veterans with dependents. Unlike the GI Bill of Rights, which paid both educational expenses and a separate subsistence allowance, the monthly benefit for the Korean GI Bill was intended to cover both. It was believed that requiring the veteran to contribute to the costs of his/her education would encourage more careful spending. In addition, partially in response to alleged incidents of fraud and abuse by for-profit (proprietary) institutions of higher education (IHEs), each veteran received a lump-sum payment from the VA instead of the VA making direct payments to IHEs. The program ended January 31, 1965.

Post-Korea and Vietnam-Era GI Bill

The Post-Korea and Vietnam-Era GI Bill was enacted in 1966 under the Veterans' Readjustment Benefits Act of 1966 (P.L. 89-358). This program was originally intended for veterans of the post-Korean War era, and was not intended to be as generous as some of the earlier programs for veterans.[5] Under this act, veterans who had been on active duty for more than 180 consecutive days were entitled to one month of educational assistance for each month of service. This was the first GI Bill that provided benefits to members of the Armed Forces while they served on active duty, as opposed to providing benefits only after the completion of active duty. The program became effective June 1, 1966, but benefits were made available retroactively to post-Korean War era veterans and Vietnam-Era veterans who had served prior to the effective date. The initial monthly benefit amount for a single veteran was $100 per month, and monthly benefit amounts were increased several times during the operation of the program — ultimately, to $376 per month in 1984. The program ended December 31, 1989.

Post-Vietnam Era Veterans' Educational Assistance Program (VEAP)

The Post-Vietnam Era Veterans' Educational Assistance Program (VEAP) was established under Title IV of the Veterans' Education and Employment Assistance Act of 1976 (P.L. 94-502). The program was made available to individuals who entered active duty after December 31, 1976, and before July 1, 1985. VEAP was designed as a recruitment incentive for the Armed Forces during peacetime. Since the benefit was established for an all-volunteer force servingduring peacetime, it was deemed appropriate to require participants, for the first time, to contribute to an education fund during their period of service in the military. Program participants had to agree to monthly pay reductions of at least $25, but not more than $100. The maximum education benefit may not exceed the sum of the amount contributed by the participant and the matching federal contribution (see **Table 1** for details); and the maximum monthly benefit amount is $300.[6] VEAP benefits must be used within ten years of discharge. VEAP participants who were on active duty on October 9, 1996 were eligible until October 8, 1997, to elect to participate in the MGIB program.

Montgomery GI Bill

The MGIB consists of two major programs: MGIB-Active Duty (MGIB-AD), for individuals serving on active duty or who have separated from active duty; and MGIB-Selected Reserves (MGIB-SR), for members of the selected reserves. These programs are described below.

Montgomery GI Bill - Active Duty (MGIB-AD)

The Montgomery GI Bill (MGIB), originally called the All-Volunteer Force Educational Assistance Program, was initially enacted as part of the Department of Defense Authorization Act, 1985 (P.L. 98-525), as a three-year pilot program.[7] The MGIB-AD program is available to individuals who entered active duty after June 30, 1985; as well as, in certain circumstances, individuals who entered active duty prior to that date.[8] To become eligible for MGIB-AD benefits, individuals must not have declined the benefit in writing, and must have had their military pay reduced by $100 per month for 12 months. MGIB-AD benefits may be used for a maximum of 36 months; and in general, benefits must be used within ten years of discharge from active duty.[9] To be eligible for benefits, individuals must have received a fully honorable discharge (or be serving on active duty); and must have a high school diploma or the equivalent, or have completed at least 12 credit hours towards a college degree. In most instances, individuals must have served for three continuous years on active duty to become eligible to receive MGIB-AD benefits; however, in certain circumstances, individuals may qualify to receive benefits after two continuous years of active duty service.

MGIB-AD benefits are paid on a monthly basis. Monthly benefit rates vary according to whether individuals have served for three continuous years on active duty; and the intensity of the training toward which the benefits are being applied. For FY2008, the maximum monthly benefit rate is $1,101 for individuals who have served for three continuous years on active duty, and who are enrolled full-time. Maximum monthly benefit amounts are adjusted annually according to the consumer price index for all urban consumers (CPI-U). Lower benefit rates apply to eligible individuals who have not served for three continuous years on active duty, and to those enrolled less than full-time. In certain instances, individuals may also be eligible to receive higher benefit amounts, referred to as a "kicker" or a "college fund" (see below).

MGIB-AD benefits may be used to pay for tuition, fees, books, supplies, and other expenses associated with enrollment in an array of approved education and training programs, including

- courses at colleges and universities leading to an associate, baccalaureate, or graduate degree;
- courses at business, vocational, and technical schools leading to a certificate or diploma;
- apprenticeship and on-the-job training, including self-employment training for ownership or operation of a franchise (for individuals not on active duty);
- flight training (for qualified individuals);
- state-approved teacher certification programs;
- preparatory courses for admission to undergraduate or graduate education programs;
- approved licensing and certification tests;
- entrepreneurship training courses for the creation or expansion of small businesses; and
- tuition assistance using MGIB as "Top-Up" (see below).[10]

MGIB "Kicker"/College Fund

The College Fund is an add-on benefit to the MGIB-AD benefit that may be made available to individuals at the time of enlistment. Individuals must elect to participate in the MGIB-AD program to become eligible for the College Fund. Each service branch elects whether to offer the College Fund benefit to recruits serving in certain critical military occupational specialities. (Currently, the Army and the Navy participate.) Veterans receive the College Fund benefit as an add-on to the MGIB-AD monthly benefit amount. While MGIB-AD monthly benefit amounts are adjusted annually according to changes in the CPI-U, no annual adjustments are made to College Fund monthly benefit amounts.

Tuition Assistance "Top-Up"

The Tuition Assistance "Top-Up" program was established under the Floyd D. Spence National Defense Authorization Act for Fiscal Year 2001 (P.L. 106-398). Through Tuition Assistance programs, military service branches may pay tuition and expenses for the education and training of active duty personnel.[11] Under Tuition Assistance Top-Up, MGIB-AD participants who have served for at least two years on active duty and who are approved for Tuition Assistance benefits may elect to receive MGIB benefits to pay for education and training expenses above the amount paid by their military service branch. If a service member's service branch will not pay 100% of tuition and fees, the servicemember may use MGIB Top-Up to pay the difference between the total cost and the amount paid by the service branch. Use of the MGIB Top-Up benefit results in a reduction of future MGIB benefits.

Montgomery GI Bill - Selected Reserve (MGIB-SR)

The MGIB-SR program is available to individuals serving in the Selected Reserves.[12] Eligibility for MGIB-SR is determined by Selected Reserve service components; and individuals must agree to a six-year service obligation. Individuals may receive up to 36 months of benefits, and these must be used within 14 years of becoming eligible. (Individuals who became eligible for MGIB-SR prior to October 1, 1992 must use benefits within 10 years of becoming eligible.) Education benefits may be used for activities that include degree programs, certificate or correspondence courses, cooperative training, independent study, apprenticeship, and vocational flight training programs. For FY2008, the maximum MGIB-SR monthly benefit amount is $317.

Reserve Educational Assistance Program (REAP)

The Reserve Educational Assistance Program (REAP) was established under the Ronald W. Reagan National Defense Authorization Act for Fiscal Year 2005 (P.L. 108-375);[13] and provides benefits for members of the Selected Reserves, Individual Ready Reserve (IRR), and National Guard who are called or ordered to active duty in response to a war or national emergency as declared by the President or Congress. In general, an individual called to active

Table 1. Selected Characteristics of Veterans' Education Benefits Programs

Criteria	GI Bill of Rights	Korean GI Bill	Vietnam- Era GI Bill	Post-Vietnam Era Veterans' Educational Assistance Program (VEAP)	Montgomery GI Bill - Active Duty	Montgomery GI Bill - Selected Reserves	Reserve Educational Assistance Program (REAP)
Year enacted	1944	1952	1966	1976	1984	1984	2004
Initial authorization	P.L. 78-346	P.L. 82-550	P.L. 89-358	P.L. 94-502	P.L. 98-525	P.L. 98-525	P.L. 108-375
Period of service	September 16, 1940, through July 25, 1947	June 27, 1950, through January 31, 1955	February 1, 1955 through August 4, 1964 (Post-Korean War); August 5, 1964, through May 7, 1975 (Vietnam-Era veterans)	December 31, 1976, through July 1, 1985	Entered active duty after June 30, 1985	July 1, 1985, to present	After September 11, 2001, to present
Period of Use	June 22, 1944, to July 25, 1956	August 20, 1952, to January 31, 1965	June 1, 1966, to December 31, 1989	January 1, 1977, to present	July 1, 1985, to present	July 1, 1985, to present	December 9, 2001, to present
Highest standard benefit amount (current dollars)	$500 per year maximum; and $75 monthly subsistence	$110 per month maximum	$376 per month	$300 per month[a]	$1,101 per month (FY2008)[b]	$317 per month (FY2008)[b]	$881 per month (FY2008)[c]
Duration of benefits	One year full-time training plus a period equal to time in service; 48 months maximum	1.5 times the duration of active service; 36 months maximum	One month of education benefits for every month of active duty service; 45 months maximum	Lesser of 36 months or number of months of contributions	Lesser of 36 months or number of months of active duty	36 months	36 months
Contribution	None	None	None	$25 to $100 per month; $2,700 maximum	Pay reduction of $100 per month for the first 12 months of pay	None	None

Table 1. (Continued)

Criteria	GI Bill of Rights	Korean GI Bill	Vietnam- Era GI Bill	Post-Vietnam Era Veterans' Educational Assistance Program (VEAP)	Montgomery GI Bill - Active Duty	Montgomery GI Bill - Selected Reserves	Reserve Educational Assistance Program (REAP)
Length of service	Minimum 90 days	Minimum 90 days	More than 180 days of active duty service	Minimum 181 continuous days of active duty service, if entered before October 16, 1981; 24 months of continuous active duty service if entered after October 16, 1981	Minimum 181 continuous days of active duty service; 24 months of active duty if enlisted after September 7, 1980	Accepted 6-year reserve obligation after June 30, 1985	Minimum 90 of consecutive service in a Contingency operation
Discharge status	Other than dishonorable	Other than dishonorable	Other than dishonorable	Other than dishonorable	Fully honorable discharge or on active duty	Must remain with Reserve unit	Must remain Reserve unit
Time limitation on use of benefits	Initiated by later of end of war or two years after discharge	Initiated by three years and completed by eight years after discharge	Within 8 years after discharge; 10 years for Vietnam veterans	Within 10 years of discharge or release from active duty	Within 10 years of discharge or release from active duty	Within 14 years of initial eligibility, if eligible on or after October 1, 1992 (for those first eligible prior to October 1, 1992, benefits must be used within 10 years of initial eligibility)	Benefits can be used after 90-day minimum service period completed — no fixed delimited date; must remain with Reserve component

Source: Table prepared by CRS based on data available from the U.S. Department of Veterans Affairs.

a. Government matches every $1 the service person contributes with $2. The maximum benefit available under the program is $8,100 ($5,400 federal contribution and $2,700 individual contribution). The total contribution (service person contribution plus government share) is then divided by the number of months the service person contributed to VEAP.

b. Amounts shown are for full-time institutional training, and are for individuals who completed a minimum of three years of service. The amounts are less for individuals who served less than three years and who attend less than full-time. The education benefits payment rate schedule is available at [http://www.gibill.va.gov/GI_Bill_Info/rates.htm].

c. The monthly amount is a percentage of the MGIB-Active Duty and is based on the number of continuous days of active duty service. The amount shown is for full-time institutional training, and is for individuals who completed at two years or more of active duty service. The amount is less for individuals who served two years or less, and who attend less than full-time.

duty who serves for at least 90 consecutive days on or after September 11, 2001, is eligible for REAP. The REAP benefit amount is based on a percentage of the MGIB-AD benefit amount and is indexed to the duration of service. Members who serve at least 90 days, but less than 1 year receive 40% of the full MGIB-AD rate; those who serve more than 1 year, but less than 2 years receive 60% of the full MGIB-AD; and those who serve 2 or more continuous years receive 80% of the full MGIB-AD rate. In general, REAP benefits may be used to pay for education programs with the exception of reimbursement for examinations and testing. REAP benefits are potentially payable from December 9, 2001.[14] A maximum of 36 months of REAP benefits are available; and benefits must be used within 10 years. For FY2008, the maximum REAP monthly benefit amount is $881.

Survivors' and Dependents' Educational Assistance Program (DEA)

The DEA program[15] was first established by the War Orphans' Educational Assistance Act of 1956 (P.L. 84-634).[16] It provides up to 45 months of education and training benefits to the spouse and children (including stepchildren or adopted children) of a veteran who

- is permanently and totally disabled, or dies, as a result of a service-connected disability that arises out of or is aggravated by active duty;
- has a permanent and total service-connected disability and diesfrom any cause;
- is missing in action or is captured in line of duty and held by a hostile force;
- is currently detained in line of duty by a foreign government or power;
- is hospitalized or receiving outpatient treatment for a service-connected permanent and total disability and is likely to be discharged for that disability.[17]

Generally, children of such veterans are eligible from the age of 18 to the age of 26, although there are some exceptions. Spouses are eligible for benefits for ten years from the date of death of the veteran or from the date of VA notification of eligibility due to the veteran's permanent and total disability, although, again, there are some exceptions. If the servicemember died on active duty, the spouse's benefits end 20 years after the date of death.

DEA benefits can be used for undergraduate and graduate degree programs at colleges and universities; cooperative training programs; certificate programs at colleges, universities, business, technical, or vocational schools; apprenticeships or on-the-job training programs offered by companies or unions; farm cooperative courses; overseas programs that lead to college degrees; preparatory courses for college or graduate school entrance examinations; highschool programs; and, for the spouse of a servicemember, correspondence courses. Other types of educational costs, including tutorial assistance, tests for course credit at colleges and universities, tests required for admission to certain programs, licensing and certification tests, may also be covered.

The FY2008 rate for those attending an institution full-time is $881 per month. Amounts are reduced for those attending less than full-time or pursuing farm cooperative training or apprenticeship or on-the-job training.

CHANGES IN THE VALUE OF VETERANS' EDUCATION BENEFITS OVER TIME

Overtime, there have been numerous changes to the veterans' education benefit programs. Periodically, programmatic eligibility criteria and benefit amounts have been amended. Several programs have expired and been replaced by successor programs. One useful way to examine veterans' education benefits is to compare the actual (real) value of the benefits made available under these different programs over time. The analysis presented here considers only the benefits available for education and living expenses. It does not factor in any individual contributions toward education benefits that servicemembers have been required to make beginning with the establishment of the VEAP in 1976, nor "kickers" provided to encourage enrollment in the Armed Forces. In addition, it only considers benefits available to full-time students with no dependents.[18] This section examines the value of the education benefits provided through the GI Bill of Rights and successor programs from 1944 through 2007 in inflation-adjusted (constant) 2007 dollars. It also examines the purchasing power of benefits made available under the MGIB-AD program — the largest of the currently active veterans' education benefits programs — with respect to the costs of obtaining a postsecondary education.

Veterans' education benefits are generally awarded for a specific number of months, depending upon the program, when the recipient enrolled, and the duration of service. For example, a recipient can receive MGIB benefits for 36 months, which could be disbursed over the course of three years (twelve monthly payments per year) or over the course of four years (nine monthly payments per 9-month academic year).[19] In the analyses presented here, it is assumed that the benefits will be disbursed over a four-year period (i.e., for four 9-month academic years). College price data are primarily from the *Digest of Education Statistics, 2007*, produced by the Department of Education (ED). Data for 2007-2008 are from the College Board because these data are not currently available from ED. The College Board bases its college price data on a sample of institutions, whereas ED includes the universe of institutions of higher education (IHEs) in its price data.

Value of Veterans' Education Benefits: 1944-2007

As previously discussed, the original GI Bill provided up to $500 annually for education expenses. This is the equivalent of $5,890 in 2007 dollars.[20] An additional $50 was provided monthly for living expenses in 1944, which in 2007 dollars is equivalent to $589 monthly, or $5,301 annually.[21] Thus, the total education benefit, including the living allowance, in 1944 would have been worth $11,191 annually, or $1,243 monthly in 2007 dollars.[22] In 1956, when the original GI Bill ended, the education benefit was $131 per month, which is equal to $999 per month in real-dollar 2007 terms. Subsequent GI Bills provided benefits on a monthly basis.[23] The monthly benefit amount for the Korean War GI Bill was $110 for duration of the program. In 1952, this was equivalent to $861 in 2007 dollars, and in 1965 when the program ended, it was equivalent to $724. When the Post-Korea and Vietnam-Era GI Bill was enacted in 1966, the monthly benefit amount was $100, which was equivalent to $640 in 2007 dollars. In 1989, when the Post-Korea and Vietnam-Era GI Bill ended, the monthly benefit amount was $376, or $629 in 2007 dollars. The maximum monthly benefit amount for the VEAP has remained constant at $300 since first becoming available in 1977. In 1977, this was equivalent to $1,026 in 2007 dollars.

When the MGIB-AD program was enacted in 1985, the maximum monthly benefit was $300, or $578 in constant 2007 dollars. The MGIB-AD benefit amount has been increased numerous times, most recently under the Veterans Education and Benefits Expansion Act of 2001 (P.L. 107-103). Since FY2004, MGIB-AD monthly benefit amounts have been adjusted annually according to the CPI. Currently, the MGIB-AD monthly benefit amount is $1,101. When enacted in 1985, the MGIB-SR monthly benefit amount was $140, which was the equivalent of $270 in 2007 dollars. The monthly benefit amount for the MGIB-SR program has also been increased numerous times; however, these increases have not kept pace with those for the MGIB-AD program. The maximum monthly benefit amount for the REAP program is a fixed proportion of the MGIB-AD benefit amount. Thus, REAP benefits have increased in concert with MGIB-AD.

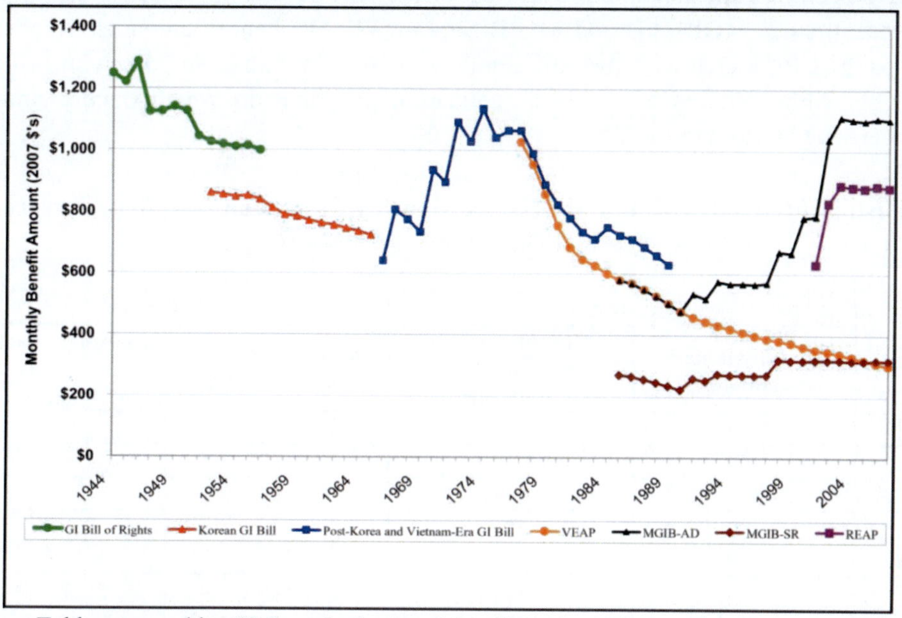

Source: Table prepared by CRS on the basis of data from the U.S. Department of Veterans Affairs and U.S. Bureau of Labor Statistics.

Note: All constant dollar calculations are based on the average Consumer Price Index-All Urban Consumers (CPI-U) for each year. Monthly education benefits include any funds available for living expenses. All dollar amounts have been rounded.

Figure 1. Veterans' Education Program Monthly Benefit Amounts: Constant 2007 Dollars, 1944-2007

Figure 1 shows the real value of the maximum monthly benefit amounts made available under the various veterans' education benefit programs that have been in effect since 1944. As can be seen, benefits were most generous in real terms in the late 1940s under the original GI Bill of Rights, in the early 1970s under the Post-Korea and Vietnam-Era GI Bill, and in the 21st century under the MGIB-AD program.

Value of Education Benefits Provided Through the Montgomery GI Bill: 1987-2007

The maximum monthly benefit amounts available under the MGIB-AD and MGIB-SR programs since their inception in 1985 are presented in **Table 2.** Monthly benefit amounts are shown at the inception of the programs, at annual intervals, and when adjustments to benefit amounts have been made. Benefit amounts are shown in both current and constant (2007) dollars.

In the initial years of both the MGIB-AD and MGIB-SR programs, benefit amounts remained stagnant. However, in real terms, benefit amounts declined slightly. Beginning in the early 1990s benefit amounts began to be increased and through most of that decade, proportionalincreases were provided for both programs. In the late 1990s and the early years of this decade, a number of substantial increases have been made to MGIB-AD benefit amounts, resulting in increases in several years that exceed the CPI. Increases for MGIB-SR benefits have been less substantial and for most of the past decade have been indexed to the CPI. At present, since MGIB-AD and MGIB-SR (and REAP) benefit amounts are adjusted according to the CPI, increases in benefit amounts are designed to keep pace with inflation. This contrasts with predecessor veterans' education programs in which benefit amounts generally were not indexed to the CPI.

Table 2. History of MGIB-AD and MGIB-SR Monthly Education Benefits: Current and Constant 2007 Dollars, 1985-2007

Date	MGIB-AD		MGIB-SR	
	Monthly Benefit (nominal dollars)	Monthly benefit (constant 2007 dollars)	Monthly Benefit (nominal dollars)	Monthly benefit (constant 2007 dollars)
July 1985	$300	578	140	270
July 1986	300	568	140	265
July 1987	300	548	140	256
July 1988	300	526	140	245
July 1989	300	502	140	234
July 1990	300	476	140	222
Oct. 1991	350	533	170	259
Oct. 1992	350	517	170	251
Apr. 1993	400	574	190	273
Oct. 1994	405	566	192	269
Oct. 1995	417	567	198	269
Oct. 1996	428	565	203	269
Oct. 1997	440	568	209	270
Oct. 1998	528	672	251	319
Oct. 1999	536	667	255	317
Oct. 2000	552	665	263	317
Nov. 2000	650	783	263	317

Table 2. (Continued)

Date	MGIB-AD		MGIB-SR	
	Monthly Benefit (nominal dollars)	Monthly benefit (constant 2007 dollars)	Monthly Benefit (nominal dollars)	Monthly benefit (constant 2007 dollars)
Oct. 2001	672	787	272	318
Jan. 2002	800	922	272	313
Oct. 2002	900	1,037	276	318
Oct. 2003	985	1,110	282	318
Oct. 2004	1,004	1,102	288	316
Oct. 2005	1,034	1,098	297	315
Oct. 2006	1,075	1,106	309	318
Oct. 2007	1,101	1,101	317	317

Sources: U.S. Department of Veterans Affairs; and Military Officers Association of America.

Note: All constant dollar calculations are based on the average Consumer Price Index-All Urban Consumers (CPI-U). All dollar amounts have been rounded.

Purchasing Power of the MGIB-AD Program

Since college prices have often increased at a rate that exceeds the CPI, it is also useful to examine what proportion of the costs of obtaining a postsecondary education may be met with MGIB-AD benefits. **Table 3** shows the percentage of tuition, fees, room, and board the MGIB-AD benefit has covered on an annual basis at four-year public and private institutions, as well as at two-year public institutions from 1985-1986 through the 2007-2008 academic years.

As shown in **Table 3**, since the inception of the MGIB-AD program in 1985, the benefits have covered only a portion of the average tuition, fees, room, and board at public and private four-year institutions.[24] In academic year 1985-1986, the benefit would have covered 70% of the average expenses at a public four-year institution, and 29.3% of the average expenses at a private four-year institution.[25] In the 2007-2008 academic year, the MGIB-AD benefit covers 72.7% of the average expenses at public four-year institutions, and 30.6% of the average expenses at private four-year institutions. **Table 3** also shows that during the 1990s, MGIB-AD benefits met just over half of the average costs of attending public four-year institutions and just over one-fifth of the average costs of attending private four-year institutions. In the early years of this decade, MGIB-AD benefits were increased substantially, and although benefits are currently indexed to the CPI-U, since college prices are increasing at a rate that exceeds the CPI-U, their purchasing power relative to college costs is again declining. MGIB-AD benefits cover a much greater proportion of the average costs of attending public two-year institutions. Public two-year institutions have typically had lower prices of attendance and smaller price increases. Since the late 1990s, the MGIB benefits have covered more than 100% of the average price for tuition, fees, room, and board at public two-year institutions.

Use of Education Benefits

Information on the number of individualsreceiving veterans' education benefits by program for FY1998 through FY2007 is shown in **Table 4**. Nearly two-thirds of individuals receiving veterans' education benefits participate in the MGIB-AD program. Most other beneficiaries are spread across the MGIB-SR, REAP, and DEA programs. Only a very small number of veterans currently receive benefits under VEAP.

Table 3. Percent of Average Price of Public and Private Four-Year IHEs and Public Two-Year IHEs Covered by the MGIB-AD Education Benefit: 1985-1986 through 2007-2008 (in current dollars)

Academic Year	MGIB-AD Benefit (Septembe r-May)	Public Four-Year IHEs		Private Four-Year IHEs		Public Two-Year IHEs	
		Average Tuition, Fees, Room, and Board	% of Price Covered by Benefit	Average Tuition, Fees, Room, and Board	% of Price Covered by Benefit	Average Tuition, Fees, Room, and Board	% of Price Covered by Benefit
1985-1986	2,700	3,859	70.0	9,228	29.3	2,981	90.6
1986-1987	2,700	4,138	65.2	10,039	26.9	2,989	90.3
1987-1988	2,700	4,403	61.3	10,659	25.3	3,066	88.1
1988-1989	2,700	4,678	57.7	11,474	23.5	3,183	84.8
1989-1990	2,700	4,975	54.3	12,284	22.0	3,299	81.8
1990-1991	2,700	5,243	51.5	13,237	20.4	3,467	77.9
1991-1992	3,100	5,693	54.5	14,258	21.7	3,623	85.6
1992-1993	3,150	6,020	52.3	15,009	21.0	3,799	82.9
1993-1994	3,250	6,365	51.1	15,904	20.4	3,996	81.3
1994-1995	3,640	6,670	54.6	16,602	21.9	4,137	88.0
1995-1996	3,741	7,014	53.3	17,612	21.2	4,217	88.7
1996-1997	3,841	7,334	52.4	18,442	20.8	4,404	87.2
1997-1998	3,948	7,673	51.5	19,070	20.7	4,509	87.6
1998-1999	4,664	8,027	58.1	19,929	23.4	4,604	101.3
1999-2000	4,816	8,275	58.2	20,706	23.3	4,720	102.0
2000-2001	5,638	8,653	65.2	21,856	25.8	4,839	116.5
2001-2002	6,666	9,196	72.5	22,896	29.1	5,137	129.8
2002-2003	8,000	9,787	81.7	23,787	33.6	5,601	142.8
2003-2004	8,780	10,674	82.3	25,083	35.0	6,020	145.8
2004-2005	9,017	11,426	78.9	26,257	34.3	6,375	141.4
2005-2006	9,276	12,108	76.6	27,317	34.0	6,492	142.9
2006-2007	9,634	12,805	75.2	28,869	33.4	6,810	141.5
2007-2008	9,883	13,589	72.7	32,307	30.6	—	—

Source: Table prepared by CRS based on data from the Department of Veterans Affairs, data available from the U.S. Department of Education, National Center for Education Statistics (NCES), *Digest of Education Statistics: 2007*, table 320, and data available from The College Board, *Trends in College Pricing: 2007*.

Notes: The annual MGIB-AD benefit shown here is based on nine months of education benefits to coincide with a nine-month (Sept. to May) academic year. See **Table 2** for monthly benefit amounts by date. All dollar amounts have been rounded.

Table 4. Recipients of Veterans' Education Benefits by Program: FY1998 - FY2007

FY	MGIB-AD	MGIB-SR	REAP	DEA	VEAP	Total
1998	276,568	121,063	0	22,223	1,023	420,877
1999	288,052	73,580	0	44,423	3,939	409,994
2000	279,948	70,299	0	44,820	2,522	397,589
2001	289,771	82,283	0	46,917	1,680	420,651
2002	323,165	85,766	0	53,888	1,340	464,159
2003	321,837	88,342	0	61,874	917	472,970
2004	332,031	88,650	0	68,920	796	490,397
2005	336,347	87,161	0	74,267	723	498,498
2006	332,184	66,105	23,747	75,460	627	498,123
2007	343,751	60,298	41,388	77,339	568	523,344

Source: Data provided to CRS by the Department of Veterans Affairs.

VETERANS' EDUCATION BENEFITS AND FEDERAL STUDENT AID AVAILABLE UNDER THE HIGHER EDUCATION ACT

Unlike when the GI Bill of Rights was enacted in 1944, veterans' education benefits are made available to veterans alongside a broad array of federal student financial aid programs under which veterans and servicemembers may also be eligible for assistance. The Higher Education Act (HEA) of 1965, as amended, authorizes the major federal student aid programs through which financial assistance is made available to individuals seeking to obtain a postsecondary education. Most programs that make available federal student aid to individual students are authorized under Title IV of the HEA. Major programs authorized under HEA, Title IV include the Pell Grant program, the American Competitiveness (AC) grant and National Science and Mathematics Access to Retain Talent grant (SMART) programs, the Teacher Quality Enhancement Grants for States and Partnerships (TEACH) Grant program, the Federal Supplemental Educational Opportunity Grant (FSEOG) program, the Federal Work-Study (FWS) program, the Federal Perkins Loan program; and the Federal Family Education Loan (FFEL) and William D. Ford Federal Direct Loan (DL) programs.[26] The FFEL and DL programs both make available subsidized Stafford Loans, unsubsidized Stafford Loans, and PLUS Loans. These and other programs authorized under the HEA make available federal student aid in numerous forms, including grants, work-study employment, and loans. The types and amounts of aid students may be eligible to receive is determined by programmatic requirements and federal need analysis provisions. As explained below, federal need analysis provisions take into account students' status as a veteran and veterans' education benefits for which they may be entitled.

Federal Need Analysis

The expected family contribution (EFC) is the amount that the federal need analysis system (HEA, Title IV, Part F) determines a family has available to contribute toward postsecondary education expenses. In calculating the EFC, consideration is given to available income (a combination of taxable and untaxed income and benefits) and, for some families, available assets. In addition, living expenses, retirement needs, and federal and state tax liability are considered. The income contribution is calculated by determining a student's (or a student's family's, where applicable) total income, next determining available income by subtracting a series of allowances from total income, and then considering a percentage of that available income as an income contribution toward postsecondary education costs. A contribution from assets is similarly calculated. The combination of the available income contribution and asset contribution, divided by the number of individuals in the family enrolled in college, constitutes the EFC.

The calculation of the EFC varies depending upon the applicant's dependency status. There are three separate dependency classifications for individual applicants: dependent student, independent student with dependents, and independent student without dependents. These distinctions are important because parental financial information is *not* considered if the applicant meets the statutory definition of an *independent student*. To be classified as statutorily independent (HEA, § 480(d)), an applicant must meet *one* of the following conditions:

- be 24 years of age or older by December 31 of the award year;
- be an orphan or ward of the court or was a ward of the court until the individual reached the age of 18;[27]
- be a veteran[28] of the Armed Forces of the United States or is currently serving on active duty in the Armed Forces for other than training purposes;
- be a graduate or professional student;
- be married;
- have legal dependents other than a spouse; or
- be a student for whom a financial aid administrator makes a documented determination of independence by reason of other unusual circumstances.

Students who do not meet any of the aforementioned conditions are considered to be financially dependent on their parents for the purposes of Title IV student aid.

Cost of attendance (COA) is determined by each higher education institution. The COA is a measure of a student's educational expenses at a specific IHE.[29] In general, it is the sum of tuition and fees; an allowance for books, supplies, transportation, and miscellaneous personal expenses; and a room and board allowance.

The financial aid administrator determines the student's need for federal aid and other sources of aid, based primarily upon the EFC and COA. This is true for all federal student aid programs except for the Pell Grant program (see below). The final outcome of this process is the financial aid award or package, which consists of the specific sources and amounts of student aid each applicant will receive.[30]

Table 5. Student Eligibility Requirements for Participation in the Federal Student Aid Programs under Title IV of the Higher Education Act and GI Bill Education Benefits

Eligibility Criteria	HEA, Title IV Programs	Veterans Education Assistance Program (VEAP)	Montgomery GI Bill-Active Duty	Montgomery GI Bill-Selected Reserve
Citizenship requirement	Generally, students must be U.S. citizens or U.S. permanent residents. Individuals with several other entrance statuses can qualify for aid	N/A	N/A	N/A
Selective Service registration	Males between ages 18-25 must register for the selective service.	N/A	N/A	N/A
Contribution	N/A	$25 to $100 per month; $2,700 maximum.	Pay reduction of $100 per month for the first 12 months of pay	None
Discharge requirement	N/A	Conditions other than dishonorable	Fully honorable	Must remain with Reserve unit
Drug conviction	Conviction for possession or sale of drugs can disqualify students for federal student aid	N/A	N/A	N/A
Duration of benefits	N/A	Lesser of 36 months or number of months they contributed	Lesser of 36 months or number of months on active duty	36 months

Table 5. (Contiuned)

Eligibility Criteria	HEA, Title IV Programs	Veterans Education Assistance Program (VEAP)	Montgomery GI Bill-Active Duty	Montgomery GI Bill-Selected Reserve
Education requirement	Students must have a high school diploma or the recognized equivalent; absent such a diploma or its equivalent, students must demonstrate an ability to benefit from postsecondary education by passing an examination approved by the Department of Education	N/A	High school diploma or equivalency, or 12 hours of college credit	High school diploma or equivalency before applying for benefits
Enrollment status	Must be enrolled or accepted for enrollment in a degree, certificate, or other program leading to a recognized educational credential	Courses must lead to an educational, professional, or vocational objective	Courses must lead to an educational, professional, or vocational objective	Courses must lead to an educational, professional, or vocational objective
Imprisonment	Students who are incarcerated in a federal or state penal institution are ineligible for Pell Grants and federal student loans, but may qualify for FSEOG and FWS aid	Only the costs of tuition and fees, necessary books, and supplies are covered	Only the costs of tuition and fees, necessary books, and supplies are covered	Benefits will be reduced
Length of service	N/A	Minimum 181 continuous days of active duty service, if entered before October 16, 1981; 24 months of continuous active duty service if entered after October 16, 1981	Served continuously for 181 days or more; 24 months of active duty if enlisted after September 7, 1980	Accepted 6-year reserve obligation after June 30, 1985

Table 5. (Continued)

Eligibility Criteria	HEA, Title IV Programs	Veterans Education Assistance Program (VEAP)	Montgomery GI Bill-Active Duty	Montgomery GI Bill-Selected Reserve
Money owed to federal government	Cannot owe a refund on a grant previously received, or be in default on any education loan	N/A	N/A	N/A
Period of service	N/A	December 31, 1976, through July 1, 1985	Entered active duty after June 30, 1985	July 1, 1985, to present
Progress while enrolled	Students have to maintain satisfactory academic progress while enrolled in postsecondary education in order to be eligible for federal student aid; satisfactory progress is delineated by policies developed by each participating higher education institution.	Satisfactory attendance, conduct and progress, as determined by the institution	Satisfactory attendance, conduct, and progress, as determined by the institution	Satisfactory attendance, conduct, and progress, as determined by the institution
Time limitation on use of benefits	N/A	Within 10 years of discharge or release from active duty	Within 10 years of discharge or release from active duty	Within 14 years of initial eligibility, if eligible on or after October 1, 1992; otherwise, benefits must be used within 10 years of initial eligibility

Source: Table prepared by CRS based on data available from the U.S. Department of Education, U.S. Department of Veterans Affairs, relevant legislation, and the Code of Federal Regulations.

Military Education Benefits, Need Analysis, and Federal Student Aid

This section describes military education benefits and how they are treated in the federal need analysis system. Military education benefits[31] are not treated as income, and therefore are not used in the calculation of the expected EFC. However, depending upon the federal student aid program, veterans' education benefits may be treated as a *resource* or *other estimated financial assistance* (to be discussed).[32] Financial need is calculated by subtracting the EFC and resources or other estimated financial assistance from the student's COA. As a result, as the amount of the EFC or estimated financial assistance/resources increases, the amount of need declines, which reduces the amount of need-based aid a student can receive.

Military Education Benefits and Pell Grants

The primary Pell Grant award rule is that a student's annual grant is the least of (a) the maximum appropriated Pell Grant, minus EFC, or (b) the cost of attendance (COA) of the institution attended, minus EFC. For nearly all Pell recipients, the Pell Grant award is calculated by subtracting the EFC from the maximum appropriated Pell Grant for the year (i.e., without regard to the COA). This is because the maximum Pell Grant minus the recipient's EFC is almost always lower than the COA minus the EFC. Because military education benefits are not considered in calculating the EFC, the receipt of these benefits does not affect a student's Pell Grant award.

Military Education Benefits and FFEL/DL Program Student Loans

Need analysis also determines the amount that students may borrow in need-based, subsidized Stafford Loans under the FFEL and DL program. Eligibility for subsidized Stafford Loans is determined by subtracting the student's EFC and other estimated financial assistance (EFA) from the COA of the institution attended. In general, EFA includes all grants, loans, scholarships, and veterans' education benefits (with the exception of MGIB-AD benefits)[33].

Slightly different need analysis rules apply to the awarding of non-need-based unsubsidized Stafford Loans and PLUS Loans. For non-need-based loans, eligibility is determined by subtracting the student's EFA from COA; and MGIB-AD benefits are included in this calculation. Students may borrow unsubsidized Stafford Loans and PLUS Loans to replace their EFC.

Military Education Benefits and Campus-Based Programs

For the FSEOG, FWS and Federal Perkins Loan programs (also commonly referred to at the campus-based student aid programs), military education benefits, including MGIB-AD benefits, are considered to be a resource. Thus, all veterans' education benefits directly affect the determination of a student's need for campus-based student aid. However, regulations for the campus-based programs permit an institution of higher education, in its determination of a student's campus-based assistance, to exclude from consideration as a resource any portion of a subsidized Stafford Loan up to the amount of a student's MGIB-AD benefits.[34] This regulatory provision permits an institution to protect — if it chooses to do so — a certain amount of the subsidized Stafford Loan assistance from having an adverse effect on the MGIB-AD benefit recipient's campus-based assistance.

Student Eligibility Requirements for Title IV Programs and Military Education Benefits

As illustrated by **Table 5**, few similarities exist between the student eligibility requirements for Title IV programs and the eligibility requirements for military education benefits. The only similarity among all of the programs is that a student must maintain satisfactory academic progress — as determined by the institution — while enrolled.

The differences between the programs are primarily eligibility-related, and are targeted to the particular program. For example, the eligibility requirements for military education benefits generally focus on the beneficiary's time and duration of service, the amount that was contributed toward the benefit, and how much the recipient is eligible to receive. Similarly, the eligibility requirements for the HEA, Title IV programs generally relate to the student having the requisite education and citizenship status, not having a drug conviction, not owing money to the federal government, and registering for the Selective Service (where applicable).

End Notes

[1] This chapter is adapted from a prior CRS report, *Montgomery GI Bill Education Benefits: Analysis of College Prices and Federal Student Aid Under the Higher Education Act*, by Charmaine Mercer. The report, now out of print, is available from the authors upon request.

[2] For additional information on college costs and prices, see CRS Report RL34224, *College Costs and Prices: Issues for Reauthorization of the Higher Education Act*, by Rebecca R. Skinner and Blake Alan Naughton.

[3] Proposals are being considered in the 110th Congress to enact expanded education benefits for veterans. These proposals are beyond the scope of this chapter. For information on legislative proposals to expand veterans' education benefits programs, see CRS Report RL33985, *Veterans' Benefits: Issues in the 110th Congress*, coordinated by Carol D. Davis; and CRS Report RL34451, *Second FY2008 Supplemental Appropriations for Military Operations, International Affairs, and Other Purposes*, by Stephen Daggett, Susan B. Epstein, Rhoda Margesson, Curt Tarnoff, Pat Towell, Catherine Dale, and Shannon S. Loane.

[4] Reliable, comprehensive data on the price of college attendance during the 1940s are not available. Based on data obtained on individual institutions, it seems likely that $500 annually would have been sufficient to cover educational costs at most institutions. For example, based on anecdotal evidence tuition and fees at Harvard University and theMassachusetts Institute of Technology were $450 and $500, respectively, in the 1940s.

[5] In 1976, at the end of the Vietnam hostilities, benefits were extended from 36 months to45 months, and the time period in which benefits could be used was extended from eightyears to 10 years following discharge.

[6] The Department of Defense could also make additional contributions, known as "kickers," to individuals in critical military fields to encourage enlistment or reenlistment in the Armed Forces.

[7] The New GI Bill Continuation Act (P.L. 100-48) permanently authorized the All-Volunteer Force Educational Assistance Program and the Selected Reserve Component. It also changed the name of the program to the Montgomery GI Bill. The MGIB-AD program is authorized under Title 38, Chapter 30, of the United States Code.

[8] There are four categories of eligibility for the MGIB-AD program. Category 1applies to the majority of individuals and is addressed here. Category 2 applies to Vietnam-Era GI Bill conversion; Category 3 applies to involuntary separation/special separation; and Category 4 applies to veterans who participated in VEAP. For additional information on the four categories of eligibility, see Department of Veterans Affairs, *Federal Benefits for Veterans and Dependents, 2008 Edition*, Chapter 4, Education and Training, at [http://www1.va.gov/ opa/vadocs/fedben.pdf].

[9] In addition, individuals may receive veterans' education and training benefits under only one program at a time; and individuals may receiveveterans' education and training benefits under all programs combined for a maximum of 48 months.

[10] Department of Veterans Affairs, *Federal Benefits for Veterans and Dependents, 2008 Edition*, p. 34.

[11] For additional information on Tuition Assistance programs, see the Defense Activity for Non-Traditional Education Services (DANTES), Tuition Assistance Programs, at [http://www.dantes.doded.mil/dantes_web/tuitionassistance/index.htm].

[12] The MGIB-SR program is authorized under Title 10, Chapter 1606 of the United States Code.

[13] The REAP program is authorized under Title 10, Chapter 1607 of the United States Code.

[14] Department of Veterans Affairs, *Reserve Educational Assistance Program (REAP)*, VA Pamphlet 22-05-1, December 2005.

[15] The DEA program is authorized under Title 38, Chapter 35 of the United States Code.

[16] Department of Veterans Affairs, *Dependents' Educational Assistance Program (DEA)*, VA pamphlet 22-73-3 Revised, January 2005, at [http://www.gibill.va.gov/pamphlets/ CH35/CH35_Pamphlet.pdf].

[17] This category is effective as of December 23, 2006.

[18] Veterans with dependents have historically received additional funding to acknowledge this added responsibility under programs prior to VEAP.

[19] Other payment distribution arrangements are possible.

[20] All constant dollar calculations were performed using Consumer Price Index-All Urban Consumers (CPI-U) data available from the U.S. Department of Labor, Bureau of Labor Statistics (BLS).

[21] This assumes that living expenses were provided for nine months each year, the length of a traditional academic year. P.L. 78-346 specifically refers to an "ordinary school year" when discussing education benefits. The monthly allowance for living expenses increased to $65 in 1946 and $75 in 1948.

[22] Details may not add to totals due to rounding.

[23] Benefits provided through the original GI Bill were converted to monthly amounts for comparison purposes.

[24] For both analyses, prices are based on in-state tuition and fees and room and board rates paid by full-time-equivalent students enrolled in degree-granting institutions. While GI Bill recipients may choose not to live on campus, roomand board for on-campus residency were used in the calculations because these prices are comparable to or higher than room and board expenses for students living off-campus (The College Board, *Trends in College Pricing: 2007*. Available online at [http://www.collegeboard.com].)

[25] Due to program eligibility requirements, including minimum time-in-service provisions, maximum benefit amounts, in general, would not be initially available.

[26] For additional information on federal student aid programs authorized under the HEA, see CRS Report RL34214, *A Primer on the Higher Education Act (HEA)*, by Blake Alan Naughton.

[27] Effective July 1, 2009, this provision is revised to "is an orphan, in foster care, or a ward of the court, at any time when the individual is 13 years of age or older." Additionally, effective July 1, 2009 a student may also be deemed to be independent upon meeting the following criteria: is an emancipated minor or is in legal guardianship as determined by a court of competent jurisdiction in the individual's State of legal residence; or has been verified as a homeless child or youth as defined by the McKinney-Vento Homeless Assistance Act. Finally, effective July 1, 2009, a financial aid administrator may make a determination of independence based upon a documented determination of independence that was previously made by another financial aid administrator in the same award year.

[28] HEA, § 480(c) defines a veteran as an individual who was engaged in the active duty in the U.S. Army, Navy, Air Force, Marines or Coast Guard; and was released under a condition other than dishonorable.

[29] See HEA Title IV, § 472 for relevant statutory language.

[30] For a more detailed description of the federal student aid need analysis system, see archived CRS Report RL33266, *Federal Student Aid Need Analysis System: Background, Description and Legislative Action*, by Charmaine Mercer.

[31] HEA, § 480(c)(2) defines "veterans' education benefits" as including, but not limited to, 10 different sources of veterans' education support. In addition to the Montgomery GI Bill benefits, these include benefits from such sources as the Dependents Educational Assistance program (U.S.C., Title 38, Chapter 35), and the Reserve Officer Training Corps program (U.S.C., Title 37, Chapter 2).

[32] The program regulations for the three campus-based programs (FSEOG, FWS, and Perkins Loans) refer to other types of aid, such as veterans' education benefits, as a resource and the federal Stafford Loan programs refer to themas estimated financial assistance. HEA Title IV, Section 480(j)(1) states that for the purpose of determining a student's eligibility for funds under this title, *estimated financial assistance* shall include all scholarships, grants, loans, or other assistance known to the institution at the time the determination of the student's need is made, including veterans' education benefits as defined in Subsection (c), and national service education awards or post-service benefits under Title I of the National and Community Service Act of 1990. According to the *Federal Student Aid Handbook, 2006-2007*, the term *resources* comprises aid from federal student aid programs, as well as grants, scholarships, loans, and need-based employment that a financial aid administrator can reasonably anticipate at the time he/she awards aid to the student, regardless of whether the assistance is awarded by the school or by an individual or organization outside the school.

[33] This exception applies only to the rules for awarding subsidized Stafford Loans.

[34] Title CFR § 673.5(c)(3).

In: Veterans' Benefits and Care
Editor: Mathew H. Bradley

ISBN: 978-1-60692-500-3

Chapter 4

THE MILITARY SURVIVOR BENEFIT PLAN: A DESCRIPTION OF ITS PROVISIONS

David F. Burrelli

SUMMARY

The military Survivor Benefit Plan (SBP) was created in 1972. Since its creation, it has been subjected to a number of substantial legislative changes. This chapter describes the basic provisions of the military Survivor Benefit Plan and all relevant changes or modifications that have occurred.

Specifically, the military Survivor Benefit Plan is described and explained in terms of its eligibility provisions, costs, benefits, and its integration with other federal programs (including social security and Veterans' Administration Dependency and Indemnity Compensation) for members and retirees of active duty military service and the Reserve Components (both the reserves and National Guard). In addition, tables and work sheets are provided to assist the reader in computing the costs and benefits available under this program.

Nearly every Congress since 1972 has, in some way, modified the provisions of the military Survivor Benefit Plan. These modifications have had a significant effect on current and prospective participants and beneficiaries. In nearly every instance, these changes have made the SBP more generous. Furthermore, these modifications involve complex issues and processes, and are, therefore, a source of numerous requests for information from constituents to their congressional representatives.

INTRODUCTION

This chapter outlines the purpose and legislative background of providing benefits to the surviving dependents of a deceased member/retiree of the uniformed services. In certain cases, individuals other than dependents can be designated recipients of survivor benefits. This chapter describes the categories of beneficiaries eligible for survivor benefits under the military Survivor Benefit Plan (SBP), the formulas used in computing the income level (including the integration of SBP benefits with other federal benefits), and the costs of SBP participation incurred by the retiree and/or the beneficiary.[1]

Under the SBP, a military retiree can have a portion of his or her monthly retired pay withheld in order to provide, after his or her death, a monthly survivor benefit (55% of base[2] amount of military retired pay at the time of the retiree's death) to a surviving spouse or other eligible recipient(s). The cost of this protection is shared by the retiree (in the form of reductions from monthly military retired pay after retirement), the government, and possibly the beneficiary (under certain types of coverage). The original intended purpose of the SBP (and its antecedents) is to "insure that the surviving dependents of military personnel who die in retirement or after becoming eligible for retirement will continue to have a reasonable level of income."[3] Coverage was later expanded to active duty personnel as well.

The Survivor Benefit Plan was created by legislation enacted on September 21, 1 972,[4] and has been modified by later legislation. The SBP replaced the Retired Serviceman's Family Protection Plan (RSFPP).[5] The RSFPP was replaced because it had a number of unpopular features that made it unattractive. The RSFPP could be expensive for the retiree; the cost was approximately $0.23 of deducted retired pay per dollar of survivor benefits for a retired member age 45 who elected to provide coverage for a spouse who was 5 full years younger. The RSFPP was intended to be actuarially neutral in terms of costs — in other words, the cost of this program was fully paid for by its participants. The decision to elect RSFPP coverage had to be made by the prospective military retiree before his or her 18th year of military service. Furthermore, the methods used in computing the RSFPP's cost and benefit could change between the time at which the servicemember elected to provide coverage and the time at which the member actually retired. Thus, the costs and benefits remained an unknown quantity, limiting the ability of the retiree to make future financial plans. During its 19-year history, participation in the RSFPP never exceeded more than 15% of eligible military retirees. It was expected — and has largely been proven — that the SBP would be a significant improvement over the RSFPP, in terms of participation rates, costs to the retiree, and benefits for the survivors. It also entails higher costs to taxpayers because the SBP costs are shared with the government in most cases.

Major Provisions of the Survivor Benefit Plan

Coverage for Military Members Retired from an Active Duty Career

Six separate types of coverage are available under the SBP for military members retired from an active duty military career, characterized according to the relationship of the beneficiary or beneficiaries to the military retiree:[6]

- Spouse Only;
- Spouse and Child(ren);
- Child(ren) Only;
- Persons with an Insurable Interest;
- Former Spouse;

- Former Spouse and Child(ren).

The type of coverage and the amount of coverage provided are factors used in determining the cost to the military retiree. Generally, a retiree is automatically enrolled in the SBP upon retirement at the maximum level of coverage to his or her respective surviving spouse and surviving dependent children, unless the retiree elects not to participate, to participate at a lesser level of coverage, elects other than spouse coverage, or is ordered by a court to provide such benefits to a former spouse. To participate at a reduced level of coverage, the retiree elects to have his or her *base* amount of retired pay — that amount of monthly retired pay the retiree selects to be used in determining the SBP benefit and cost — be less than his or her total retired pay subject to a $635 minimum. The maximum SBP benefit is 55% of base amount of military retired pay, when the base amount and total retired pay are the *same*. Reduced coverage consists of 55% of the base amount of retired pay when the retiree elects a base amount that is *less* than total retired pay.[7]

If a retiree elects not to participate, or to participate at a reduced level of coverage, the retiree's spouse must be notified, and in the case of such an election made on or after March 1, 1986, the spouse must concur with the election for it to be effective.[8] Any decision not to participate or to participate at a reduced level is usually irrevocable. However, under certain circumstances, a retiree who is unmarried at the time of his or her retirement and who elects not to participate in the SBP, but who marries after his or her retirement, may elect within one year of marriage to provide SBP benefits for the new spouse. This election takes effect only after a one-year waiting period. With the enactment of P.L. 99-145 (November 8, 1985, effective March 1, 1986), the spouse of a post-military-retirement marriage must be notified if the retiree does not elect to provide an SBP benefit, or elects to provide an SBP benefit at a reduced level.

Spouse Only Coverage

In order to be eligible for Spouse Only coverage, the intended SBP beneficiary must be a widow or widower who was (1) married to the retiree at the time of retirement, (2) married to the deceased retiree for at least one year prior to the retiree's death, or (3) the parent of a child born of a post-retirement marriage. The benefit (considering income from all federal sources — including social security and veterans' benefits — attributable to military service) was intended to be at least 55% of the base amount of retired pay the retiree was receiving at the time of death — which, for maximum coverage, is the same as total retired pay.

Computational Formulas

The computational formula for determining the amount of retired pay withheld is based on the date the member entered the service and/or the type of retirement the service member is entitled to receive. The formulas are discussed below as the "Original Computational Formula" and the "Flat-Rate Formula." Military personnel who entered the service on or after March 1, 1990, *and* who are not entitled to retired pay under either Chapter 61 of title 10 U.S. Code (Retirement or Separation for Physical Disability), or Chapter 67 (Retired Pay for Non-Regular Service), i.e., "Disability Retired Pay" or "Reserve Retired Pay," will have their withholdings computed under the "Flat-Rate" method. Those military personnel who first became a member before March 1, 1990, or those who have their retired pay computed under either Chapter 61 or 67 (regardless of the date of retirement) will have their SBP withholdings computed under whichever alternative (Original or Flat-Rate) is more financially advantageous.[9] The reduction in retired pay does not apply during any month in which there is no eligible spouse (or former spouse) beneficiary. (Reductions to retired pay are not considered taxable income.)

Original Computational Formula

Under this method, the retiree's contribution to the total cost of providing the SBP benefit is computed as 2.5% of the first $635 of the base amount of retired pay plus 10% of the remaining base amount of retired pay. This contribution is withheld from the retiree's total monthly retired pay.[10] For example, a hypothetical retiree (E-5, with 20 years of service in 2006) receives a monthly base amount of military retired pay of $1,263 (see **Table 1**). The cost of providing survivor protection for this retiree is $78.68. In other words, $78.68 is deducted from this hypothetical retiree's base amount of monthly retired pay of $1,263 to insure that upon the retiree's death, his or her surviving spouse will receive a monthly survivor benefit of 55% of his or her base amount of retired pay, or $694 per month, if the retiree dies while receiving the $1,263 amount. If the retiree received more than $1,263 per month in total military retired pay — say as an E-8 with 20 years of service, or $2,035 — but elected to provide less than the maximum coverage (by using $1,183, rather than total retired pay, as the base amount), the computation of costs and benefits would remain the same. If an individual's retired pay increases as the result of cost-of-living adjustments (COLAs), the amount deducted from his or her retired pay, and the potential SBP benefit to his or her designated survivor (in this case, his or her spouse), usually will increase proportionately as well. The costs of SBP protection and benefits are computed on the basis of retired pay rates at the time of retirement [including any adjustments made to the base ($635) amount]. All subsequent post-retirement changes are a result of cost-of-living adjustments to retired pay.[11]

Line six is the cost of survivor protection under the Spouse Only coverage. The payment to the beneficiary is 55% of base amount military retired pay, or $694. The base $635 is indexed for inflation. *Worksheets are at the end of this chapter.*

Table 1. Computation of Survivor Benefit Plan Costs to a Hypothetical Retiree for Spouse Only Coverage

1.	Enter base amount of retired pay.	$1,263.00
2.	Enter $635, or total retired pay if less than $635 (see fn. 10).	$635.00
3.	Multiply the figure in line two by 2.5%.	$15.88
4.	Subtract $635 from line one. If line one is less than $635 enter zero.	$628.00
5.	Multiply line four by 10%.	$62.80
6.	Add lines three and five.	$78.68

Flat-Rate Formula

P.L. 101-189 (November 29, 1989, 103 Stat. 1577 et seq.) revised and simplified the computational formula for determining SBP withholdings.[12] Under this new formula, SBP withholdings are computed to be 6.5% of the base amount of retired pay. A retiree who used $1,263 (E-5, 20 years of service) as the amount of thc basc amount of retired pay would have $82.83 ($1,263 x 0.065) withheld in order to provide the same level of protection under the Flat-Rate method.

The basic benefit is not affected by the type of computational formula used. (See *Computational Formulas* section for an explanation of who is eligible to use the Flat-Rate method.)[13]

Remarriage

Regardless of which formula is used, a surviving spouse (or eligible former spouse) may become ineligible to receive SBP benefits if he or she remarries. Eligibility for SBP benefits when remarriage occurs is dependent upon the age at remarriage and the date that such a remarriage occurs. A surviving spouse (or eligible former spouse) becomes ineligible to receive SBP benefits if he or she remarries prior to reaching age 60, if such a remarriage took place **prior to** November 14, 1986 (remarriage after age 60 does not affect receipt of an SBP benefit). A surviving spouse (or eligible former spouse) becomes ineligible to receive SBP benefits if he or she remarries prior to reaching age 55 if such a remarriage took place **on or after** November 14, 1986 (remarriage after age 55 for these beneficiaries does not affect receipt of SBP payments). If the second marriage is terminated (by death, annulment, or divorce), the original SBP benefit can be reinstated (subject to certain restrictions). The surviving spouse of two or more deceased military retirees (each a participant in the SBP) may select and receive the more financially advantageous benefit.

"Paid-Up" Provisions

In 1999, Congress further expanded the generosity of the SBP by enacting the so-called "paid-up" provision. Under this language, reductions in retired pay made to cover the retiree's share cease when two conditions are met: (1) the retiree reaches age 70, and (2) the retiree has participated in the SBP for 360 months. As enacted, these provisions become effective October 1, 2008.[14] Language was included in the Senate version of the National Defense Authorization Act for Fiscal Year 2006 to move the effective date of this provision to October 1, 2005. This language was dropped by the Conference Committee.[15] Again, language was included in the Senate version of the National Defense Authorization Act for Fiscal Year 2007 to move the effective date of this provision to October 1, 2006. This language, too, was dropped by the Conference Committee.[16]

Spouse and Child(ren) Coverage[17]

Under Spouse and Child(ren) coverage, upon the retiree's death, SBP benefits are first paid to the surviving spouse. If the surviving spouse predeceases the retiree, dies after becoming eligible to receive SBP benefits, or becomes ineligible to receive SBP benefits (through remarriage, for example), the SBP benefits will then be paid directly to the designated child or children. If there is more than one child, the SBP benefits are paid in equal shares to each child for as long as he or she remains eligible.

The cost of this coverage is additive to that of Spouse Only coverage, and is determined on an actuarial[18] basis, taking into account the age of the retiree, the spouse, and the youngest child. For example, a retiree who is 45 years old, with a spouse who is 40 years old (i.e., 5 full years younger than the retiree) and a child age 10, would have to pay an additional 0.10% of the base amount of retired pay in order to cover a child or children in addition to the amount paid for Spouse Only coverage. The hypothetical retiree mentioned above under Spouse Only coverage who has $82.55 per month withheld from his or her retired pay (see Flat-Rate formula, p. 5) to provide an SBP benefit for his or her spouse, would thus have an additional $1.26 ($1,263 x 0.10%) withheld per month in order to provide Spouse and Child(ren) coverage.[19] The reduction in retired pay that represents the cost of child protection continues only for as long as there is at least one eligible child.

A child becomes ineligible for an SBP benefit upon reaching age 18 (or 22, if a full-time student).[20] A child who marries becomes ineligible to receive SBP benefits regardless of age.[21] An eligible child who becomes incapacitated (either physically or mentally) may continue to receive SBP benefits for the duration of the incapacitation if the condition existed prior to the child's 18th birthday.

Child(ren) Only Coverage

Under Child(ren) Only coverage, SBP benefits are paid directly to the surviving child(ren) of a deceased military retiree regardless of whether or not there is a surviving spouse. Eligibility under this coverage is subject to the same restrictions as a child is, or children are, under Spouse and Child(ren) coverage. (Under certain circumstances, spouse coverage can be restored if a spouse later becomes eligible.) The cost of this coverage is also computed on an actuarial basis (and therefore subject to modification). For example, a military retiree who is 45 years old, has a child age 10, and elects maximum coverage, would have approximately 2.5% of his or her base amount of retired pay withheld in order to provide, at the time of his or her death, an SBP survivor benefit for the surviving child. In other words, in the example mentioned above under Spouse Only coverage, $31.58 ($1,263 x 2.5%) would be withheld from a retiree's retired pay in order to provide his or her surviving child(ren) with a benefit of $694 per month. (Child Only coverage is less expensive due to the limitation on the number of years — until age 18 or 22 under most circumstances — a beneficiary remains eligible to receive SBP benefits.)

Persons with an Insurable Interest

Insurable Interest coverage may be selected only if there is neither a spouse nor a dependent child at the time of retirement. Under this coverage a beneficiary is defined as "a natural person with an insurable interest"[22] in the retiree. Included in this category are relatives of the retiree, such as a parent, sibling, or a child who may not qualify for SBP beneficiary status under Spouse Only, Spouse and Child(ren), or Child(ren) Only provisions.

Non-relatives, such as a business partner, may also be covered. Unlike other SBP options, Insurable Interest must be elected at the maximum level.

The cost of Insurable Interest coverage is (1) 10% of the base amount of military retired pay *plus* (2) 5% of total base amount of retired pay for each *full* 5 years that the named beneficiary is younger than the retiree. Insurable Interest coverage is thus more expensive than other types of coverage. However, the total cost to the retiree of this coverage cannot exceed 40% of total military retired pay. In other words, a retiree who wishes to provide Insurable Interest coverage to a person 30 or more years younger would have the maximum of 40% of the base amount of military retired pay withheld.

For example, a retiree who is 50 years old and receives $1,263 per month as the base amount of military retired pay, elects to provide protection to a person 10 full years younger. This retiree would have the cost of this protection computed as follows: 10% of the base amount of retired pay (or $126) plus 5% for each full 5 years the beneficiary is younger (in this case the beneficiary is age 40) than the retiree. The SBP costs would thus be $252 (see **Table 2**).

According to language contained in the National Defense Authorization Act for FY1995, Insurable Interest coverage could be voluntarily discontinued (except in those cases where a former spouse is being covered). Retirees discontinuing this coverage, who later remarry or acquire dependents, may again participate in the SBP under another allowable beneficiary category.[23]

Line 11 is the cost of survivor protection under the Persons with an Insurable Interest category of coverage. The payment to the beneficiary is 55% of the base amount of military retired pay less the premium, or ($ 1,263-252) x 55%=$556. *Worksheets are at the end of this chapter.*

Table 2. Computation of SBP Costs under Persons with an Insurable Interest Coverage

1.	The amount of base military retired pay.	$1,263.0 0
2.	Multiply line one by 10%.	$126.00
3.	Age of the retiree at his/her last birthday.	50
4.	Age of prospective beneficiary as of the date of the retiree's last birthday.	40
5.	Subtract line three from line four. (If line three is less than line four, enter 0.)	10
6.	Divide the sum in line five by the number 5 and round the quotient to the lower whole number.	2
7.	Multiply 5% by line six.	10%
8.	Multiply line one by line seven.	$126.00
9.	Add line two and line eight.	$252.00
10.	Multiply line one by 40%.	$505.00
11.	Compare lines nine and ten: enter the lesser.	$252.20

Former Spouse Coverage[24]

A military member may choose, or may be required by a court order, to provide SBP coverage for a former spouse, depending on when the divorce occurred. This election can occur as part of or incident to a divorce-related property settlement. For divorces occurring before November 14, 1986, federal law explicitly states that *no court was authorized to order* a member or retiree to provide SBP protection to a former spouse. If a retiree voluntarily decides, *in writing*, to provide benefits to a former spouse, this decision must be honored by the retiree. The retiree who elected Spouse Only or Spouse and Child(ren) coverage, and was subsequently divorced before November 14, 1986, may switch to Former Spouse coverage for the (now) ex- spouse. This latter change in coverage must be elected within one year of the date the divorce decree becomes final.

If a divorce occurs on or after November 14, 1986, however, *a court may order* a member or retiree to provide SBP protection as part of or incident to a divorce. According to changes in law implemented by the FY1 987 DOD Authorization Act (P.L. 99-661, November 14, 1986), "A court order may require a person to elect (or to enter into an agreement to elect) ... to provide an annuity to a former spouse (or to both a former spouse and child)."[25] This language does not require courts to make such an order but gives them the freedom to do so.

The FY 1986 DOD Authorization Act (P.L. 99-145, November 8, 1985) included a change in Former Spouse coverage which provided that military retirees and "former spouses ... covered under the insurable interest category (could) ... elect jointly to switch to spouse coverage at the maximum level within one year (and it provided) current participants who had the option of electing Former Spouse coverage in the past and chose not to do so, the option of electing Former Spouse coverage."[26] Those electing Former Spouse coverage after March 1, 1986, have the cost of this coverage and benefit amount computed in the same manner as in the case of Spouse Only coverage.

Because a retiree may provide only one type of SBP coverage for one category of beneficiary, election of coverage for a former spouse can have the effect of denying SBP protection to a second or future spouse. However, it is not clear whether courts have the authority to divide SBP benefits between a former spouse and current/subsequent spouse. In other words, although the services will provide SBP benefits to only one category of beneficiary (former spouse, for example), it is not clear whether or not a court, as part of an equitable divorce property settlement, has the authority to divide SBP benefits between a former spouse (designated to receive them in this example) and a current/subsequent spouse.

The FY2000 National Defense Authorization Act provided for the "effectuation of intended SBP annuity for [a] former spouse when not elected by reason of [the] untimely death of [the] retiree."[27] This language pertains to any retiree who, on or after August 21, 1983, agreed to (or was required by a court to) provide SBP coverage to a former spouse, but who died within 21 days of making such an agreement (or being so required). Under this language, the former spouse of such a retiree is deemed to have been covered effective November 5, 1999.

Former Spouse and Child(ren) Coverage

Coverage for a former spouse and child(ren) became available on March 1, 1986.[28] This coverage is provided on the same terms as Spouse and Child(ren) coverage described above.

Coverage for Military Members Retired from the Reserve Components

As with the Survivor Benefit Plan for active duty retirees, retirement eligible members of the reserves (Army Reserve, Naval Reserve, Marine Corps Reserve, Air Force Reserve and Coast Guard Reserve) and National Guard (Army National Guard and Air National Guard) may elect to provide SBP protection for their survivors. However, because members of the Reserve Components[29] are not eligible to receive Reserve Component retired pay until age 60, regardless of the age at which they actually retire, the structure of the Reserve Component SBP (RCSBP) is different from that applicable to active duty members.

Prior to 1978, Reserve Component personnel could not provide survivor protection for an eligible beneficiary until they were eligible to draw retired pay at age 60. Legislation passed in 1978[30] allows Reserve Component members to decide whether or how they will participate in the RCSBP when they are notified of retirement eligibility (not yet eligible to receive retired pay) — in almost all cases, many years before reaching age 60.

Reserve Component members who are not yet 60 years old and who are retirement eligible may elect to provide SBP protection under one of three options. The costs and amount of coverage available depend on the option selected and the category of beneficiary. A prospective Reserve Component retiree must select one of the following RCSBP options within 90 days of being notified of retirement eligibility:

> **Option A** - The retiree may decline RCSBP protection. Should the retiree die before reaching age 60, no RCSBP benefit will be paid. The retiree will again be offered the opportunity to participate in the SBP upon reaching age 60.
>
> **Option B** - The retiree may elect RCSBP coverage such that survivor payments will begin on (1) the date of the retiree's death of (2) the date the retiree would have turned 60, whichever is later.
>
> **Option C** - The retiree may elect, under this option, to provide an RCSBP benefit that would begin immediately following the death of the retiree, regardless of the retiree's age at the time of death.

Under option A, the costs and types of coverage available once the retiree reaches age 60 are the same as under the active duty SBP. Under options B and C, the cost of RCSBP protection is shared by the retiree, the Government, and the beneficiary. The retiree's portion is paid through deductions in retired pay beginning at age 60. The beneficiary's or beneficiaries' share is paid through benefit reductions. The costs under options B and C are dependent upon the type of coverage (see active duty retirees), as well as the age of the retiree and selected beneficiary(ies).

Under certain circumstance, an RCSBP benefit may be paid to the eligible surviving spouse, dependent child(ren), or former spouse of a member of the Reserve Components who dies

(1) before being notified that he or she had completed the years of service required to be eligible for Reserve Component retired pay; or

(2) during the 90-day period beginning on the date of notification that the member had completed the years of service required for eligibility for Reserve Component retired pay, if he or she had not already rejected participation in the RCSBP.

The income payable is equal to 55% of retired pay which the member would have been entitled to receive had the service member been retired and at least age 60 at the time of death (less any Veterans Affairs Dependency and Indemnity Compensation payable, see below).

"Forgotten Widow" Coverage

In 1997, Congress created a special annuity of then-$165, now $205.61, (subject to cost of living adjustments) payable monthly to certain surviving spouses. These widows were married to certain retired or retirement-eligible members who died without electing SBP coverage. Subject to certain restrictions on remarriage and the receipt of certain other government-sponsored compensation, the eligible surviving spouse must have been married to a member who

(A) became entitled to retired or retainer pay before September 21, 1972, died before March 21, 1974, and was entitled to retired or retainer pay on the date of death; or
(B) died before October 1, 1978, and at the time of his death would have been entitled to retired pay under chapter 67 [Retired Pay for Non-Regular Service] of title 10, United States Code (as in effect before December 1, 1994), but for the fact that he was under 60 years of age.[31]

Coverage for Military Members Serving on Active Duty

Under the original SBP, an SBP benefit may be paid to an eligible spouse, dependent child(ren), eligible former spouse, or eligible former spouse and dependent child(ren) following the death of an active duty member. This benefit will be paid if the deceased active duty service member, at the time of death,

(1) was eligible to receive retired pay; or
(2) was a commissioned officer, had completed 20 years of service, but was not yet eligible to retire as a commissioned officer.[32]

The SBP benefit payable to the survivor of such a deceased active duty member is equal to 55% of the amount of retired pay (less any amount received on the basis of Department of Veterans Affairs (VA) Dependency and Indemnity Compensation or DIC; see section below on VA DIC) that the deceased service member would have been eligible for had he or she elected maximum coverage and retired on the day of his or her death.

Recent legislation[33] has expanded the coverage to the survivors of individuals who die while on active duty and who are *not* retirement-eligible, effective September 10, 2001. Under these provisions, the surviving spouses of active duty personnel who die are provided an annuity. This annuity for an active duty (nonretirement-eligible member) is determined by assuming the individual would have been eligible to retire under Sec. 1201, Title 10 USC,[34] with a total disability. The surviving spouse's annuity is based on the amount of disability retired pay the servicemember would have received under Sec. 1201. The spouse's share is 55% of that amount of the member's disability retired pay if the surviving spouse is under age 62, and 35% if age 62 or over. Depending on when the individual entered the service, the amount used may be either the terminal monthly basic pay (for those who entered service on or before September 7, 1980) or the average basic pay for the 36- month period (i.e., "high three" years) the member earned the highest rate of basic pay (for those who entered the service after September 7, 1980).[35] The amount of monthly disability pay is computed either by multiplying the determined amount of basic pay by the percentage disability or by computing 2.5% of basic pay times the member's years of service up to 75%, whichever is higher. Since the legislation assumes the level of disability is 100%, the amount of basic pay (or "high three") used would be multiplied by 75%. In 2003, Congress allowed for these benefits to be paid to the surviving children, if any, of an active member who dies.[36] This provision was made effective November 23, 2003. As part of the National Defense Act for Fiscal Year 2007, Congress replaced the November 23, 2003 effective date with October 7, 2001.[37] With the children as the SBP beneficiaries, the surviving spouse avoids any offsets from the receipt of Dependency and Indemnity Compensation (see the sec. entitled "Survivor Benefit Plan and Veterans' Affairs Dependency and Indemnity Compensation").

SURVIVOR BENEFIT PLAN AND SOCIAL SECURITY

The relationship between benefits received from the Survivor Benefit Plan and social security is complicated and has been subjected to periodic changes. For this reason, the following three sections describe how military personnel are covered under social security, the relationship between SBP and social security benefits (**integration**) that existed before enactment of the FY1 986 DOD Authorization Act,[38] and the changes in the SBP which affected the interaction of the two benefit systems that were made by this latter act and others.

Social Security Coverage for Military Personnel

Active duty military personnel have been fully covered by social security and have paid social security taxes since January 1, 1957. In addition to providing monthly benefits to civilian retirees and retired military personnel age 62 or older, social security provides benefits to the widows or widowers of deceased military and civilian retirees.

The surviving spouse or former spouse of a military retiree is entitled to receive social security survivor benefits based on the deceased retiree's active duty basic military pay.[39]

Persons eligible for social security survivor benefits may *also* be entitled to social security retirement benefits based on *their own* employment. However, this "dual entitlement" is *prohibited under social security law*. People always receive social security benefits that they themselves earned as a result of their own employment. If those benefits *exceed* the amount of social security survivor benefits, the latter are not payable. However, if the survivor's own social security retirement benefits are *less than* the social security survivor benefits, the difference between the two is paid in addition to the survivor's own social security retirement benefits.

For example, assume that A and B are both surviving spouses of military retirees and are both entitled to social security benefits — based on the military service of their deceased spouses — of $400 per month.[40] Assume further that both surviving spouses have been employed and are entitled to their own social security retirement benefits based on that employment. Survivor A is entitled to $450 per month in social security retirement benefits based on his or her own employment. Because survivor A's own social security retirement benefit of $450 per month *exceeds* the social security survivor entitlement of $400 per month, only the $450 retirement benefit is payable. Survivor B, on the other hand, is entitled to $350 per month in social security retirement benefits based on his or her own employment. Because B's social security retirement benefit ($350) is *less than* the social security survivor benefit ($400), the full $350 retirement benefit is payable, plus the $50 difference between the two, for a total of $400 per month in social security benefits.

Social security survivor benefits based on a spouse's or former spouse's employment (including military service) are first payable at age 60 (at age 50, if the surviving spouse is totally disabled, or at any age if and as long as there are children under the age of 16), and social security retirement benefits based on one's own employment are first payable at age 62.

Integration of the Survivor Benefit Plan and Social Security Benefits

The SBP was (and for certain beneficiaries, is) "integrated" with social security: SBP benefits are reduced or "offset" when the survivor reaches age 62. The **rationale for this integration** was (1) the SBP was intended to provide a specific portion of a deceased military retiree's retired pay to the retiree's surviving spouse or former spouse, and (2) to recognize the government's employer contribution under both social security and SBP. It was, therefore, considered appropriate by the Congress that *all* sources of survivor benefits attributable to military service — DOD and non-DOD — be considered in the computation of this specific portion of a deceased retiree's retired pay. The cost of the SBP as well as the benefit received by the survivor(s), therefore, reflect this offset.[41] The offset occurs at age 62 regardless of when the survivor actually begins to draw social security benefits.[42]

The 1972 legislation which established the SBP provided that those social security survivor benefits which a surviving spouse or former spouse of a deceased retiree is eligible to receive, based solely on the military service of the retiree, are subtracted from the survivor's SBP payment. The legislative history of the SBP statute indicates that the sum of (1) the reduced SBP payments, plus (2) social security benefits earned as a result of the retiree's military service (computed assuming the retiree lived to age 65 and the surviving spouse begins to draw social security survivor benefits at age 62), and other sources as well, would provide the desired 55% of the base amount of retired pay. The aggregate of these integrated benefits are used in determining the 55%. In other words, this plan was designed to provide coverage at a rate no less than what the survivor was entitled to on the basis of social security survivor benefits earned as a result of military service. However, the eligible survivor may be too young to receive social security survivor benefits at the time the member or retiree dies. Therefore, the SBP provides a larger benefit until the eligible survivor reaches age 62 (in recognition of eligibility for social security benefits regardless of the age when a survivor begins to draw such benefits).

The Comptroller General has noted that it was the intention of Congress that the combined total of the offset SBP benefit and the social security survivor benefit would not be less than the pre-offset SBP benefit. The Comptroller General, noting congressional intention, stated that:

> The method of computing the offset was intended to be a "most generous formula ... to assure that a widow will receive at least 55 percent of the man's military retired pay." H.Rept. 92-481, 92d Cong., 1st Sess., September 16, 1971, accompanying H.R. 1067, at page 14. Similar statements appear on pages 30, 31 and 53 of S.Rept. 92-1089, 92d Cong., 2d Sess., September 6, 1972.
>
> It is clear, therefore, that Congress did not intend to authorize an offset which would amount to more than the comparable social security benefit. We do not find that the statutory language of the Survivor Benefit Plan requires or permits that result.[43]

Thus, it was the intent of Congress that (1) the SBP benefit alone, or (2) the offset SBP benefit and social security survivor benefit combined, would be at least equal to 55% of the base amount of retired pay.

However, the amount of social security survivor benefits can vary based on a variety of factors. These include (1) the survivor's age when he or she begins to receive benefits, (2) the age of the military retiree at the time of death, and (3) whether or not the retiree had begun to receive social security benefits before death. The actual social security benefit due to some or all of these factors may therefore be less than the hypothetical benefit computed under the assumptions of the SBP statute, and on which the SBP offset is based.

As an example of the integration of the SBP and social security, assume a survivor is receiving an SBP income of $600 per month. The survivor is also entitled to social security survivor benefits of $ 100 (based on the military service of his or her deceased spouse or former spouse). Because of the survivor's own employment, this same survivor is eligible to receive social security retirement benefits of $150 per month (see **Table 3**). Because the social security survivor benefit is *less than* the social security retirement benefit (and therefore not payable) the survivor only receives his or her own earned social security retirement benefit of $150. However, because the survivor was entitled to a social security survivor benefit of $100 based on the military service of the deceased spouse, the SBP payment is reduced or offset by $100 when the survivor reaches age 62. Thus, the survivor's final monthly income is computed as follows:

Table 3. Breakdown of Pre-Integration Monthly Benefits of a Hypothetical SBP Beneficiary

SBP benefit	$600
Social Security Survivor Benefits	$100
Social Security Benefits based on the Survivor's own employment	$150

(The SBP benefit minus the social security survivor benefit) plus the social security retirement benefit equals the total sum received from both social security and the SBP, or

($600 - $100) + $150 = $650.

In 1980, legislation was enacted that limited the reduction of SBP income due to social security benefits to 40%.[44] For example, assume a survivor receives a monthly SBP benefit of $600 and becomes entitled to social security survivor payments (based on the member's military service) of $300 per month. The social security survivor benefit is therefore 50% of the SBP income. However, because the offset can be no more than 40% of the SBP income, the SBP benefit will be offset or reduced, at age 62, by the maximum of 40% ($600 x 40% = $240) and not by the entire $300 from social security. The total amount the survivor will receive is $660, or (1) $300 of social security benefits plus (2) $600-$240=$360 of the reduced SBP income.

Two-Tier Survivor Benefit Plan

In title VII of the FY1986 DOD Authorization Act (P.L. 99-145, November 8, 1985),[45] Congress modified the Survivor Benefit Plan so that retirees and their prospective spouse survivors would know the exact amount of the SBP benefit that would be paid upon the retiree's death. Congress did this by eliminating the integration with social security. The House Armed Services Committee report on the legislation stated the rationale for such a change regarding the social security offset:

> The principal problems associated with the social security offsets are twofold:
> (1) the offset is not calculated until the time of death; hence military members cannot predict the impact of the offset at the time of retirement when the decision to participate in the plan is made;
> (2) the provision is difficult to explain and to understand; hence many perceive that an earned benefit is unfairly taken away.[46]

The new plan was labeled the "two-tier" SBP. Under the two-tier SBP, a surviving spouse of a deceased military retiree will receive 55% of the base amount of military retired pay as a survivor benefit (as was the case under the original plan). Upon reaching age 62, the SBP benefit will be reduced *automatically* to 35% of the base amount of military retired pay for any surviving spouse or former spouse covered under the two-tier SBP. Since it is expected that benefits for those eligible for the two-tier plan would have been subjected to the full 40% social security offset (i.e., a reduction from 55% to 33% in SBP benefits at age 62), 35% was considered an appropriate approximation. Under the two-tier SBP, a spouse or former spouse who becomes a widow or widower *after* age 62 will receive an SBP payment equal to 35% of the base amount of military retired pay. For example, assume a military retiree receives $1,183 per month in military retired pay at the time of his or her death and has elected to provide the maximum SBP coverage of 55% of total — and base — retired pay (see **Table 1**). The retiree's surviving spouse or former spouse will receive a $650 per month SBP payment if under age 62 at the time the retiree dies, as was the case before enactment of the two-tier system. When the surviving spouse or former spouse reaches age 62, the SBP payment will be reduced to $414 per month (or 35% of the original base amount military retired pay of $1,183 per month). This reduction from 55% to 35% occurs at age 62 and is not affected by the receipt of social security benefits.[47] The two-tier plan thus allowed retirees and their prospective surviving spouses or former spouses to predict what their survivors' future SBP payments will be upon a retiree's death and/or when the survivors reach age 62.

Two selected groups will have their SBP payments calculated under *either* the pre-two-tier plan (including the social security offset) *or* the two-tier plan, depending upon which is more financially advantageous to the survivor. The first group includes those beneficiaries (widow or widowers) who were receiving an SBP benefit on October 1, 1985. The second group includes the spouses or former spouses of military personnel who were qualified for or were already receiving military retired pay on October 1, 1985.[48] The spouses or former spouses of military personnel who were *not* qualified to receive military retired pay on October 1, 1985 (i.e., those who had not been on active duty with 20 or more years of service or completed 20 or more years of creditable Reserve Component service as of October 1, 1985) will have their SBP payments computed using the two-tier method.

Participation rates have increased since the introduction of the two-tier plan. Of those retiring in FY1 984, 54% elected to participate in the SBP. Of those retiring in FY1990 and FY1993, 60 and 58% elected to participate, respectively. (Some of those retiring in FY1990 may be eligible to have the benefits for there survivors calculated under either the two-tier or social security offset method.)[49] In other words, the change to the two-tier benefit has been associated with an increase in participation over the social security offset method.

Comparison of the Social Security Offset and Two-Tier SBP

The complicated nature of the social security offset was not fully understood by many servicemembers, retirees, or widow(er)s. Thus, when the two-tier SBP was introduced, with its straight forward reduction of benefits at age 62, many felt that the two-tier SBP represented a reduction in their benefits or potential benefit over what was available under the social security offset SBP. **Table 4** provides a comparison of both plans computed for an active duty service member (E-7) who retires from the military at age 42 with 20 years of service. Upon retirement from the military, the retiree is enrolled in the SBP and selects coverage for a base pay amount equal $1,670. This retiree then accepts civilian employment (including social security deductions) for another 15 years. In this case, the hypothetical retiree has SBP withholdings computed under the Flat-Rate formula, $1,670 x 6.5%=$108.55.

(For the purposes of this example, cost of living adjustments are not used. All numbers represent reasonable approximations.)

At age 59, the retiree dies. The surviving spouse begins receiving a military Survivor Benefit equal to 55% of base military retired pay or $1,670 x 55%=$918 per month.

In addition, the retiree's spouse was employed and earned social security benefits of $500 per month from this employment. Since the military retiree made social security payments both in the service and in the subsequent civilian employment, the surviving spouse is eligible to receive social security survivor benefits of $631 per month based on the retiree's entire career. For the sake of this example, $378 of the $631 are attributed to the social security contributions made during military service. (It is this $378 per month that will be taken into account under the offset plan.)

As described above, a person (in this case the surviving spouse) receives his/her own earned social security benefits first. Thus, this spouse will receive $500 per month in social security benefits. In addition, since the social security survivor benefit is greater ($631) than the spouse's earned benefit ($500), the spouse will also receive the difference ($631 - $500=$ 131) added to his/her own earned benefit ($131 + $500) for a total social security benefit of $631 per month. In this example, the spouse begins receiving these benefits at age 62.

Under the two-tier formula, the military SBP amount is reduced from 55 to 35% of base military retired pay or from $918 to ($1,670 x 35%=) $584 per month at age 62. When the social security benefit is added, the surviving spouse's income is ($584 + $63 1=) $1,215 per month. In other words, prior to age 62, the surviving spouse receives $918 per month from the military Survivor Benefit Plan. Assuming the spouse begins receiving social security benefits at age 62, total income for the spouse (from both the reduced military SBP and social security) increases to $1,215 per month.

Table 4. Comparison of Monthly SBP and Social Security Benefits Computed Using the Two-Tier and Offset Formulas

	Social Security Offset	Two-Tier
Base retired pay (1994, E-7, with 20 years of service)	$1,670	$1,670
SBP monthly withholdings (Flat-Rate or 6.5% of base pay)	$108.55	$108.55
SBP benefit for a spouse under age 62 (55% of base pay)	$918	$918
Social security benefits of the surviving spouse		
Based on the surviving spouse's career	$500	$500
	$631	$631
Based on the retiree's civilian and military career	($378 attributable to military service only)	
Total social security benefit (spouse's $500 plus $131 [631-500] from the member's career	$631	$631
SBP benefits at age 62	$550 ($918 - $378 or 40%, whichever is less)	$584 (35% or base)
Total survivor income from both SBP and social security	$1,181 ($550 + $631)	$1,215 ($584 + $631)

Turning to SBP benefits computed under the offset method, prior to age 62, this spouse receives the same SBP benefit of 55% of base military retired pay ($918 per month). At age 62, however, the SBP is offset — reduced — by social security benefits attributable to the member's military service, ($378), subject to the 40% limit on the offset. Under law, this offset occurs regardless of whether or not the spouse is actually receiving these benefits. Since the $378 of social security benefits based on the service member's career is greater than 40% of the SBP (40% of $918 is rounded to $367), the SBP is offset by 40% or $367 rather than by entire social security benefit attributable to the member's military service (i.e., $918 - $367= $551). Thus, at age 62, the surviving spouse's SBP benefit is reduced from $918 to $551 per month. When the total social security benefit is added in, the surviving spouse's total income is $551 + $631 for a total of $1,182 per month.

In other words, prior to age 62, a spouse receives the same SBP benefit under either the two-tier or original offset formula SBP ($918). However, as this example shows, at age 62, monthly benefits from both SBP and social security are greater under the two-tier method ($1,215) than under the offset formula ($1,182).

This example can only allude to some of the possible effects and interactions of the SBP and social security. The amount of SBP benefits and the final income of the surviving spouse are dependent upon a number of factors including, but not limited to, the retiree's years of service, rank at retirement, year in which the retirement occurred, social security payments made by the retiree, the work history of the surviving spouse and the eligibility for VA benefits (as described below).

SUPPLEMENTAL SURVIVOR BENEFIT PLAN

Established under Public Law 101-189,[50] the Supplemental Survivor Benefit Plan provides SBP participants an opportunity to avoid or limit any reductions in SBP benefits that would occur at age 62 for a spouse or former spouse. This legislation also created an open season that would allow certain retirees to enroll in the SBP, increase SBP coverage, and opt to participate in the new Supplemental SBP.

Participation in the Supplemental SBP is voluntary and not automatic. In order to be eligible, retirees must be participants in the two-tier SBP. Those eligible to have their benefits computed under either the Social Security offset method or the two-tier method had an opportunity to make an irrevocable switch to the two-tier method in order to participate in the Supplemental SBP. (Such a shift may not be a wise change for all retirees — particularly for those who retired before or around 1957 or who may also be civil service retirees. In certain instances, the social security offset would be less than that which would occur under the two-tier plan. Such a limited reduction may negate the need for purchasing supplemental benefits.) Members who are retirement-eligible may elect to participate in the Supplemental SBP prior to actually retiring. Should the member die while retirement-eligible (but before actually retiring) that member's designated spouse or former spouse would be provided benefits under SBP without the Supplemental. Actual eligibility for Supplemental benefits begins only after retired pay is withheld. Should a retirement-eligible member elect to participate in the Supplemental before retiring and later refuse SBP participation at retirement, the Supplemental SBP would be voided. Those members who are participants without an eligible spouse and who remarry, may elect to participate in the Supplemental SBP. Such an election is irrevocable and must be made within one year of the remarriage.

An eligible participant may voluntarily elect to provide Supplemental coverage for a former spouse. The service secretary concerned must be provided with a statement (in a manner prescribed by the secretary) setting forth whether such an agreement is part of or incident to a divorce settlement and, if so, whether it has been voluntarily incorporated in the court order. This documentation must be provided to the secretary within one year of the date of the court order or filing invoice. With the receipt of the appropriate documentation, such an election is deemed to have been made.

Costs and Benefits of Supplemental Coverage

Under current two-tier SBP rules, 6.5% of pre-tax base amount retired pay is withheld (as described above under "Flat-Rate"). A surviving spouse or former spouse is eligible to receive 55% of the base amount of retired pay until reaching age 62 when benefits are reduced to 35%. Under the Supplemental SBP, the change that occurs at age 62 can be reduced or eliminated. The cost of this coverage depends on the age of the retiree at sign-up time, as well as the amount of coverage to be provided to the survivor at age 62.

Table 5 provides a breakdown of costs by level of coverage. According to this breakdown, a retiree who enrolls in the SBP under the two-tier option (benefits of 55% of the base amount of retired pay until age 62, then reduced to 35%) will have 6.5% of the base amount of retired pay withheld regardless of the retiree's age at the time of enrollment. Should this same retiree enroll at age 46 and opt to limit the age62-reduction to 45% of the base amount of retired pay, 9.48% of the base amount of retired pay will be withheld. Conversely, a retiree who enrolls at age 45 and opts to eliminate entirely the age-62-reduction will have 12.22% of the base amount of retired pay withheld.[51]

Elimination of the Two-Tier and Social Security Offset Computational Formulas

The FY2005 National Defense Authorization Act[52] contained language that made a substantial change in the computation of the SBP benefit for those age 62 and over. Simply stated, this law phased out the two-tier and Social Security offset formulas discussed above. The actual mechanics of this process depend on various scenarios.

Generally speaking, this language raised the minimum SBP benefit for those age 62 and over as follows: On October 1, 2005, the minimum SBP benefit for those survivors age 62 and older was increased to 40%. This amount will increase to 45% on April 1, 2006, 50% on April 1, 2007, and 55% on April 1, 2008. In other words, a survivor who is age 62 or over and receiving 35% of base retired pay under the two-tier method will see the benefit increase over the next few years to 55%. This increase occurs without any additional cost to the retiree or the survivor and therefore represents a substantial increase for many.

Table 5. SBP Supplemental Benefits and Costs by Age

Sign Up Age	Percentage Coverage at Age 62				
	35%	40%	45%	50%	55%
37	6.5	7.62	8.74	9.86	10.98
38	6.5	7.63	8.76	9.89	11.02
39	6.5	7.67	8.84	10.01	11.18
40	6.5	7.72	8.94	10.16	11.38
41	6.5	7.77	9.04	10.31	11.58
42	6.5	7.78	9.06	10.34	11.62
43	6.5	7.81	9.12	10.43	11.74
44	6.5	7.87	9.24	10.61	11.98
45	6.5	7.93	9.36	10.79	12.22
46	6.5	7.99	9.48	10.97	12.46
47	6.5	8.06	9.62	11.18	12.74
48	6.5	8.12	9.74	11.36	12.98
49	6.5	8.17	9.84	11.51	13.18
50	6.5	8.24	9.98	11.72	13.46
51	6.5	8.30	10.10	11.90	13.70
52	6.5	8.38	10.26	12.14	14.02
53	6.5	8.47	10.44	12.41	14.38
54	6.5	8.57	10.64	12.71	14.78
55	6.5	8.67	10.84	13.01	15.18
56	6.5	8.77	11.04	13.31	15.58
57	6.5	8.87	11.24	13.61	15.98
58	6.5	8.98	11.46	13.94	16.42
59	6.5	9.10	11.70	14.30	16.90
60	6.5	9.12	11.74	14.36	16.98
61	6.5	9.37	12.24	15.11	17.98
62	6.5	9.52	12.54	15.56	18.68
63	6.5	9.66	12.82	15.98	19.14
64	6.5	9.81	13.12	16.43	19.74
65	6.5	9.96	13.42	16.88	20.34
66	6.5	10.12	13.74	17.36	20.98
67	6.5	10.30	14.10	17.90	21.70
68	6.5	10.45	14.40	18.35	22.30
69	6.5	10.63	14.76	18.89	23.02
70	6.5	10.80	15.10	19.40	23.70
71	6.5	11.00	15.50	20.00	24.50
72	6.5	11.24	15.98	20.72	25.46
73	6.5	11.45	16.40	21.35	26.30
74	6.5	11.68	16.86	22.04	27.22
75	6.5	11.88	17.26	22.64	28.02
76	6.5	12.14	17.78	23.42	29.06
78	6.5	12.63	18.76	24.89	31.02
79	6.5	12.92	19.34	25.76	32.18
80	6.5	13.18	19.86	26.54	33.22

A survivor who turns 62 during the scheduled increase will have the benefit computed to the amount that is applicable in the above schedule. For example, consider a covered widow receiving 55% of base retired pay prior to reaching age 62. If this widow turns 62 on April 30, 2007, the benefit will be reduced to 50% of base retired pay. On April 1, 2008, according to the schedule, the SBP benefit will be returned to the 55% level.

For those individuals who purchased Supplemental SBP coverage prior to the enactment of this law, they will see their benefits increase as well after reaching age 62. For example, a 62 year old widow who is receiving 45% of base retired pay (i.e. 35% under the two-tier computation plus 10% in supplemental coverage), had the benefit increase to 50% on October 1, 2005 and finally to 55% on April 1, 2006. (Note: Effective October 28, 2004, reductions in retired pay used to cover the supplemental benefit were terminated; however, the supplemental coverage remained in effect.)

As noted, certain individuals had the opportunity to remain under the Social Security offset computational formula. These individuals will likewise see their benefits increase under the above schedule, ultimately reaching 55% on April 1, 2008. The increase in these benefits will occur when the scheduled increases pass their current benefit level. For example, a widow receiving say 48% of base retired pay (as computed under the Social Security offset method) will see no change in benefits until April 1, 2007 when the benefit will increase in 50%, and again to 55% on April 1, 2008. In other words, these beneficiaries will have their benefits computed either under the Social Security offset method or according to the above schedule, depending on which is more financially advantageous.

In enacting the above language, Congress also created an open-enrollment period or "open season" to allow certain retirees to begin SBP participation or to increase their current level of coverage. The open season began on October 1, 2005 and lasted one year. Those who took advantage of the open season must have participated for at least two years from the date of making such an election in order to qualify their survivors for these new benefits. If the retiree dies before the end of this two-year period, amounts deducted from retired pay to effectuate the benefits resulting from the open season will be returned to the designated survivor. Premiums charged "would be calculated based on the total amount of the premium, plus interest, by which the members' retired pay would have been reduced if they had elected to participate in the SBP at the first opportunity that they had been afforded."[53]

In addition, those opting for supplemental coverage during the open season will see the supplemental premiums phased out by April 1, 2008. Critics have raised doubts about the wisdom of participating in this open season supplemental coverage given the two-year participation minimum imposed under law. Critics note that a retiree who signs up for supplemental coverage on the first day of the open season (October 1, 2005) must contribute to the supplemental for two years. Should the retiree die two years after making the election (on October 1, 2007), the SBP benefit will already be increased to 50% under the above schedule for those survivors over age 62, and will reach the 55% level 6 months later. In other words, a retiree will make 2 or more years worth of supplemental payments in order to effectuate a 6- month or less benefit. Furthermore, a retiree who waited until April 1, 2006 of the open season (or later) to sign up for supplemental coverage, or one whose survivor will not turn 62 until after April 1, 2008, will see no benefit in electing the supplemental coverage during the open season. For these reasons, it has been suggested that retirees consider the limited benefits and additional costs of such an election before deciding to participate in the supplemental SBP during the open season and for the same reasons, DOD may elect not to offer supplemental coverage during this period.

SURVIVOR BENEFIT PLAN AND VETERANS' AFFAIRS DEPENDENCY AND INDEMNITY COMPENSATION

Department of Veterans Affairs (VA) Dependency and Indemnity Compensation (DIC) was established in 1956 by the Servicemen's and Veteran's Survivor Benefit Act.[54] "Under this Act, as amended, DIC is paid to the survivors ... of servicemen or veterans who died on or after January 1, 1957, from: (1) a disease or injury incurred or aggravated in line of duty while on active duty or active duty training; or (2) an injury incurred or aggravated in line of duty while on inactive duty training; or (3) a disability compensable under laws administered by the VA."[55]

A service member can, for example, (1) contract a disease or incur an injury during active duty or active duty training, (2) recover and return to active duty, (3) retire from an active duty or Reserve Component military career and participate in the SBP, and (4) subsequently die because of complications resulting from the original service-related disease or injury. The surviving spouse or former spouse of the retiree is then entitled to DIC payments from the VA. In this situation, however, the surviving spouse or former spouse of the retiree is **not entitled to receive the combined total of full SBP and DIC benefits**. Instead, the SBP benefit is offset by the amount of DIC received (with certain limitations).[56] This offset occurs regardless of the retiree's enrollment in the SBP Supplemental.

The total of DIC and offset SBP payments combined is, at least, equal to the full SBP benefit. A surviving spouse or former spouse who remarries loses his or her entitlement to Dependency and Indemnity Compensation payments. Upon losing Dependency and Indemnity Compensation, however, the remarried spouse or former spouse has his or her full SBP benefit restored, provided the remarriage — in accordance with SBP restrictions — occurs after age 60 or age 55 if the remarriage occurs after November 14, 1986. Also, if the DIC is paid to an SBP-eligible surviving spouse or former spouse, a percentage of the deceased retiree's original contributions to the SBP offset by DIC will be returned to the surviving spouse or former spouse. In other words, if the SBP is offset by DIC, that proportion of deductions from the deceased retiree's retired pay which financed the offset portion of the SBP will be refunded to the surviving spouse or former spouse. SBP payments can be restored, if the beneficiary becomes ineligible for DIC and remains eligible for SBP, provided that the refunded SBP payments are returned.

"Concurrent Receipt"

In recent years, Congress has addressed an issue concerning the payment of military retired pay to retirees who qualify for disability compensation from the Department of Veterans Affairs (VA). In 1891, Congress passed language prohibiting what it regarded as "dual compensation" for either past or current service and a disability pension.[57] As modified in 1941, the law prevented the concurrent receipt of both military nondisability retired pay and VA disability compensation. For those eligible for both, military retired pay was offset or reduced, dollar for dollar, by VA disability benefits.

Numerous attempts to address this issue over the past few years or so resulted initially in the creation of "Combat Related Special Compensation" for certain disabled military retirees whose disability was a direct result of military combat operations or training and whose disability is rated at 10% or more.

Later, in FY2004, Congress authorized concurrent receipt for all retirees with at least a 50% disability, regardless of the cause of the disability.[58] However, 100% disabled retirees were entitled to immediate concurrent receipt effective January 1, 2005.[59]

Although such changes do not affect the receipt of an SBP annuity, some have claimed that if concurrent receipt or "special pays" for military retirees is allowed, such should also be afforded their survivors. Under this reasoning, if a military retiree is allowed to receive both military retired pay and VA disability payments or other "special pay", it is only fair that the surviving spouse also receive both the SBP annuity and DIC benefits. Critics contend that concurrent receipt was originally barred because Congress viewed it as "double dipping" or paying someone twice for the same period of service. These critics reason that allowing concurrent receipt to the retiree or the retiree's survivor are forms of "double dipping" that are inherently unfair to the taxpayer.

In order to avoid this SBP-DIC offset, surviving spouses of active duty personnel are allowed to designate their children, if any, as the recipient of the SBP benefit. Unlike retirees, active duty personnel do not designate a beneficiary. (As stated earlier, children remain eligible to receive SBP until they reach age 18 or 22; or for life if mentally of physically incapacitated and if the incapacitating condition existed prior to age 18. Eligibility terminates if the child marries.)[60]

The Senate version of the National Defense Authorization Act for Fiscal Year 2006 contained a provision that would eliminate the SBP-DIC offset entirely. This language was dropped by the Conference Committee prior to final passage.[61] Again, the Senate version of the National Defense Authorization Act for Fiscal Year 2007 contained a provision that would eliminate the SBP-DIC offset entirely. This language was, too, dropped by the Conference Committee prior to final passage.[62]

Retiree and Government Contributions to SBP

As noted above, the cost of the SBP is shared by the government and the retirees. The amount paid by a particular retiree varies depending on level of coverage, years of payments, years the survivor receives an annuity, etc. For active duty personnel who make no contributions, the benefit is essentially free. Certain retirees and organizations representing their interests have claimed that, as originally structured, withholdings from retired pay for SBP were expected, on average, 40% of the cost of this benefit. Further it is claimed that since retirees are living longer and since the government has manipulated the withholdings formula, the retirees' share has increased to more than 73%.[63] These claims are made in an effort to increase government payments into the SBP in hopes of increasing benefits (particularly with regard to the apparently successful effort of eliminating the reduction in benefits that occurs when the surviving spouse reaches age 62).

In reviewing these claims, a number of points may be considered. First, as noted, there is no legal mandate for any ratio of retiree to government contributions. Second, such claims of a shift in the retiree/government share appear to be based on a selective use of retiree data. Third, the claim that retirees are living longer and paying more ignores the obvious point that survivors, too, are living longer and collecting more. Fourth, the above history of this benefit shows that Congress has expanded eligibility (including 'free' benefits to "forgotten widows" and active duty survivors), increased benefits, reduced costs, will eliminate withholdings under the "paid-up provision" afforded supplemental coverage, etc. At no time did Congress reduce the benefit. As such, the claims that the government's contribution to SBP have been reduced are unreliable. Nor do such claims rationalize the increase of benefits at age 62 for surviving spouses (a change that arguably creates a superior benefit relative to those available to the survivors of other federal employees).

It is noteworthy that after the SBP was introduced, the FY1 973 cost to retirees was $36,145,000 with a fiscal year payment to families of only $5,700,000. This is due to the relatively small number of participants who died shortly after signing up. Ten years later, as more retirees signed up and more died, the FY1 983 cost to retirees grew to $652,536,000 while the payment to families grew to $406,887,000. In FY1 993, as participant deaths increased, the cost to retirees was $822,955,000 with payments to families reaching $1,177,185,000. Finally, in FY2005, costs to retirees was reported to be $1,099,363,000 while payments to families surged to $2,253,728,000. From 1973 through 2005, the cumulative cost to retirees was $22,597,064,000 while cumulative payments to families was $30,923,249,000. Considering the cumulative payments by retirees and to military families, the government paid $8,326,185,000 more in benefits to families than it received. The cost to retiree/family payment gap will grow as the age 62 reduction is phased out and the "paid-up provision" is implemented.[64] From this perspective, if the cost/benefit share has shifted, the shift has been in the favor of recipients with taxpayers assuming an increasing cost of the program.

The National Defense Authorization Act for Fiscal Year 2006 directed Comptroller General to report on the actuarial soundness of the Survivor Benefit Plan. [65]

On July 26. 2006, the Government Accountability Office issued its report.[66] The foregoing is verbatim from that report:

Results in Brief

The significant statutory SBP program changes implemented within the past 7 fiscal years that we reviewed have resulted in increased DOD normal cost payments and annual Treasury amortization payments to the Fund in order to maintain the actuarial soundness of the Fund. When changes are made to SBP coverage or benefits, the DOD OOA [Office of the Actuary] calculates the necessary DOD and Treasury contributions to ensure that sufficient moneys are available to make all benefit payments to eligible recipients each year, and that sufficient Fund assets will be available in the future to liquidate all current unfunded liabilities.

According to the DOD OOA estimates, the significant SBP program changes[67] we reviewed have resulted in the following:

- Eliminating the reduction in surviving spouses' SBP benefits when such spouses are also eligible for Social Security benefits at age 62 and thereafter increased the SBP liability by an estimated $25.2 billion as of September 30, 2004. Of this amount, Treasury and DOD will be responsible for an estimated $23.7 billion and $1.5 billion, respectively. DOD's $1.5 billion liability includes $1.3 billion in normal costs for current active duty and full-time reservists (full-time employees) and $0.2 billion in normal costs for current part-time reservists (part-time employees). Periodically, Congress has allowed an open season for SBP enrollment, the most current one being during fiscal year 2006. Although the total effects of the SBP open season cannot be fully estimable for at least 2 years, the estimated increase in the SBP liability will likely range from $31 million to $86 million.
- Eliminating further SBP premiums to be paid by retirees who are aged 70 or older and who have paid such premiums for 30 years increased the SBP liability by an estimated $2.5 billion.[68] Of this amount, Treasury will be responsible for an estimated $2.4 billion, and DOD will be responsible for $0.1 billion in normal costs related to current full-time employees.
- Extending SBP surviving spouse or child benefits for all personnel who are killed in the line of duty and are not eligible for retirement at the time of their deaths increased the SBP liability by an estimated $72 million as of September 30, 2001. Of this amount, Treasury will be responsible for an estimated $28 million, and DOD will be responsible for $44 million in normal costs related to current full-time employees.

The two potential changes to SBP benefits mentioned in Section 666 of the National Defense Authorization Act for Fiscal Year 2006 would likely also result in increases to the DOD normal cost payments and the annual Treasury amortization payments to the Fund as follows.

- Currently, an unmarried DOD retiree without dependent children may elect to have another person with an insurable interest as the SBP beneficiary; however, if that beneficiary dies, designation of another insurable interest is not allowed. Using conservative assumptions, the DOD OOA calculated that the SBP liability would increase by an estimated $2.2 million if retirees were allowed the option of choosing a second insurable interest. Of this increase, Treasury would be responsible for $2 million and DOD for $231,000. Of DOD's $231,000, $211,000 would be for normal costs related to current full-time employees and $20,000 for normal costs related to current part-time employees.
- The survivors of veterans who die because of complications resulting from a service-connected disease or injury are entitled to DIC benefits from the Department of Veterans Affairs (VA).[69] Under current law, SBP benefits for survivors of retired veterans are offset by any DIC payments received. The DOD OOA calculated that eliminating the current offset requirement would increase the SBP liability by an estimated $12.9 billion. Of this amount, Treasury and DOD would be responsible for $12.3 billion and $645 million, respectively. Of DOD's $645 million, $617 million would be for normal costs related to current full-time employees and $28 million for normal costs related to current part-time employees.

Enactment of these legislative changes would require the Board of Actuaries and the DOD OOA to adjust DOD and Treasury payments, subject to future appropriations, by amounts necessary to offset any increased costs related to expanded benefits; for this reason, enactment of these changes should not negatively affect the actuarial soundness of the Fund.

Table 6A. Computation of Original Survivor Benefit Plan Cost to the Retiree for Spouse Only Coverage (Work Sheet)

1.	Enter base amount of retired pay. If base amount is $1,275 or more, use Table 6B below.	$_______
2.	Enter $595 or total retired pay if less than $595 (see fn 10). Do not enter less than $300.	$_______
3.	Multiply the figure in line two by 2.5%.	$_______
4.	Subtract $595 from line one. If line one is less than $595, enter 0.	$_______
5.	Multiply line four by 10%.	$_______
6.	Add line three and line five.	$_______

Note: Line 6 is the cost of survivor protection under Spouse Only coverage.

Table 6B. Computation of Flat-Rate Survivor Benefit Plan Cost to the Retiree for Spouse Only Coverage (Work Sheet)

1.	Enter base amount of retired pay	$_______
2.	Multiply line one by 6.5%.	x0.065
3.	Cost of Basic SBP protection.	$_______
	****To compute supplemental coverage cost, please continue****	
4.	Enter the factor that corresponds to the retiree's age and level of coverage desired at age 62 (see **Table 5**).	_______
5.	Divide the factor from line four by 100.	_______
6.	Multiply line one by line five.	$_______

Note: Line 6 is the cost of survivor supplemental protection under Spouse Only coverage.

Table 7. Computation of SBP Costs under Persons with an Insurable Interest Coverage (Work Sheet)

1.	The amount of base military retired pay.	$_____
2.	Multiply line one by 10%.	$_____
3.	Age of the retiree at his/her last birthday.	$_____
4.	Age of prospective beneficiary as of the date of the retiree's last birthday.	_____
5.	Subtract line three from line four. (If line three is less than line four, enter 0.)	_____
6.	Divide the sum in line five by 5 and round the quotient to the lower whole number.	_____
7.	Multiply 5% by line six.	_____%
8.	Multiply line one by line seven.	$_____
9.	Add line two and line eight.	$_____
10.	Multiply line one by 40%.	$_____
11.	Compare lines nine and ten: enter the lesser.	$_____

Note: Line 11 is the cost of survivor protection under the Persons with an Insurable Interest category of coverage.

In responding to a draft of this chapter, DOD did not have any objections or substantive comments. DOD separately provided some technical suggestions, which we incorporated as appropriate

End Notes

[1] Retirees of the uniformed services (Army, Navy, Marine Corps, Air Force and Coast Guard), as well as retirees of the Public Health Service (PHS) and the National Oceanic and Atmospheric Administration (NOAA) are eligible to participate in the Survivor Benefit Plan. This chapter emphasizes the provisions of the SBP as they relate to members or retirees of the Armed Forces.

[2] Base retired pay is that amount of retired pay that the retiree selects to be used in determining the SBP benefit and cost. This amount may not be greater than total monthly retired pay and may not be less than (1) $635 monthly as of January 1, 2006, or (2) total retired pay, if smaller than $635 monthly. This 55% maximum may include amounts received from other federal sources.

[3] U.S. Department of Defense, Office of the Secretary of Defense, Military Compensation Background Papers, *Compensation Elements and Related Manpower Cost Items: Their Purposes and Legislative Backgrounds*, 6th Ed., April 2005: 902.

[4] P.L. 92-425, 10 U.S.C. 1447 et seq.

[5] Originally known as the Uniformed Services Contingency Option Plan of 1953, P.L. 83- 239, 67 Stat. 501, 1953; name changed by P.L. 87-381, 75 Stat. 810, 1961.

[6] In certain instances, the annuity may be paid to the representative of a legally incompetent survivor (P.L. 102-190; 105 Stat. 1389; Dec. 5, 1991).

[7] The maximum coverage of 55% of base retired pay is subject to a reduction when certain survivors reach age 62. An explanation of these reductions is provided in the sections below entitled "The Integration of the Survivor Benefit Plan and Social Security Benefits" and "The Two-Tier Survivor Benefit Plan." Use of the "55% maximum coverage" in this chapter applies to those survivors discussed in the sections below who have not reached age 62.

[8] P.L. 99-145; Nov. 8, 1985; 99 Stat. 676, 677.

[9] Members with base amounts of $1,275 or more who retire on or after January 1, 2004, will have their contributions determined using the "Flat-Rate" method.

[10] If total retired pay is less than $635 per month — i.e., $7,620 per year — the base amount must be equal to total retired pay. As of September 30, 2003, only 6.5% of military retirees received less than $7,000 gross yearly (FY2003 DOD Statistical Report on the Military Retirement System, Office of the Actuary, Defense Manpower Data Center: 177-178). Sec. 714 of P.L. 99-145, the FY1 986 DOD Authorization Act, provided that the then-$300 base shall be increased by the same percentage amount and at the same time as across-the-board increases in military basic pay after October 1, 1985. The basic pay index will apply only to retirees whose retired pay is computed on the basis of basic pay rates in effect on or after the date of the basic pay increase. As of January 1, 2006, the base amount had been indexed to $635. Amounts are rounded to the lower dollar.

[11] The Omnibus Budget Reconciliation Act (OBRA) of 1993 delayed nondisability retirees' COLA until April 1, 1994. The OBRA did not delay the increase in SBP costs to each nondisability retiree enrolled in the SBP. Therefore, SBP premiums were increased for the three months of retired pay payable on January 1, February 1, and March 1, 1994. Because DOD could not reprogram its retired pay computers to accommodate the new law by January 1, 1994, the three months' of increased SBP premiums were taken out of the retired pay received on April 1, 1994.

[12] This legislation also provided for the recomputation of survivor annuities in the case of a member who dies on active duty while qualified to apply for retired pay, or who serves at least 20 years, but is not eligible to receive retired pay as a commissioned officer because he/she has not served at least 10 years as a commissioned officer. Under this language, effective March 1, 1990, the survivor annuity would be computed based on the grade in which the member was serving at the time of death, unless he/she would have been entitled to be retired in a higher grade.

[13] For those individuals retiring on or after January 1, 2004 with base amounts of $1,275 or greater, their premiums are computed using the more generous 6.5% method, regardless of when they entered the service.

[14] P.L. 105-261, 112 Stat. 2045 Oct. 17, 1998. P.L. 106-65; 113 Stat. 667; Oct. 5, 1999; This law extended this provision to participants in the RSFPP. Furthermore, P.L. 105-261; 112 Stat. 2045, Oct. 17, 1998, created an open enrollment that allowed persons not currently participating in the SBP to enroll subject to certain restrictions. P.L. 106-65 extended the paid-up provision to these "late" enrollees, provided they paid the total premiums that would have been withheld from their retired pay, had they been participating since they first

became eligible. In addition, from April 1, 1992 through March 31, 1993, retirees who initially rejected coverage were afforded a one-year opportunity to enroll. This late enrollment required greater withholdings on retired pay. (See P.L. 102-190; 105 Stat. 1388; Dec. 5, 1991) Lastly, P.L. 105-85; 111 Stat. 1797; Nov. 18, 1997, created a one-year opportunity for participants to discontinue SBP coverage, subject to certain restrictions.

[15] U.S. Congress. Conference Committee, National Defense Authorization Act for Fiscal Year 2006, H.Rept. 109-360, 109th Cong., 1st Sess., H.R. 1815, December 18, 2005: 738.

[16] U.S. Congress. Conference Committee, National Defense Authorization Act for Fiscal Year 2007, H.Rept. 109-720, 109th Cong., 2nd Sess., H.R. 5122, September 29, 2006: 755-6.

[17] The term "child" includes an adopted child, a stepchild, foster child, or recognized natural child who lived with the participant in a regular parent-child relationship. It may be necessary for the child to prove dependency in order to be eligible to receive an SBP annuity.

[18] Costs that are actuarially determined are based on probabilities of known life expectancy rates, as well as interest and inflation assumptions.

[19] Since the cost of coverage is computed on an actuarial basis, the cost used in this example is subject to change. Actuarial figures provided by L. Giesecke, Office of the Actuary, Defense Manpower Data Center, Mar. 31, 1992.

[20] A child who becomes ineligible because he or she reaches age 18 and then later becomes a full-time student prior to reaching age 22 may become eligible to receive SBP benefits while a full-time student.

[21] A married child who, prior to being married, was eligible to receive SBP benefits will not become eligible to receive these benefits anew if the marriage ends by divorce. If, however, the marriage is terminated as the result of an annulment, SBP eligibility may be reinstated.

[22] 10 U.S.C. 1448(b)(1).

[23] U.S. Congress, House Conference Committee, National Defense Authorization Act for Fiscal Year 1995, H.Rept. 103-701, 103rd Cong.2nd Sess., S. 2182, Aug.12, 1994: 132-133. (P.L. 103-336) It is expected that this change will affect approximately 3,000 of the more that SBP 900,000 participants. Rick Maze,"Survivor Benefit Plan ...," *Air Force Times*, Sept. 12, 1994: 20.

[24] For more information on issues affecting former spouses, see CRS Report RL31663, *Military Benefits for Former Spouse: Legislation and Policy Issues*, by David F. Burrelli.

[25] 10 U.S.C. 1550(f)(4).

[26] U.S. Congress, House Conference Committee, *Department of Defense Authorization Act*, 1986. S.Rept. 99-235, S. 1160. 99th Cong., 1st Sess., July 29, 1985: 443. (Hereafter cited as Conference Committee, DOD 1986 Authorization.)

[27] P.L. 106-65; 113 Stat. 668; Nov. 5, 1999.

[28] Conference Committee, DOD 1986 Authorization: 96.

[29] "Reserve Components" refers to both Reserve and National Guard personnel.

[30] P.L. 95-397, 92 Stat. 843, Sept. 30, 1978.

[31] P.L. 105-85; 111 Stat. 1800; Nov. 18, 1997 as amended by P.L. 106-65; 113 Stat. 668; Nov. 5, 1999 as amended by P.L. 107-314; sec. 634; Dec. 2, 2002.

[32] Former enlisted personnel or warrant officers who are commissioned must complete at least 10 years of active duty as commissioned officers before they are allowed to retire as commissioned officers. Section 523, P.L. 101-5 10, Nov. 5, 1990, reduced the ten-year minimum to eight years, through Oct. 1, 1995, to assist in the drawdown of the Armed Forces.

[33] P.L. 107-107, 115 Stat. 1151 et seq.; Dec. 28, 2001.

[34] Under these provisions, the member's disability may not be the result of intentional neglect of misconduct.

[35] P.L. 108-375, sec. 641, Oct. 28, 2004 modified the computation of retired pay for reservist who die on active duty "by calculating the average monthly basic pay for purposes of ... annuity payments as if they had been entitled to basic pay for the 36 months preceding their retirement [or active duty death] regardless of whether the member served the entire period on active duty." Congressional Record, Oct. 8, 2004: H9544.

[36] P.L. 108-136, Nov. 24, 2003.

[37] U.S. Congress. Conference Committee, National Defense Authorization Act for Fiscal Year 2007, H.Rept. 109-720, 109th Cong., 2nd Sess., H.R. 5122, September 29, 2006: 748.

[38] P.L. 99-145; 99 Stat. 666 et seq.; Nov. 8, 1985.

[39] The surviving spouse might also be entitled to additional social security benefits based on any civilian employment of the deceased retiree. For ease of explanation, however, this chapter only discusses the entitlement to survivor benefits based on the retiree's military service.

[40] All amounts are hypothetical and used only for purposes of example.

[41] In the legislative history of P.L. 92-425, (S.Rept. 92-1089), it was noted that "Adding a survivor benefit plan, similar to the one available to civil service retirees, on top of the survivor benefits available from social security would provide a plan superior to plans available to other government employees . . . [T]he proposed benefit program is designed to build upon the income-maintenance foundation of the social security system."

[42] A surviving spouse or former spouse who is the parent of a child of the deceased may also receive social security mother's or father's benefits at any age, as long as the child is under age 16. The SBP offset also applies to these mother's or father's benefits if there is only one such child, but does not apply if there are two or more children under age 16.

[43] Office of the Comptroller General of the United States. Vol. 62, B-203393, Matter of: Dora M. Lambert, June 15, 1983: 472-473.

[44] P.L. 96-402, Oct. 9, 1980. See U.S. Congress, Senate, *Uniformed Services Survivor Benefits Amendment of 1980*, S.Rept. 96-748, 96th Cong., 2nd Sess., Sept. 29, 1980.

[45] See Conference Committee, DOD 1986 Authorization: 88-100.

[46] U.S. Congress, House Committee on Armed Service, Department of Defense Authorization Act, 1986. H.Rept. 99-81, H.R. 1872, 99th Cong., 1st Sess., May 10, 1985: 251.

[47] Under the social security offset the benefit of a spouse or former spouse in this example could be reduced from $650 per month to $690 per month at age 62 (i.e., a 40% offset).

[48] "Retirement qualified" includes those members of the Reserve Components who are qualified to receive military retired pay except for the fact that they are under age 60 and, therefore, may not begin to draw reserve retired pay.

[49] Department of Defense, Office of the Actuary, RCS No. DDM (A) 1375, *DOD Statistical Report on the Military Retirement System, FY1984*: 215 and RCS No. DD-FM&P (Q) 1375, FY1990: 233; *DOD Statistical Report, FY1993*: 247.

[50] 103 Stat. 1577, et seq., Nov. 29, 1989; as amended by P.L. 101-510, 104 Stat. 1580, Nov. 5, 1990.

[51] Rick Maze, "Face-lift yields five SBP options," *Army Times*, Oct. 28, 1991: 10.

[52] P.L. 108-375; 118 Stat. 1811; Secs. 644-645; Oct. 28, 2004.

[53] Congressional Record, Oct. 8, 2004: H9544.

[54] P.L. 84-88 1, 70 Stat. 862, 867.

[55] Military Compensation Background Papers: 457.

[56] The amount of DIC payable to a surviving spouse is contained in one section of law — title 38 U.S.C. 411(a). Under three other sections — 38 U.S.C. if, for example, the spouse 1) is supporting a dependent child or children, 2) is in a nursing home, blind or requiring aid or assistance from another person, or, 3) is, because of a disability, housebound or institutionalized in a ward or clinic. SBP annuities are only offset by the amount of DIC received under 38 U.S.C. 411(a) and not by any increase to this amount as a result of eligibility under 38 U.S.C. 41 1(b)-(d).

[57] See CRS Report 95-469, *Military Retirement and Veterans' Compensation: Concurrent Receipt Issues*, by Robert L. Goldich and Carolyn L. Merck.

[58] See CRS Issue Brief IB85 159, *Military Retirement: Major Legislative Issues*, by Charles A. Henning.

[59] See CRS Issue Brief IB85 159, *Military Retirement: Major Legislative Issues*, by Charles A. Henning.

[60] P.L. 108-136; sec. 645; November 24, 2003.

[61] U.S. Congress. Conference Committee, National Defense Authorization Act for Fiscal Year 2006, H.Rept. 109-360, 109th Cong., 1st Sess., H.R. 1815, December 18, 2005: 738.

[62] U.S. Congress. Conference Committee, National Defense Authorization Act for Fiscal Year 2007, H.Rept. 109-720, 109th Cong., 2nd Sess., H.R. 5122, September 29, 2006: 755.

[63] Mike Lazorchak, " SBP still a good program, but ratio has changed," *Navy Times*, Jan. 15, 2001: 18.

[64] 2006 Retired Military Almanac, (Falls Church, Virginia: Uniformed Services Almanac, Inc., 2004) p. 218.

[65] P.L. 109-163, 119 Stat. 3136, January 6, 2006, sec. 666.

[66] U.S . GAO, Actuarial Soundness of the DOD Survivor Benefit Plan, GAO-06-837R, July 26, 2006.

[67] The DOD OOA estimates the cost of each significant SBP program change as of a specific valuation date. Subsequent to that date, the costs of each SBP program change become part of the baseline actuarial model and are not separately identified. According to the DOD OOA, there have been no significant cost reestimates after the valuation date for the three program changes we reviewed.

[68] The liability estimate for this legislative change was determined as of September 30, 2001, and will be effective on October 1, 2008.

[69] VA's DIC was established in 1956 by the Servicemen's and Veterans' Survivor Benefits Act, P.L. 84-88 1, 70 Stat. 857, 862 (Aug. 1, 1956) (*codified, as amended, at* 38 U.S.C. ch. 13).

In: Veterans' Benefits and Care
Editor: Mathew H. Bradley

ISBN: 978-1-60692-500-3

Chapter 5

VETERANS AFFAIRS: BENEFITS FOR SERVICE-CONNECTED DISABILITIES

Douglas Reid Weimer

SUMMARY

Congress provides various benefits to American veterans and their dependents through the United States Department of Veterans Affairs (VA). One of these benefits is *disability compensation*, which is a monthly cash benefit program for veterans currently impaired from past service-connected activities.

A claim for disability compensation is initially analyzed by the VA at the local level to determine: 1) whether the claimant is considered a "veteran" (eligible for benefits); 2) whether the veteran qualifies for disability compensation (entitled to benefits); 3) the extent of the impairment and the "rate" of the disability; and 4) the effective date for the compensation.

Three requirements to qualify for disability compensation are: 1) medical diagnosis of the current impairment; 2) evidence of an in-service occurrence or an aggravation of the disease or injury; and 3) medical proof of a connection between the in-service incident or aggravation of an injury or illness and the current disability. The requisite standard of proof and certain medical presumptions are set by statute. The VA is required to provide assistance to the veteran in his/her case preparation by providing records and medical examinations. Special rules have been established for certain specific situations involving combat veterans, prisoners of war, and veterans exposed to Agent Orange.

If the veteran is found eligible for disability compensation, the VA then uses the Schedule for Rating Disabilities (SRD) to set the amount of earnings impairment on a percentage basis; the higher the percentage, the greater the compensation will be. Certain complications arise with the use of the rating system. A veteran's rating may be increased or decreased over time — depending on his/her medical condition. Rating decisions may be appealed administratively.

Legislation passed in the First Session of the 110th Congress increased the 2008 monthly disability compensation payments. Other legislation has been introduced that would provide veterans a cost-of-living (COLA) for their VA benefits equal to the COLA for Social Security benefits. The 110th Congress has considered additional legislation that may affect service-connected disabilities. One bill would change the manner in which disabled veterans could qualify to receive Social Security Disability Insurance (SSDI) benefits. Several bills have been introduced to deal with the claims processing backlog at the VA and issues related to the receipt of disability benefits.

INTRODUCTION

Veterans' Disability Programs

Congress, through the United States Department of Veterans Affairs (VA), provides a wide variety of services and benefits to veterans and to certain members of their families.[1]

Two disability programs are administered by the VA. These programs pay monthly cash benefits to certain disabled veterans.[2] *Disability compensation*, the focus of this chapter, provides a monthly cash benefit if the veteran is at least 10% disabled[3] as a consequence of his/her military service — which is considered to be a *service-connected disability*. A veteran applying for service-connected disability compensation does not need to be totally disabled, have low income, or wartime military service. In contrast, a *disability pension* may be paid to a *wartime*[4] veteran with limited income, who is no longer able to work, or is at least age 65. A disability pension is not related to a service-connected injury or medical condition and takes into account the material needs of the veteran; it is a "needs-based" pension.[5]

The "Local Determination"

The VA analyzes each veteran's claim for disability compensation at the VA regional office closest to the veteran's residence, called the "local determination." This determination involves a four-step adjudication process of the veteran's claim.

First, the VA determines the claimant's basic eligibility to receive VA benefits. A determination is made as to whether the claimant was discharged or separated under other than dishonorable conditions,[6] whether the claimant had "active service,"[7] and whether the claimant's condition is based upon the veteran's willful misconduct.[8]

Second, if the claimant is found eligible for benefits,[9] the VA then determines whether the veteran qualifies for in-service disability compensation.

Third, if the VA determines that the veteran is entitled to disability compensation, the VA then evaluates the extent of the disability and makes a determination of the percentage of the disability based upon the "Schedule for Rating Disabilities,"[10] which is sometimes referred to as the "SRD" and/or the "VASRD." Findings adverse to the interests of the veteran may be appealed administratively.

Fourth, the VA establishes the effective date for the award.

Requirements for Disability Compensation[11]

The purpose of disability compensation is to assist currently disabled veterans whose injury is connected to military service, and to that end, a veteran[12] must meet three basic criteria to the VA's satisfaction.

- *One:* A recent medical diagnosis of a *current* impairment, disability, or disease.
- *Two:* Medical or, on occasion, lay evidence of an *in-service* occurrence or aggravation of the disease or injury.
- *Three:* Medical proof of a *connection* between the in-service occurrence or aggravation of an injury or illness and the current disability.

Each of these requirements is examined below.

Medical Evidence of the Current Impairment or Disability

Disability compensation is available only to veterans with current disabilities.[13] Although a veteran may have had an illness or injury during his/her service time, the mere fact that this occurred is not compensable.

To provide evidence of the current medical problem, the veteran may submit medical records of the current diagnosis and/or treatment. Letters from physicians may be added to the record. Generally speaking, lay evidence of a medical condition is not sufficient. The VA has certain duties to assist veterans in the application process.[14] The VA must assist by providing the veteran with the appropriate records.[15] Usually, the VA is required to provide veterans with a medical exam in order to diagnose a current medical condition.[16] However, certain circumstances may exist under which the VA may not be required to provide such an examination or assistance to the veteran.[17] In addition, the VA must advise veterans of incomplete applications[18] and evidence which is needed to evaluate the veteran's claim.[19]

Evidence of an In-Service Occurrence or Aggravation of the Disease or Injury

The veteran's second requirement for disability compensation is that there is medical or, under certain circumstances, lay evidence of an in-service occurrence or aggravation of a disease or injury. The in-service requirement is construed broadly. A disability incident or onset of disability is not required to be related to the veteran's military responsibilities and is covered even if it occurred during leave.[20] Further, the evidence submitted on the record must only demonstrate that it is as likely as not that there was an in-service aggravation or occurrence of a disease or injury. When there is nearly equal positive and negative evidence regarding a material issue, the Secretary is required to give the benefit of the doubt to the veteran.[21]

The veteran must submit corroborating evidence of the incident.[22] He/she must prepare and submit a statement describing the occurrence, disease, or injury in detail, along with the circumstances surrounding the event. The type of evidence that the veteran must submit may depend upon the type of injury or disease which is being connected to the time of service. For example, a veteran who sustained a fall while in-service might produce evidence of medical treatment for the fall at the time of its occurrence and evidence from military personnel who witnessed the fall.

Medical Proof of a Connection between the In-Service Incident or Aggravation of an Injury/Illness and the Current Disability

This third element requires that there must be a *link* between the current injury or illness (requirement 1) and that the disease, injury, or event happened during a period of military service (requirement 2). This requirement is sometimes known as service-connected, the "service connection," or the nexus requirement.

Statutes and regulations require proof of one of five types of connections. *One:* there is a direct connection between the current disability and an incident that happened during the period of military service.[23] *Two:* the current medical condition existed prior to service but was exacerbated during service.[24] *Three:* the current medical problem did not appear during military service, but is presumed to have begun or be connected with something that occurred during service, either by statute or by VA regulation.[25] *Four:* the present problem is the result of a primary medical condition, and that condition is connected to a period of military service.[26] *Five:* the condition is the result of an injury caused by VA health service, VA training/rehabilitation services, or by participation in a VA sponsored work therapy program.[27]

In order to establish this connection, it is necessary to have adequate medical evidence in the claim.[28] What this signifies is that for the in-service connection to be approved, the veteran is required to have medical proof that the disease, injury, or event which occurred during service *actually caused* the veteran's current disability.

The VA's Obligations in the Preparation/Presentation of the Veteran's Case and Certain Presumptions

The VA is required by law to use certain standards in the review of a veteran's claims, and the VA has certain statutory obligations in the preparation of the veteran's case. In addition, statute and regulations provide for certain presumptions of disability as a result of certain occurrences. These standards, requirements, and presumptions are summarized below.

Standard of Proof

As explained, to receive disability benefits evidence is required to prove a connection between an in-service incident and a current disability, but in assessing evidence on these elements the veteran is to be given the "benefit of the doubt."[29] The statute provides that "When there is an approximate balance of positive and negative evidence regarding any issue material to the determination of a matter, the Secretary shall give the benefit of the doubt to the claimant."[30] Regulations provide that when reasonable doubt arises, such doubt will be resolved in favor of the claimant.[31] Hence, in order to satisfy this element, the submitted medical evidence generally needs to show that it is as likely as not that there is a connection between the in-service injury, occurrence, or illness and the current disability.

Assistance in Case Preparation

The VA has a responsibility to assist the veteran in developing a claim. Among other things, the VA is required to advise the veteran of the type of evidence that will need to be submitted to substantiate the claim.32

The VA also must make service and medical records available to veterans for the preparation of their cases.[33] Such records are often crucial in proving the veteran's claim. In many instances, the VA is required to provide veterans with a *medical examination* in order to diagnose the current medical condition.[34] However, under certain circumstances the VA may not be required to provide assistance to the veteran.[35]

Certain Presumptions

In its analysis of certain claims, the VA is required by statute and/or regulation to make certain presumptions.

Presumption of Medical Soundness

In evaluating a veteran's claim, the VA generally presumes that the veteran entered the service in sound medical condition.[36] This may assist the veteran in proving a claim by making it difficult for the VA to claim that the condition or disease existed prior to service. However, if the medical impairment was noted at the time of entry into service, the veteran may have to prove that the condition was exacerbated in-service. If the VA is able to prove by "clear and unmistakable evidence" that the disease or injury was in existence prior to service, and that it was not worsened during service, the veteran's claim will be denied.

Special Rules for Certain In-Service Occurrences

Special rules exist under which the VA is required to consider a service-connected problem by presumption. For example, certain diseases associated with exposure to Agent Orange will be presumed to be service-related in the case of Vietnam veterans. [37]

A similar regulation holds that veterans who were held prisoners of war, or who served in combat, can be presumed to have suffered traumatic, stressful events during their military service.[38] Similarly, combat veterans have special rules applicable to them in proving an in-service injury, or other incident.[39] Usually, if a combat veteran states that he/she suffered a disease, injury, or other event during combat, the VA will usually accept that statement as fact. This is the case even if there are no service records to substantiate the claim.

THE VA RATING SYSTEM

Congress has established by statute a rating system to categorize a veteran's degree of disability for in-service injuries.[40] This system is implemented by the VA through a series of complex regulations and procedures.

After the VA determines that a disability is service-connected, the VA regional office goes through a review process (the "rating activity") to determine the disability rating (on a percentage basis). As used by the VA, the term "disability" is defined as "the average impairment in earning capacity" that results from diseases, injuries, or their resultant aftermath.[41]

Schedule for Rating Disabilities (SRD)

By authority of Congress the VA set up the Schedule for Rating Disabilities ("SRD"), which rates various disabilities on a percentage basis.[42] The statute provides for ten grades of disability,[43] and the higher the disability determination, the higher is the monthly compensation that the veteran receives. The VA determines the disability level for an eligible veteran, and Congress sets the compensation rates for veterans based on ratings.[44]

Again, in making individual determinations, the VA and the Board of Veterans' Appeals (BVA) apply the various ratings of the SRD.[45] The SRD is detailed: various sections deal with injuries or diseases that impact particular body functions/parts, including the musculoskeletal system,[46] eyes,[47] and other functions such as hearing, infectious diseases, respiratory system, cardiovascular system, digestive system, genitourinary system, gynecological conditions, and other functions. Each of these sections of the SRD (dealing with a particular body part or function) has a series of medical diagnoses with a numerical diagnostic code (dc) that breaks down percentages of disability[48] based upon the severity of the disability. Each degree of disability under each dc has a description of the symptoms that the claimant veteran must have in order to qualify for that rating. The disability degree increases with the increase in the severity of the symptoms.

Application of the Rating System[49]

Applying this rating system, the VA examines the veteran's medical records to determine the medical diagnosis for the veteran's service-connected disability. The VA then finds the applicable diagnostic code for the disability and finds the degree of disability that is appropriate to the symptoms and diagnosis of the veteran's condition. If a rating falls between two ratings, and the symptoms are closer to the higher rating, then the higher rating will be selected.[50] In makings its determination, the VA examines all of the available evidence, including service records, lay statements, and medical records and other evidence.[51]

Complications in the Use of the Rating System

When the VA applies the diagnostic code(s) to veterans' claims, a number of variables come into play, some of which may be quite complex. And while every rating has unique circumstances, VA ratings in similar cases may not always seem consistent. Having to make fine distinctions within an intricate rating system based on a reading of a veteran's symptoms inevitably leads to some claims that a rating is "wrong" or "underrated."

Another complication in the rating process is that a medical condition may be able to be rated under more than one diagnostic code, sometimes to the detriment of the veteran. In addition, not all disabilities and their symptoms and complications are listed on the rating chart, in which case an analogous condition may be used for the rating. [52]

A further complication in the rating system occurs when a veteran has two or more service-connected disabilities. In such a circumstance, the overall percentage of disability is determined by combining the individual ratings, but *not by adding them up together.* To calculate the appropriate combined rating, the VA makes a determination by considering each impairment in the order of its severity. Direction on how to make these determinations is contained in the "Combined Rating Table" in the VA regulations.[53]

Changes in Veterans' Ratings

Should the severity of the service-connected disability increase over time, the veteran may apply for an increase in the rated percentage of disability.[54] Similarly, should the condition improve, the ratings percentage may be decreased, and the monthly payments would decrease.

Special Monthly Compensation (SMC)

If a veteran has severe disabilities,[55] he/she may be entitled to special monthly compensation (SMC) which provides compensation payments at a rate higher than the 100% rate.[56] In addition to the SMC, certain veterans with severe disabilities that require daily assistance or regular health services may be eligible for extra compensation.[57]

Zero Percent Evaluation

If the degree of disability from a service- connected incident does not impair earning capacity, a veteran may receive a 0% rating.[58] However, even a noncompensable evaluation under certain circumstances may entitle the veteran to preferences in federal or state employment and VA health care. A noncompensable evaluation may also be used to document a medical condition if it subsequently worsens.

Periodic Examinations

Following the award of compensation benefits, the VA may require periodic examinations to determine whether the condition is constant in its severity and that continued payment of disability compensation is warranted.[59] The VA is authorized to reexamine veterans receiving compensation benefits at any time. However, under certain circumstances — if the condition is static — the VA may not schedule review examinations.

Appeals from Ratings

Some veterans may not be satisfied with their disability rating, and may wish to appeal. Such an appeal is first undertaken at the local VA level and may eventually proceed to the Court of Veterans Claims ("Court").[60] The Court examines whether the VA considered all of the appropriate facts and set forth a satisfactory explanation for its choice and application of the diagnostic code.

Evaluation of the Rating System

A 2005 Government Accountability Office (GAO) study, *Veterans' Disability Benefits — Claims Processing Challenges and Opportunities for Improvements*[61] evaluated certain aspects of the disability compensation process. GAO noted that the VA provided $30 billion in cash disability benefits to more than 3.4 million veterans and their survivors in FY2004.[62] GAO found that the VA has continuing challenges in the disability compensation process, including large numbers of pending claims and long processing times.[63]

Another issue that GAO highlighted is the lack of consistency and accuracy of rating decisions at and among the VA's 57 regional offices.[64] Consequently, veterans with similar disabilities may receive different evaluations, and hence may receive significantly different compensation from the different VA regional offices. GAO also noted that the VA's evaluative process has not kept pace with recent developments in medical technology.[65]

GAO uncovered another issue — that more recent veterans with severe injuries would appear to favor a lump sum compensation payment, as opposed to monthly compensation payments over an extended period of time.[66]

CURRENT LEGISLATION[67]

Veterans' COLA (Cost-of-Living Adjustment)

Congress typically has passed legislation annually to provide a COLA in veterans disability compensation equal to the COLA automatically provided under permanent law to recipients of Social Security disability. However, this COLA is not automatic, and must be enacted annually. The Veterans' Compensation Cost-ofLiving Adjustment Act of 2007[68] increased, effective December 1, 2007, the rates (dollar amounts) of veteran's disability compensation (as well as for additional compensation for dependents, the clothing allowance for certain disabled veterans, and the dependency and indemnity compensation for surviving spouses and children).[69]

S. 161 (sponsored by Senator John Thune),[70] **H.R. 402** (sponsored by Representative Joe Knollenberg),[71] and **S. 1315** (sponsored by Senator Daniel K. Akaka)[72] would create an automatic veterans' COLA based on the Social Security adjustment.

Social Security Disability Insurance (SSDI) Benefits

H.R. 2943 (introduced by Representative John P. Sarbannes)[73] would change the manner in which disabled veterans could qualify to receive SSDI benefits. If enacted, the bill would permit veterans with service-connected disabilities that are rated and certified by the VA as total, to be eligible for SSDI benefits without having to be evaluated by the Social Security

Administration (SSA) if they meet the other requirements for SSDI benefits. At the present time, SSA evaluates all applicants (veterans and non-veterans) to determine their eligibility for SSDI benefits.[74]

Veterans' Claims Backlog and Related Issues

Presently, there is a large number of pending veterans' claims before the VA. According to the VA, which tracks these figures, for the week ended May 3, 2008, there were 396,898 rating cases pending.[75] This compares to a backlog of 405,248 rating cases from the same time period in 2007.[76] Concern over this backlog has been expressed by legislators and veterans' groups.

In response to this backlog, several bills have been introduced in the 110th Congress that would impact disability determinations by the VA. The proposed Wounded Warrior Assistance Act of 2007 is pending in the House, **H.R. 1538** (introduced by Representative Ike Skelton),[77] and in the Senate, **S. 1283** (introduced by Senator Mark Pryor).[78] Both bills address disability evaluations, a study by the DOD and VA concerning their evaluation systems, and the possibility of combining the two systems.

H.R. 653 (sponsored by Representative Thomas M. Reynolds)[79] would have the Secretary of Veterans Affairs accept that an injury or disease is service-connected (if there is no clear and convincing proof to the contrary), based upon the sworn affidavit of a veteran who served in combat on or before July 27, 1953 (prior to or during the Korean War).

H.R. 797 (sponsored by Representative Tammy Baldwin), which was enacted into law,[80] expands disability compensation for veterans who are visually impaired in both eyes by using a standard definition of blindness used by other federal agencies.

H.R. 1435 (sponsored by Representative Joe Baca)[81] would direct the VA to conduct a pilot program with County Veterans Services Officers (CVSOs) in certain states. Certain claims requiring further development would be referred to the CVSOs. The CVSOs would be required to act as claimant advocates in developing such claims and have access to client information contained in the VA's Benefits Delivery Network.

H.R. 1444 (sponsored by Representative John Hall),[82] although not specifically addressing the backlog, would provide some benefits for those veterans awaiting their rating/appeal. The bill would require the Secretary of the VA to pay an interim benefit of $500 per month when a claim for veterans' benefits is remanded (referred back) by either the U.S. Court of Appeals for Veterans Claims or the Board of Veterans' Appeals, and the Secretary does not make a decision on the matter within 180 days of the date of the remand.

H.R. 1490 (sponsored by Representative Joe Donnelly)[83] would create a presumption of service-connectedness in claims for service-connected benefits unless the Secretary of the VA determines that there is positive evidence to the contrary. The bill would require the claimant to support the claim with proof of service in a conflict referred to in the claim, as well as a brief description of the nature, including the service connection, of the disability or claim. The Secretary would be required to redeploy, for the purpose of assisting veterans applying for benefits, those employees who are no longer needed to evaluate claims due to this presumption.

H.R. 1538 (sponsored by Representative Ike Skelton)[84] deals primarily with improving the management of medical care, personnel actions, and quality of life issues for members of the Armed Forces. The bill addresses disability evaluations, a study by DOD and the VA concerning their individual evaluation systems, and the possibility of combining the two systems. The bill would also streamline record keeping and the transfer of records from DOD to the VA. Some of the bill's provisions are similar to those of S. 1283, discussed below.

H.R. 2257 (sponsored by Representative Peter Welch)[85] would require the Secretary of the VA to increase the number of benefits claims representatives. The bill would require that no fewer than two claims representatives be located at each "vet center"[86] to provide readjustment counseling and related mental health services.

H.R. 2855 (sponsored by Representative Ciro Rodriguez)[87] would establish a Wounded Heroes Independent Review Board ("Board") to review certain cases involving a member of the Armed Forces or a veteran who was severely injured on or after September 11, 2001, while on active duty. Upon the request of a "Wounded Hero," the Board would expeditiously review the decision or determination of the VA or other federal department or agency relating to the eligibility for or scope of benefits, including health care or vocational rehabilitation benefits. Following a review, the Board would render a written advisory opinion relating to such eligibility or provision of such care or benefits. The advisory opinion would be "considered as evidence" by the BVA and the CAVC in any case with respect to the "Wounded Hero." An advisory opinion rendered by the Board would not be reviewed by any other official or by any court, whether by an action in the nature of mandamus or otherwise.

H.R. 3047 (sponsored by Representative Doug Lamborn)[88] would direct the Secretary of the VA to establish a work credit system for evaluating regional offices of the Veterans Benefits Administration (VBA) regarding veterans' claims processing. The Secretary would be required to develop and maintain an electronic claims processing system for processing veterans' disability compensation claims that utilizes medical and military service date to generate disability rating recommendations. The Secretary would also be required to maintain a regional office at which all such claims are exclusively processed electronically. The bill would direct the Secretary to contract with a private entity to evaluate the training and assessment programs for VBA employees.

H.R. 4084 (sponsored by Representative John Hall)[89] would direct the Secretary of the VA to contract with the Institute of Medicine, or other appropriate entity, to conduct a study analyzing the extent to which the Department of Veterans Affairs schedule for rating disability accounts for or should be amended to account, measure, and compensate for loss of quality of life to veterans due to a disability resulting from a personal injury suffered, or disease contracted, in the line of duty. The bill would also provide that if a veteran who is a claimant dies before completing the submission of a claim for benefits, the person who would receive any accrued benefits due to such veteran would be treated as the claimant for purposes of completing submission of the claim.

H.R. 5089 (sponsored by Representative John Barrow)[90] would propose to reform the veterans' disability determination process by requiring the Secretary of Veterans Affairs to pay disability compensation to certain veterans based on the concurring diagnosis of two physicians.

H.R. 5576 (sponsored by Representative Steve Buyer)[91] would make various improvements to the claims processing system of the VA. Among these improvements would be training for agents/attorneys representing veterans, quality control assessment for regional offices of the Veterans Benefits Administration (VBA), the electronic processing of claims, treatment of beneficiaries in the event of the death of the veteran before claim determination, evaluation of training and assessment programs for employees of the VBA, electronic monitoring of claim status, a pilot program permitting the submission of claims to any regional office of the VA, and other programs.

H.R. 5892 (sponsored by Representative John J. Hall)[92] would amend title 38 of the U.S. Code to direct the Secretary of the VA to modernize the disability benefits claims processing system of the VA to ensure the accurate and timely delivery of compensation to veterans and their families and survivors. Various disability benefit issues are covered in the bill.

S. 1283 (sponsored by Senator Mark Pryor)[93] deals primarily with improving the management of medical care, personnel actions, and quality of life issues for members of the Armed Forces. The bill addresses disability evaluations, a study by the DOD and the VA concerning their individual evaluation systems, and the possibility of combining the two systems. Some of the bill's provisions are similar to those of H.R. 1538, discussed above.

S. 1363 (sponsored by Senator Hillary Rodham Clinton),[94] the proposed Bridging the Gap for Wounded Warriors Act, would improve health care for severely injured members and former members of the armed forces. The bill would create a Department of Defense — Department of Veterans Affairs Office of Transition ("Office").[95] Among the functions of this Office would be to "develop uniform standards, to be applicable across the military departments and to the Department of Veterans Affairs, for the rating of disabilities incurred or aggravated by members of the Armed Forces during service in the Armed Forces."[96] The bill would also provide for the reform of the disability ratings system of the Department of Defense and the Department of Veterans Affairs.[97]

S. 2737 (sponsored by Senator Daniel K. Akaka),[98] the proposed Veterans' Ratings Schedule Review Act, would amend title 38 of the United States Code to grant jurisdiction to the U.S. Court of Appeals for Veterans Claims to review compliance of ratings for disabilities under the schedule of 38 U.S.C. § 1151 with the statutory requirements applicable to entitlement to disability compensation.

End Notes

[1] See generally *Federal Benefits for Veterans and Dependents*, published by the Departments of Veterans Affairs (2008 edition). (Hereinafter cited as "*Federal Benefits.*") See [http://www1 .va.gov/opa/vadocs/fedben.pdf] for the publication online. See CRS Report RL33 113, *Veterans Affairs: Basic Eligibility for Disability Benefit Programs*, by Douglas Reid Weimer (cited to afterward as "RL33 113"). This chapter deals with the fundamental requirements for disability benefit programs.

[2] *Id.*

[3] The severity of the veteran's disability is evaluated by the VA and a determination is made as to what percentage of employment capacity is impaired. See discussion below.

[4] See CRS Report RL33113.

[5] For further discussion of a disability pension or a non-service-connected pension, see CRS Report RL33113.

[6] See CRS Report RL33113.

[7] *Id.* at 4-5.

[8] *Id.* at 7-8.

[9] Hence, the claimant becomes a "veteran" for purposes of benefits.

[10] 38 U.S.C. § 1155; 38 C.F.R. § 4. See discussion below.

[11] See Barton F. Stichman et al., *Veterans Benefits Manual* at § 3.1.5. (Hereinafter cited as "*Veterans Benefits Manual.*")

[12] For the purposes of this chapter, it is assumed that the claimant/applicant has met the very basic eligibility requirements for VA benefits. The claimant/applicant will be referred to as the "veteran" for the remainder of this chapter.

[13] 38 U.S.C. §§ 1110, 1131. These provisions deal with the basic entitlement for disability compensation.

[14] 38 U.S.C. § 5103A.

[15] 38 U.S.C. §§ 5103A(b),(c).

[16] 38 U.S.C. § 5103A(d).

[17] 38 U.S.C. § 5103A(a)(2).

[18] 38 U.S.C. § 5102(b).

[19] 38 U.S.C. § 5 103(a).

[20] For example, a veteran may receive compensation for a medical condition that resulted from a sports injury incurred during in-service time. See *Veterans Benefit Manual* at §3.1.1.1.

[21] 38 U.S.C. § 5107(b).

[22] 38 C.F.R. § 3.303.

[23] 38 C.F.R. §§ 3.303(a), 3.304, 3.305. See also 38 U.S.C. § 1154. In determining whether the current condition relates to the in-service problem, the VA determines whether the problem is *acute* or *chronic*. An acute problem is considered to be a problem of relatively short duration. A chronic condition is of lengthy duration and may return.

[24] 38 U.S.C. § 1153; 38 C.F.R. § 3.306(a). If the disability existed prior to service, the VA must ascertain whether there was an *increase in the disability during service*. The preexisting problem will not be considered to be aggravated by service if the VA determines that the exacerbation resulted from the natural progression of the disease.

[25] 38 U.S.C. §§ 1112, 1116, 1133; 38 C.F.R. §§ 3.307-3.309; 38 C.F.R. § 3.313(b). If the disability claimed is a disease which was not diagnosed or recorded on the veteran's service record, the VA is required to ascertain whether the *incubation time* for the disease could have started during in-service time (38 C.F.R. § 3.03(d)).

[26] 38 C.F.R. § 3.310(a). If the disability claimed cannot be determined to be in-service, either directly or by exacerbation, the VA will then decide whether the problem may be *service-connected on a secondary basis*. This reasoning is based on the theory that it was proximately caused by a service-connected condition. For instance, a primary disease is contracted in-service. A related, secondary disease develops as a result of the primary disease.

[27] 38 U.S.C. § 1151.

[28] 38 U.S.C. § 5107.

[29] 38 U.S.C. § 5107(b).

[30] *Id.*

[31] 38 C.F.R. § 3.102.

[32] 38 U.S.C. § 5 103(a).

[33] 38 U.S.C. §§ 5103A(b), (c).

[34] 38 U.S.C. § 5103A(d).

[35] 38 U.S.C. § 5103A(a)(2).

[36] 38 U.S.C. § 1111.

[37] 38 C.F.R. § 3.307(a)(6)(iii).

[38] 38 C.F.R. § 3.304(f).

[39] 38 U.S.C. § 1154(b); 38 C.F.R. § 3.304(d),(f).
[40] 38 U.S.C. § 1155.
[41] 38 C.F.R. § 4.1.
[42] 38 U.S.C. § 1155.
[43] 10% through 100%.
[44] The current monthly rates, effective on December 1, 2007, are as follows: an unmarried veteran without dependents and with a 10% disability receives $117 per month. The rates increase to a 100% disability payment of $2,527 per month (for an unmarried veteran without dependents). For rate tables and a compensation calculator, see [http://www.vba.va.gov/bln/2 1/rates/comp0 1 .htm]. *The payment rates are not automatically adjusted for inflation, and are only increased if Congress passes enabling legislation.* Congress usually grants an increase based on the consumer price index or the cost-of-living formula used to determine the Social Security old age increase. The 2008 rates were set by P.L. 110-111, 110th Cong., 1st Sess. (November 5, 2007), the Veterans' Compensation Costof-Living Adjustment Act of 2007.
[45] 38 C.F.R. § 4.1.
[46] 38 C.F.R. §§ 4.40 to 4.73.
[47] 38 C.F.R. §§ 4.75 to 4.84a.
[48] See 38 C.F.R. § 4.84a for an example of the ratings and diagnostic codes chart for impairment of vision.
[49] See CRS Report RL3399 1, *Disability Evaluation of Military Servicemembers*, by Christine Scott, Sidath Viranga Panangala, Sarah A. Lister, and Charles A. Henning.
[50] 38 C.F.R. § 4.7.
[51] 38 C.F.R. § 3.103(d).
[52] 38 C.F.R. § 4.20. However, if a case when a veteran's disability is so extraordinary or unusual that an analogy cannot be made through use of the rating charts, an "extraschedular rating" for a veteran may be made (38 C.F.R. § 3.321(b)).
[53] 38 U.S.C. § 1157; 38 C.F.R. § 4.25.
[54] See "Compensation and Pension Benefits Page" at VA website; *A Summary of VA Benefits: Putting Veterans First*, VA Pamphlet 2 1-00-1 (January 2006); see also [http://www.va.gov] (click on "Benefits," and then go to "Compensation and Pension Benefits Page").
[55] Such disabilities may involve anatomical loss or the loss of use of a hand or foot.
[56] 38 U.S.C. § 1114(k); 38 C.F.R. § 3.350.
[57] 38 U.S.C. § 11 14(r)(2); 38 C.F.R. § 3.352.
[58] Many conditions listed within the ratings tables are rated as 0. See also 38 C.F.R. § 4.31.
[59] 38 C.F.R. § 3.327(a).
[60] See CRS Report RS2256 1, *Veterans Affairs: The U.S. Court of Appeals for Veterans Claims — Judicial Review of VA Decision Making*, by Douglas Reid Weimer.
[61] GAO-06-283T, Testimony before the Committee on Veterans' Affairs, House of Representatives; Statement for the Record by Cynthia A. Bascetta, Director, Education, Workforce, and Income Security Issues (GAO) (December 7, 2005).
[62] *Id.* at 1.
[63] *Id.* at 2, 4-6.
[64] *Id.* at 5-7.
[65] *Id.* at 8-9.
[66] *Id.* at 9-10.
[67] See CRS Report RL33985, *Veterans Benefits Issues in the 110th Congress*, by Carol D. Davis, Coordinator, Shannon S. Loane, Meredith Peterson, Christine Scott, Libby Perl, and Douglas Reid Weimer.
[68] P.L. 110-111, 110th Cong., 1st Sess (November 5, 2007).
[69] This law amended 38 U.S.C. § 1114 and established increased monthly payments.
[70] S. 161, 110th Cong., 1st Sess (2007). The bill was introduced and was referred to the Senate Committee on Veterans' Affairs on January 4, 2007.
[71] H.R. 402, 110th Cong., 1st Sess (2007). The bill was introduced on January 11, 2007, and was referred to the House Subcommittee on Disability Assistance and Memorial Affairs on March 2, 2007.
[72] S. 1315, 110th Cong., 1st Sess (2007). The bill was introduced on May 7, 2007, and passed the Senate and was received in the House on April 24, 2008.
[73] H.R. 2943, 110th Cong., 1st Sess (2007). The bill was introduced and was referred to the House Committee on Ways and Means on June 28, 2007.
[74] See CRS Report RL32279, *Primer on Disability Benefits: Social Security Disability Insurance (SSDI) and Supplemental Security Income (SSI)*, by Scott Szymendera.
[75] The VA breaks these figures down in very detailed "workload reports." For more information, go to the VA website, [http://www.va.gov], and search under "workload reports." Then go to "Monday Morning Workload Report" and access for the current statistics.
[76] *Id.*

[77] H.R. 1538, 110th Cong., 1st Sess (2007). The bill was introduced on March 15, 2007, passed the House on March 28, 2007, and passed the Senate with an amendment by Unanimous Consent on July 25, 2007. The Senate ordered the measure printed as passed on September 5, 2007.

[78] S. 1283, 110th Cong., 1st Sess (2007). The bill was introduced and was referred to the Senate Committee on Armed Services on May 3, 2007.

[79] H.R. 654, 110th Cong., 1st Sess (2007). The bill was introduced on January 24, 2007, and was referred to the House Subcommittee on Disability Assistance and Memorial Affairs on March 2, 2007.

[80] P.L. 110-157, 110th Cong., 1st Sess (December 12, 2007).

[81] H.R. 1435, 110th Cong., 1st Sess (2007). The bill was introduced on March 9, 2007, and the House Subcommittee on Disability Assistance and Memorial Affairs held hearings on April 17, 2007.

[82] H.R. 1444, 110th Cong., 1st Sess (2007). The bill was introduced on March 9, 2007, and the House Subcommittee on Disability Assistance and Memorial Affairs held hearings on April 17, 2007.

[83] H.R. 1490, 110th Cong., 1st Sess (2007). The bill was introduced on March 13, 2007, and the Subcommittee on Disability Assistance and Memorial Affairs held hearings on April 17, 2007.

[84] H.R. 1538, 110th Cong., 1st Sess (2007). The bill was introduced on March 15, 2007, passed the House on March 28, 2007, and passed the Senate with an amendment by Unanimous Consent on July 25, 2007. A message on Senate action was sent to the House on July 26, 2007. On September 5, 2007, the Senate ordered the measure to be printed as passed.

[85] H.R. 2257, 110th Cong., 1st Sess (2007). The bill was introduced on May 9, 2007, and was referred to the House Subcommittee on Disability Assistance and Memorial Affairs on May 11, 2007.

[86] These "centers" provide readjustment counseling and related mental health services to veterans (38 U.S.C. § 1712A(i)(1)).

[87] H.R. 2855, 110th Cong., 1st Sess (2007). The bill was introduced on June 25, 2007, and was referred to the House Subcommittee on Military Personnel on July 25, 2007.

[88] H.R. 3047, 110th Cong., 1st Sess (2007). The bill was introduced on July 16, 2007, and the House Subcommittee on Disability Assistance and Memorial Affairs held hearings on November 8, 2007.

[89] H.R. 4084, 110th Cong., 1st Sess (2007). The bill was introduced on November 6, 2007, and the House Subcommittee on Disability Assistance and Memorial Affairs held hearings on November 8, 2007.

[90] H.R. 5089, 110th Cong., 2nd Sess (2008). The bill was introduced and was referred to the House Committee on Veterans' Affairs on January 22, 2008.

[91] H.R. 5576, 110th Cong., 2nd Sess (2008). The bill was introduced on March 11, 2008, and was referred to the House Subcommittee on Disability Assistance and Memorial Affairs on March 14, 2008.

[92] H.R. 5892, 110th Cong., 2nd Sess (2008). The bill was introduced and was referred to the House Committee on Veterans' Affairs on April 24, 2008. On April 30, 2008, the Committee held a mark-up session and the bill was ordered to be reported.

[93] S. 1283, 110th Cong., 1st Sess (2007). The bill was introduced and was referred to the Senate Committee on Armed Services on May 3, 2007.

[94] S. 1363, 110th Cong., 1st Sess (2007). The bill was introduced and referred to the Senate Committee on Armed Services on May 10, 2007.

[95] S. 1363, § 3.

[96] *Id.* § 3(c)(5).

[97] *Id.* § 4.

[98] S. 2737, 110th Cong., 2nd Sess (2008). The bill was introduced and was referred to the Senate Committee on Veterans' Affairs on March 10, 2008.

In: Veterans' Benefits and Care
Editor: Mathew H. Bradley

ISBN: 978-1-60692-500-3

Chapter 6

Disability Evaluation of Military Servicemembers

Christine Scott,Sidath Viranga Panangala and Charles A. Henning

Summary

On February 18, 2007, the *Washington Post* published the first in a series of articles describing problems with outpatient medical care and other services provided at the Walter Reed Army Medical Center (WRAMC). The series noted, among other things, concerns about the processes used to evaluate disability in injured military servicemembers. Both the Department of Defense (DOD) and the Department of Veterans Affairs (VA) conduct disability evaluations and assign disability ratings to servicemembers or veterans under their respective authorities. An individual's disability rating, from either department, affects the scope of pay and benefits for which he or she is eligible, and the cost to the respective department of providing such benefits.

There are significant differences between the disability evaluations performed by DOD and VA, as well as civilian disability evaluations conducted by the Social Security Administration (SSA) and workers' compensation programs. Most notably, the DOD disability evaluation is focused on the effect of any disabling condition on the performance of the servicemember's duties in the military, while the other three systems evaluate the impact of a disability on gainful employment in the civilian economy.

Congress has followed recent news reports with interest, and several legislative initiatives are under consideration. For example, H.R. 1538, the Wounded Warrior Assistance Act of 2007, passed unanimously in the House on March 28, 2007. The bill includes numerous provisions to improve or streamline medical care and benefits processing for returning injured servicemembers. Title XVI of the National Defense Authorization Act for FY2008 (H.R. 4986, P.L. 110-181), contains Wounded Warrior provisions related to the care and transition of injured servicemembers.

This chapter is intended as a primer to describe disability evaluation in general, including evaluations used by DOD and VA, as well as civilian evaluations used by the SSA and by workers' compensation programs. Next, the DOD and VA disability rating processes are described, respectively, in greater detail. Finally, recent congressional and executive actions and recommendations regarding DOD and VA disability evaluations are described. This chapter emphasizes the disability evaluation systems at DOD and VA, with illustrative comparisons made to civilian systems when appropriate. It will be updated as warranted.

BACKGROUND

On February 18, 2007, the *Washington Post* published the first in a series of articles describing problems with outpatient medical care and other services provided at the Walter Reed Army Medical Center (WRAMC).[1] WRAMC, a Department of Defense (DOD) facility in Washington, DC, is one of several Military Treatment Facilities (MTFs) providing medical care to injured servicemembers returning from combat theaters in Iraq and Afghanistan in support of Operation Enduring Freedom (OEF) and Operation Iraqi Freedom (OIF).

Intense media scrutiny followed the *Washington Post* series. News reports have, in general, observed that medical care provided to returning servicemembers is good or excellent, but noted evidence of problems with infrastructure and cleanliness in both DOD and Department of Veterans Affairs (VA) facilities. In addition, reported problems have included complex administrative systems, delays and errors in DOD's processing of retirement and other benefits for those servicemembers who separate from the armed forces, the transitioning of eligible servicemembers to veteran status, and VA's processing of veterans' benefits. Reports have also mentioned understaffing and inadequate training of case workers who assist servicemembers and veterans with benefits processing and other aspects of their return to civilian life. Some reports have, however, been problematic in their descriptions of the respective roles of DOD and VA in providing health care and other benefits to injured servicemembers, or in their descriptions of the health care and other benefits systems in the two departments.[2]

Recent reports have spotlighted problems faced by some returning injured OEF/OIF servicemembers. However, DOD and VA do not apply their disability evaluations differently to OEF/OIF servicemembers than to other servicemembers and veterans. Also, less than half of each department's disability evaluation caseloads involve OEF/OIF personnel. Nonetheless, the added number of OEF/OIF cases and, in particular, their complexity, do appear to have strained the capacity of the disability evaluation systems in the two departments.

WHEN IS A DISCHARGED SERVICEMEMBER CLASSIFIED AS A "VETERAN" FOR THE PURPOSES OF VA BENEFITS?

Not all discharged servicemembers are considered "veterans" for the purposes of Veterans Administration (VA) benefits and programs. In order to be eligible for most VA benefits, it is necessary for the discharged servicemember to be classified as a "veteran," or in some circumstances, the survivor of a veteran.

Federal statutes define "veteran" as a "person who served in the active military, naval, or air service, and who was discharged or released therefrom under conditions other than dishonorable." [38 U.S.C. § 101(2); 38 C.F.R. § 3.1(d)]. The VA largely bases its determination of veteran status upon military department service records. In addition to the member's service records, other factors affect his or her classification as a "veteran" and may affect future benefits. These factors include:

Discharge criteria: (38 U.S.C. § 101(2); 38 C.F.R. § 3.1(d)).

Active military, naval or air service: (38 U.S.C. § 101(2); 38 C.F.R. § 3.1(d)).

Whether the service was during "time of war:" (38 U.S.C. § 101(6)-(1 1); 38 C.F.R. § 3.2).

Minimum active-duty service requirement: (38 U.S.C. § 5303A 38, C.F.R. § 3.1 2A).

After it has been proved that the discharged servicemember meets these criteria, he or she is considered to be a "veteran," and may be eligible for certain benefits relating to health care, education, and other services provided by the VA.

See the **Appendix** for definitions of U.S. military servicemembers and veterans.

(Information provided by Douglas Reid Weimer, Legislative Attorney, American Law Division, CRS.)

Some news reports and other sources have asserted that the DOD underrates disability. In both the DOD and VA systems, disability ratings range from zero (least severe) to 100% (most severe), in increments of 10%. Generally, if an injured servicemember has served in the military less than 20 years, a DOD disability rating of 20% or less entitles the servicemember to a single lump-sum severance payment and no additional military benefits, while a rating of 30% or greater may, subject to certain other conditions, make the individual eligible for certain lifelong military benefits such as retirement pay and health insurance for the servicemember and his or her family. Hence, in most cases, a disability rating of 30% or greater yields a more favorable benefits package for the servicemember, and a higher and longer-term cost for the department. For veterans under the VA system, in comparison, a service-connected disability rating of 10% or more provides a monthly disability compensation payment whereas a disability rating of 30% or more provides additional disability compensation for a spouse and dependents. (The amount of monthly disability compensation depends on the disability percentage rating.) In addition, unlike the DOD disability evaluation, VA disability ratings may, over time, be revised as a veteran files a claim (or claims) for changes in disability status related to prior military service.

This chapter describes disability evaluation in general, including evaluations used by DOD and VA, as well as civilian evaluations used by the Social Security Administration and by workers' compensation programs. Next, the DOD and VA disability rating processes are described, respectively, in greater detail. Finally, recent congressional and executive branch actions and recommendations regarding military disability evaluation are described. This chapter emphasizes the disability evaluation systems at DOD and VA, with illustrative comparisons made to civilian systems when appropriate.

Overview of Disability Evaluation

There are significant differences between the disability evaluations performed by the DOD, the VA, the Social Security Administration (SSA), and workers' compensation programs (WC). There are differences in process and, more importantly, fundamental differences in the basis for evaluation in each of the systems. This may result in different rating outcomes from each system, which can affect the financial condition of the disabled applicant and the future costs incurred by the benefits provider. A brief overview and comparison of the four systems is provided below. More detailed descriptions of the DOD and VA systems are presented later in this chapter.

Some have proposed combining or linking different disability evaluation programs to improve outcomes or other problems with program performance. (For example, proposals to consolidate the DOD and VA disability systems, or to have the VA conduct disability evaluations of DOD personnel, are discussed in the final section of this chapter, "Recent Congressional and Executive Actions.") However, attempts to combine or link existing disability evaluation systems may be difficult and may not be desirable, given the different purposes of each system.

The Government Accountability Office (GAO) has designated as *high-risk* the federal disability programs at SSA and VA, which rate disability based on civilian employability. GAO says that these systems are based upon outmoded concepts of disability, and fail to optimize opportunities that would allow disabled beneficiaries to return to productive work.[4]

Department of Defense (DOD) Disability Evaluation

The DOD disability evaluation is focused on the effect of any disabling condition on the performance of the servicemember 's duties in the military. The evaluation can be viewed as a two-step process. The first step is to determine if the applicant (servicemember) is fit for military duty. The second step, for applicants found to be unfit, is the rating of service-connected disability.

Several factors are taken into account to determine a servicemember's fitness for duty, including

- whether or not the servicemember can perform his or her required duties (based on office, grade, rank, or rating);
- whether or not the servicemember is medically prevented from taking the required physical fitness test;
- the impact on deployability of the servicemember and his or her unit; and
- whether or not an alternative job specialty for the servicemember is feasible.

If a servicemember is found unfit for duty, the servicemember can be placed on the Temporary Disability Retired List (TDRL, which requires a reevaluation in the future), or permanently released from military service. Prior to release, DOD examines those service-connected physical impairments that rendered the soldier unfit, and provides a disability rating. For soldiers with multiple diagnosed physical impairments, each is potentially ratable, provided that DOD finds each physical impairment to be separately unfitting.[5] DOD and VA use the same rating table, the Veterans Administration Schedule for Rating Disabilities (often referred to as VASRD or SRD, described in the **Text Box** below) to determine the disability percentage. This disability percentage is one factor used to determine if the service member receives a lump-sum payment upon discharge (based on a rating of 20% or lower), or an annual pension and possibly other lifelong benefits (based on a rating of 30% or higher).

Once the ratings determination is made and accepted by the servicemember, no further changes to the evaluation, percentage rating, lump-sum payment, or pension are made in the future. The military disability evaluation process does not look at the individual servicemember's current, future, or potential earnings or earnings capacity in evaluating disability.

THE VETERANS ADMINISTRATION SCHEDULE FOR RATING DISABILITIES (VASRD)

A schedule of ratings was first officially developed in 1921. In 1924, a schedule was adopted that attempted to incorporate a veteran's occupation, with ratings in 1% increments. However, because the only job held by many veterans was their military occupation, the schedule was deemed unworkable. Two editions of a ratings schedule were published in 1933, with different levels or grades of disability (the first had 25%, 50%, 75%, and 100%, while the second had 10 grades from 10% to 100%). The current basic schedule is the 1945 Schedule for Rating Disabilities, which was reprinted in 1957. When several laws related to veterans were combined in 1958 by P.L. 85-857, which created the Veterans Administration, the Administrator was given the authority to develop a schedule of ratings for disability, and to periodically update the schedule based on experience. The VASRD last underwent a thorough review and revision for all body systems in the early 1 990s (revisions for 11 of the 15 body systems were finalized as of April 2007).

The VASRD is contained in 38 C.F.R. Chapter 1, Part 4. While some sections are descriptive of the injury and the ratings, others are schedules. For example, for removal of ribs (diagnostic code 5297), the scheduled rating percentage is as follows:

- More than six: 50%
- Five or six: 40%
- Three or four: 30%
- Two: 20%
- One, or resection of two or more ribs without regeneration: 10%

Department of Veterans Affairs (VA) Disability Evaluation

The VA evaluates a qualified individual's disability based on the likely prognosis — the progression of severity of the disability over time — and the effect of the disability on employability within the civilian job market. A qualified individual is generally a former servicemember with active-duty service in the military who has been discharged under conditions other than dishonorable.[6] The DOD's central consideration in disability evaluation, namely, fitness for military duty, is not relevant for the VA's evaluation.

The VA evaluates all medical conditions or illnesses that the veteran (the former servicemember) incurred during military service, *and* preexisting medical conditions or illnesses that were aggravated by military service.[7] The resulting disability percentage rating (based on the VASRD) determines the level of monthly disability compensation, eligibility for other benefits and also plays a role in determining the veteran's position in the priority system for VA medical care. In order to receive disability compensation, an individual must be rated at least 10% disabled.[8] In contrast to the DOD system, the veteran can be reevaluated if new or newly recognized medical conditions or illnesses occur and are determined to have been caused or aggravated by military service. A veteran may, upon reevaluation, receive a different percentage ranking than he or she received initially. (Though such a reevaluation may yield a disability payment that is a larger or smaller, the former outcome is much more common.)

Social Security Administration (SSA) Disability Evaluation[9]

The Social Security Administration (SSA) evaluates individuals to determine their eligibility for Social Security Disability Insurance (SSDI) and Supplemental Security Income (SSI) benefits. SSDI benefits are available to persons with disabilities who are below the retirement age and who have paid into the Social Security system through payroll taxes, while SSI benefits are available to children and adults with disabilities who have limited assets and income.[10] In order to qualify for either SSDI or SSI benefits based on disability, a person must have a medically determinable impairment that is expected to last at least one year or result in death, and that renders the person unable to perform his or her previous work or any other work that exists in significant numbers in the national economy.

There are no percentage ratings or partial disability determinations for SSDI or SSI benefits. SSDI benefit amounts are based on an individual's career earnings covered by Social Security. All SSI recipients receive the same basic monthly federal benefit; this benefit is reduced by any earned or unearned income the recipient receives in a month, and is augmented by any supplement paid by the recipient's state.[11]

Workers' Compensation (WC) Disability Evaluation[12]

Workers' compensation (WC) is an employer-provided benefit. Generally, an employer, under state laws, must purchase WC insurance to provide medical care and compensation for the work-related injuries or illnesses of employees. In general, WC provides, subject to limitations in state laws, medical coverage and payments for lost wages. State laws specify a percentage of the worker's usual wage (66 and two-thirds percent, in most cases) to be paid during periods of work-related total, but not necessarily permanent, disability.[13] In addition, for all work injuries, the employer is responsible for full payment of all necessary medical treatment until the point of "maximum medical improvement" is reached.[14] Various forms of cost control (e.g., utilization review) may be used, and disputes can be referred to an administrative proceeding conducted by the state labor department or equivalent agency.

Medical evaluations for WC may be done by the employee's personal physician or one specified by the insurance carrier, with disputed results again appealable to a state agency. As noted, *total* disability is compensated by a percentage of lost wages for as long as the disability persists (though with some time limits or reductions in amount at retirement age in some states). The various jurisdictions evaluate *partial* disability in many different ways, which have been classified by some analysts into three basic models:

- Impairment rating: An assessment is made of the worker's proportionate loss of general physical and/or mental functioning compared to a hypothetical "whole person."
- Loss of earning capacity: An estimate is made of the maximum level of earnings the worker can attain in his or her present condition compared to his or her previous earnings. This takes into account education, age, state of the local job market and other particulars of the case.
- Actual wage loss: Post-injury earnings are subtracted from the pre-injury rate of earnings. However, additional criteria are usually applied in order to assure that the loss of earnings is fully caused by the injury.[15]

Most jurisdictions also make distinctions among types of injury. For example, there may be benefit limitations applied to mental injury versus physical injury, or occupational disease versus traumatic injury. Most states also list specific types of injuries (called "scheduled" injuries) — usually loss of body parts or functions such as vision or hearing — and specify a standardized benefit. For example, loss of an arm could be compensated by six years of payment at two-thirds of one's normal wage.

State governments, insurers and employers generally place a high priority on *return to work*, whether it is to the original job, a light duty assignment, or with a new employer. This strategy is usually the most cost-effective, and, arguably, preferred by most workers. Accordingly, vocational rehabilitation is included in all WC systems and, indeed, a worker may lose his or her WC payments if not participating in a prescribed rehabilitation program.

In addition to WC, some employers offer private disability insurance to cover disabilities that may not be caused by work injuries. Under these policies, the employee makes premium payments (the employer may or may not contribute to the premiums) for insurance to provide a replacement for lost income in the event of an injury or illness that prevents him or her from working.[16]

THE DOD PHYSICAL DISABILITY EVALUATION SYSTEM

Initial Medical Treatment of Injured Servicemembers

In general, when a solider is injured on the battlefield, such as in the OEF/OIF conflict theaters, he or she is stabilized in theater by a combat medic/lifesaver and then moved to a battalion aid station. If the servicemember has serious injuries, he or she is transferred to a forward surgical team to be stabilized, and then moved to a combat support hospital and further stabilized for a period of about two days. If the servicemember needs more specialized care, he or she is evacuated from OEF/OIF conflict theaters and brought to Landstuhl Regional Medical Center (LRMC) in Germany for treatment. Most patients arrive at LRMC 12 to 48 hours after injury. In general, servicemembers remain in Germany for a period of about four to five days.[17] Length of stay at in-theater medical facilities is determined by the stability of the patient and the availability of medical evacuation aircraft.

After further stabilization at LRMC, seriously injured soldiers are evacuated to the United States. They arrive at an Echelon V (highest level of care) Military Treatment Facility (MTF), such as WRAMC, or the National Naval Medical Center (NNMC) in Bethesda, Maryland. Catastrophic burn patients are flown to the Brooke Army Medical Center (BAMC) at Fort Sam Houston, Texas. BAMC has also established a specialized amputee rehabilitation center.

Injured servicemembers remain hospitalized as inpatients as long as required for optimal medical care and treatment. When hospitalization is no longer required and the patient is ambulatory, the servicemember may transition to outpatient status. Depending on the severity of the servicemember's injuries, lengths of stay in inpatient and/or outpatient facilities may be considerable, lasting months or sometimes years. Nonetheless, the individual remains a member of the military — not a veteran — unless or until he or she separates from military service. Generally, servicemembers do not undergo medical assessments for disability evaluation until it is felt that the progression of their medical condition has reached a plateau. Until this occurs, active-duty servicemembers whose injury or illness prevents them from working in their assigned unit during recovery and rehabilitation are placed on "Medical Hold" status.[18]

Steps in the Disability Evaluation Process

Overview

The DOD has well-established criteria for the medical qualifications and physical aptitude of those desiring to enlist or be appointed in the military.[19] For servicemembers who become potentially unfit for further service due to injury or disease, DOD has a process to evaluate their fitness for retention in the Armed Forces. DOD has granted the Army, Navy and Air Force some latitude in tailoring disability processes to their specific requirements.[20] The determination of fitness is individualized and based, in addition to medical criteria, upon a soldier's ability to perform the duties of his or her primary military occupation speciality (MOS) or officer speciality at a minimum level of competence, taking into consideration rank and current duty position. *Consequently, two servicemembers with comparable medical conditions, but different MOSs, may receive different fitness determinations if the medical condition affects duty requirements in different ways.*

In general, if a military commander or physician determines that an active or reserve military servicemember may be physically unfit for return to duty, the servicemember is referred to a Medical Evaluation Board (MEB). If the MEB finds that the individual does not meet medical fitness standards, the case will be referred to a Physical Evaluation Board (PEB). The PEB's role is to determine whether a soldier can reasonably perform his or her military duties, and if not, to determine the severity of the soldier's physical or mental disability and rate it accordingly. The disability rating determines if the soldier is retained in the service, separated with or without separation pay, permanently retired, or placed on the Temporary Disability Retired List (TDRL). (These outcomes are discussed in greater detail later in this chapter.) The PEB process incorporates informal, formal, and appeals procedures. Throughout the process, military personnel must be provided with trained counselors to advise and assist. The steps in this process — MEB, PEB, and appeal — are referred to as the Physical Disability Evaluation System (PDES), which is diagramed in **Figure 1.** Each branch of the Armed Forces oversees its own PDES processes and procedures.

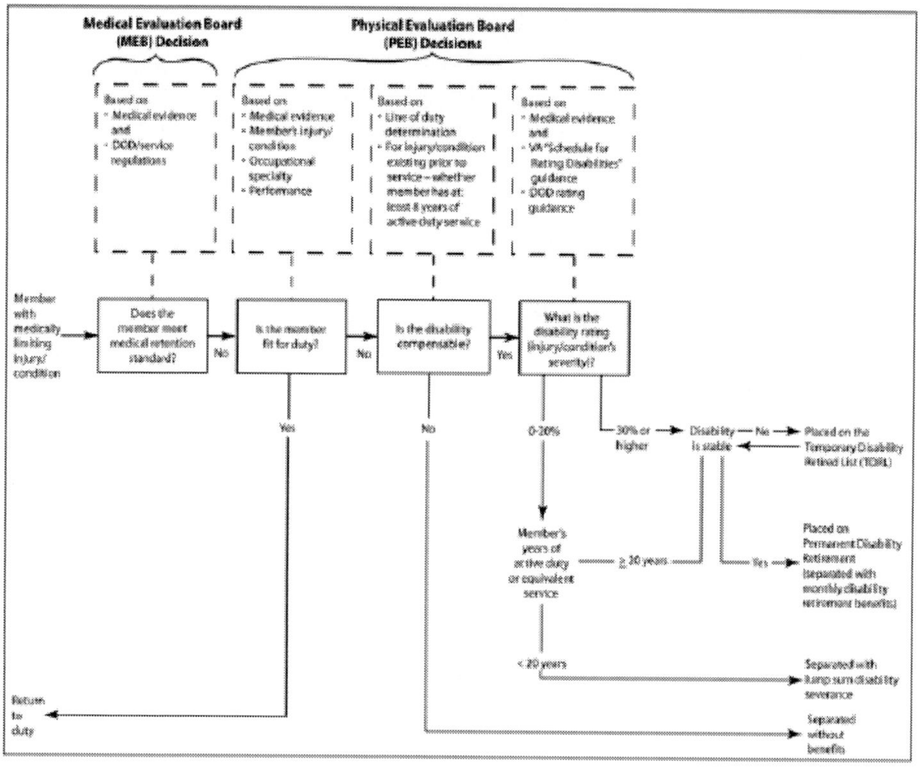

Note: The DOD Physical Disability Evaluation System also includes an appeals process, not depicted in this figure.

Source: Adapted from GAO, Military Disability System: Improved Oversight Needed to Ensure Consistent and Timely Outcomes for Reserve and Active Duty Service Members, GAO-06-362, p. 7, March 31, 2006, derived from DOD documents.

Figure 1. Steps in the DOD Physical Disability Evaluation System

Medical Evaluation Board (MEB)

The MEB, usually composed of two to three physicians, is conducted to first document the medical status and duty limitations of servicemembers referred to it. The board reviews medical information and the determination of whether an injury is service-connected. MEBs may be formal or informal, and may permit appeals based on service guidelines. Importantly, the MEB does not make a conclusion of unfitness, recommend a disability percentage rating, or make a determination regarding separation or retention in the service. MEB results are forwarded to the Physical Evaluation Board (PEB) for disability rating and retention or separation decisions.

Physical Evaluation Board (PEB)

The PEB is usually composed of both physicians and officers within the servicemember's chain of command. PEBs can also be conducted on a formal or informal basis. The informal PEB is used if the servicemember has not requested a personal appearance and only a documentary review is required. The formal PEB is required when the servicemember has requested a personal appearance before the board, with or without legal representation or other advisory assistance.

Using the medical assessment provided by the MEB, the PEB first determines whether the servicemember meets medical standards for retention in the service. The determination has a presumption of fitness. That is, the servicemember is presumed to have been fit until the injury or illness occurred. This is because the servicemember was examined prior to entering the service, and periodically afterward, including prior to deployment. If a servicemember is deemed unfit for duty, the PEB determines if the disability is service-connected and assigns a disability rating based on fitness for military service. Formal PEBs require a written record that is made available to the servicemember, and servicemembers can appeal the findings and recommendations of the PEB. Final results are forwarded to appropriate personnel authorities for final approval, as delegated by the secretary of the respective service branch.

Assistance to Servicemembers During Disability Evaluation

DOD provides trained counselors for servicemembers being evaluated in the disability process to assist with the MEB, PEB, and other required processes. These individuals are commonly referred to as Physical Evaluation Board Liaison Officers, or PEBLOs. However, the GAO recently noted inconsistencies among the military services (Army, Air Force, and Navy) in when the PEBLOs entered the disability process and the adequacy of their training.[21] Assistance is also available from new programs established by DOD and the services to support severely disabled OIF/OEF servicemembers.[22]

Outcomes of the DOD Disability Process

For the injured servicemember, there are five potential outcomes from the disability process. These are described below. For those who are separated as a result of a disability, benefits provided will vary depending on years of service, a determination of whether the disability is service-connected, and the percentage disability rating. Servicemembers with less than 20 years of service who are separated with disability ratings of 30% or greater may be eligible for lifelong benefits, including retirement pay and health insurance for the servicemember and his or her family. Servicemembers separated with disability ratings of

20% or less do not receive lifelong benefits, but instead receive a single lump-sum severance payment.

The possible outcomes of the military disability process are as follows:

1. ***Retained.*** Servicemembers may be found fit for duty and retained. In some cases, based on the physical limitations resulting from an illness or injury, a servicemember may be reclassified into a different job category.

2. ***Placed on Temporary Disability Retired List (TDRL).*** Servicemembers who are found unfit but whose condition is unstable (i.e., the condition may improve or worsen over time) may be placed on the TDRL for a maximum of five years. While on the TDRL, periodic reexaminations are required (normally every 18 months). Based on the reexaminations and a determination of stable condition, the retiree could be found fit for duty, could have his or her disability rating lowered and be separated with severance pay, or could be permanently retired. While on the TDRL, servicemembers receive monthly retired pay (not to exceed 50% of base pay), and are eligible for all retiree benefits and programs, but are not required to perform any military duties.

3. ***Separated from Service with No Benefits.*** Disability benefits are not available if the injury or illness was incurred while not on duty (i.e., is not service- connected), or as a result of willful misconduct.

4. ***Separated with Severance Pay.*** Eligibility for this outcome is based on a finding of unfitness and a disability rating of less than 30%. The amount of severance pay is determined by multiplying the monthly basic pay at the time of discharge by twice the number of years of active service. The maximum payment is two years of basic pay.

5. ***Permanently Retired with Physical Disability Benefits.*** Servicemembers who are determined to be physically unfit and have a disability rating of 30% or greater generally will be retired, even though they may have less than 20 years of active duty. The disability retirement pay calculation differs somewhat from the normal longevity retirement calculation. It is computed by multiplying the basic pay of the retired grade by the greater of the percentage of the disability, or 2.5% multiplied by the number of years of service. The maximum benefit under either computation cannot currently exceed 75% of basic pay.[23]

Retired servicemembers with service-connected disabilities may also be eligible for VA disability compensation. Until recently, military retired pay was offset by any VA compensation received. However, the FY2004 National Defense Authorization Act now allows some military retirees to receive both VA and military retirement compensation, if the individual was retired with more than 20 years of service.[24] Generally, military retired pay is taxable. Exceptions are (1) if the disability pay is for combat-related injuries or (2) if the servicemember was in the military, or so obligated, on September 24, 1975.

Issues of Timely and Consistent Processing

The goal of DOD disability policy is that the physical disability evaluation process will be conducted in a "consistent and timely manner."[25] However, DOD has given the services the latitude to set up their own processes, so inconsistencies would appear to be inevitable. While standards or common schedules such as the VASRD are used, these may be subject to interpretation and/or misapplication.

DOD has also established timeliness standards for case initiation and processing. All servicemembers must be referred for evaluation within one year of the diagnosis of their condition if they are unable to return to duty. In addition, DOD allows 30 days to complete the MEB process and 40 days to complete the PEB process. GAO has found that DOD has not monitored compliance by the services with DOD directives on disability evaluation, or exercised oversight over the training of disability program staff.[26] The Army Inspector General, in a recent inspection of the Army disability system, found that the Army was not meeting the DOD timeliness standards.[27]

VA DISABILITY EVALUATION

In general, once DOD separates a servicemember from active military service,[28] the servicemember becomes eligible to obtain various benefits administered by the VA.[29] This section of the report provides information about the veterans disability evaluation process.

The veterans disability evaluation process begins with application for veterans' disability compensation payments. The VA disability rating determines the level of monthly disability compensation payments available to the veteran and his or her spouse and children. In addition, the priority system for veterans' health care services is based in part on the VA disability rating.

An application for disability compensation requires information related to the veteran's military service and medical condition. A veteran must have been in active service and be discharged under conditions other than dishonorable. The veteran must also have a current medical condition that is service-connected (i.e., in general, incurred as a result of, or aggravated by, active service).[30]

For servicemembers who have been discharged from the military, the VA has access to DOD discharge data to determine veteran status, as well as access to military medical records. However, a veteran making an initial claim for disability compensation some years after discharge, or making a claim for an additional disability some time after an initial disability rating, may encounter more problems in providing the required documentation. For example, a veteran filing a claim for a disability 15 years after service may need to contact, or have the VA contact, several physicians who have treated the veteran for the medical condition over the period (15 years) since the veteran was discharged from the military. In addition, a veteran out of the military for a number of years may have to rely on the VA or DOD to conduct a search of stored paper documents for the needed discharge or medical documentation.

Once all of the documentation needed for the application is complete, a veteran may undergo a compensation and pension examination at a VA facility at the veteran's convenience (some examinations are done under contract outside of VA facilities). The compensation and pension examination is not a complete examination of all body systems and is not focused on diagnosis and treatment. The focus of the examination is the body system(s) covered by the veteran's claim for disability or pension and is designed to provide information specific to determining a disability rating. The information gathered during the examination is then reviewed by a ratings specialist using the Veterans Administration Schedule for Rating Disabilities (VASRD) to determine the disability rating for the veteran. The VA ratings are done in increments of 10%, with a scale of 0% to 100%.[31] The finding is then reviewed by a different rating specialist as a means of confirming the rating. A letter is sent to the veteran explaining the rating and the basis for the rating. The veteran has the right to appeal a rating determination.[32]

The veteran's disability evaluation is based on the impact of the disability on civilian employability. The VASRD rating can be viewed as a measure of the average impact on civilian employment of the disability. However, the evaluation does not take into account a veteran's current earnings or potential future earnings in determining disability payments. The evaluation may take into account the individual unemployability of a veteran if the veteran claims that he or she cannot work as a result of the disability, or if the disability is of such a nature that there is a presumption of unemployability. The payment levels are established in law based on the disability percentage and whether the veteran has a spouse or dependents. An additional payment can be made, if needed, for aid and attendance.

Problems have been noted with the veterans disability evaluation process. Because the evaluation is done at the local level, the VA Inspector General has noted that there are unwarranted geographic variations in disability ratings.[33] Also, GAO has recommended that the department do more monitoring with respect to the process, particularly of the regional medical centers reports, to ensure consistency in disability determinations.[34]

The VA's claims process also has a large backlog. Currently OIF/OEF servicemembers, particularly those recuperating in MTFs, are the VA's first priority in claims processing.[35] This may extend the processing time for claims by other veterans. The size of the claims backlog is related to the increase in the number of claims. According to the VA, the number of disability claims has increased from 578,773 in FY2000 to 806,382 in FY2006. The department attributes the increase in claims to several factors, including (1) the large size of the military's active-duty force; (2) the aging of the veteran population; and (3) increases in the number and complexity of conditions claimed. The department has also expanded outreach efforts that have contributed to the increase in claims.[36]

Recent Congressional and Executive Actions

Congress has followed recent news reports with interest, and several legislative initiatives are under consideration. For example, H.R. 1538, the Wounded Warrior Assistance Act of 2007, passed unanimously in the House on March 28, 2007. The bill includes numerous provisions to improve or streamline medical care and benefits processing for returning injured servicemembers. Several provisions address disability evaluation. These include (1) a requirement that DOD standardize training and caseload limits for staff who are involved in its disability evaluation system;[37] (2) assurance of the availability of medical personnel to advise servicemembers who are undergoing DOD disability evaluation; (3) criteria to clarify certain aspects of the DOD disability evaluation; and (4) a joint DOD/VA study and report to Congress on the disability evaluation systems used by each department, recommendations for improvement, and the feasibility of consolidating the two systems. Title XVI of the National Defense Authorization Act for FY2008 (H.R. 4986, P.L. 110-181), contains Wounded Warrior provisions related to the care and transition of injured servicemembers.

The Veterans' Disability Benefits Commission, established by Congress in 2004, is charged with, among other things, evaluating the DOD and VA disability evaluation and compensation systems.[38] Following the *Washington Post* series, the commission's Chairman, Retired Lieutenant General James Terry Scott, testified before Congress regarding preliminary findings of the commission's work. He noted that he was testifying as an individual and not on behalf of the commission, and that the commission had not reached conclusions at that time.[39] Scott's testimony included preliminary data on outcomes of DOD and VA disability ratings, as well as preliminary analyses of variations in ratings between services within DOD and between DOD and VA ratings. Scott posited possible explanations for variations, noting that the DOD services and the VA each tailor their disability evaluation standards to different missions, and, consequently, comparability of ratings is not necessarily expected. Scott also testified that the DOD has an incentive to assign disability ratings at less than 30% because they avoid lifetime payment of benefits, and made a number of recommendations, including a long-term realignment of responsibilities in which the VA is responsible for rating the disability of injured servicemembers.

The Commission issued its final report on October 11, 2007. In its report, the Commission made 113 recommendations, designating 13 of them as priority recommendations.[40] Recommendations were made in the following broad categories:

- disability evaluation and compensation;
- determining eligibility for benefits;
- appropriateness of the benefits;
- appropriateness of the level of benefits;
- survivors and dependents;
- disability claims administration;
- transition; and
- establishing an executive oversight group to implement recommendations.

In response to the news stories about WRAMC and other problems experienced by returning servicemembers, Secretary of Defense Robert Gates formed an Independent Review Group (IRG), established as a subcommittee of the Defense Health Board, to review and, within 45 days, report upon and provide recommendations regarding any critical shortcomings and opportunities to improve rehabilitative care, administrative processes, and the quality of life of patients.[41] The IRG issued its final report on April 12, 2007.[42] The report commented on the complexity of the DOD Physical Disability Evaluation System and the widespread perception that it is unfair to service personnel. The IRG recommended, among other things, a statutory remedy that would, for all personnel, place DOD in charge of fitness-for-duty determinations and VA in charge of disability assessments.[43] On May 2, 2005, Secretary Gates announced the formation of an internal oversight committee, chaired by

Deputy Defense Secretary Gordon England, that will ensure that recommendations of the Independent Review Group are implemented.[44]

On March 6, 2007, President George W. Bush directed VA Secretary Jim Nicholson to establish an interagency task force on returning servicemembers to examine the range of federal services available to these individuals, gaps in those services, and possible corrective actions. The Task Force report was submitted to the President on April 19, 2007.[45] Among other recommendations, the Task Force advised the development of a joint DOD/VA disability evaluation process.

Also on March 6, 2007, the President issued an executive order establishing the President's Commission on Care for America's Returning Wounded Warriors.[46] The Commission was charged, among other things, with evaluating the coordination, management, and adequacy of disability benefits provided to returning injured servicemembers by federal agencies, as well as by the private sector. The President named former Senator Bob Dole and former Department of Health and Human Services Secretary Donna Shalala to co-chair the Commission. The Commission issued its report on July 30, 2007. In its report, the Commission made six broad recommendations, each with several specific action steps directed to the Congress, DOD and/or VA, and published a matrix of the 23 action steps in its main report.[47] The six broad recommendations are as follows:

1. implement comprehensive recovery plans for returning injured servicemembers;
2. restructure the military and veterans disability and compensation systems;
3. improve care for people with post-traumatic stress disorder (PTSD) and traumatic brain injury (TBI);
4. strengthen support for families;
5. transfer patient information across the DOD and VA systems; and
6. support Walter Reed Army Medical Center (WRAMC) until its closure.[48]

On March 12, 2007, the U.S. Army Inspector General provided congressional committees with a report on the Army Physical Disability Evaluation System, detailing findings of military medical and personnel policies, procedures, and services for injured soldiers.[49] The inspection — which was requested by the Secretary of the Army in April 2006 — found that policies varied between VA, DOD, and Army regulations; that training for personnel assisting soldiers was not standardized; and that current information-management databases were inadequate. The report also noted that cases are often more complicated than in the past because of the types of combat injuries soldiers now sustain, and found that because of this and an increased patient volume, the Army currently does not meet its own case-processing time standards or those of the DOD.

In November 2007, the VA and DOD announced that they had begun a one-year pilot program for a single physical for disability evaluations. The pilot program is being conducted at the three MTFs (Walter Reed Army Medical Center, the National Naval Medical Center in Bethesda, and the Malcolm Grow Medical Center at Andrews Air Force Base) in the Washington, D.C. area. Under the pilot program, the VA will be conducting the physical examination used by both the VA and DOD for disability ratings. Both the VA and DOD will use the results of the single physical examination to independently (according to their regulations) determine their respective disability ratings.

APPENDIX. DEFINITIONS OF U.S. MILITARY SERVICEMEMBERS AND VETERANS[50]

Members of the U.S. Military Service

Federal statutes define various components of, and types of service in, the United States military — for those currently serving and for those discharged or released from service. This section provides a list of relevant definitions. Different services and benefits provided by the federal government (such as medical, educational, and financial) may be available to the servicemembers based upon the type of military service that the servicemembers provide or have provided.

Armed Forces

The term "armed forces" means the Army, Navy, Air Force, Marine Corps, and the Coast Guard.[51]

Reserve Components.[52]

National Guard

"National Guard" means the Army National Guard and the Air National Guard.[53]

Army National Guard

The term "Army National Guard" means that part of the organized militia of several states and territories, active and inactive, that is a land force, is trained and has its officers appointed under Article 1, § 8, cl. 16 of the Constitution, and is supported by federal funds and federally recognized. The Army National Guard is a state rather than a federal entity.

Army National Guard of the United States

The term "Army National Guard of the United States" means the reserve component of the Army, all of whose members are members of the Army National Guard.[54]

Air National Guard

The term "Air National Guard" means that part of the organized militia of the several states and territories, active and inactive, that is an air force, is trained and has its officers appointed under Article 1, § 8, cl. 16 of the Constitution, and is supported by federal funds and federally recognized.[55] The Air National Guard is a state rather than a federal entity.

Air National Guard of the United States

The term "Air National Guard of the United States" means the reserve component of the Air Force, all of whose members are members of the Air National Guard.[56]

Reserve

The term "reserve," with respect to an enlistment, appointment, grade, or office, means enlistment, appointment, grade, or office held as a reserve of one of the armed forces.[57]

Reserve Active-Status List

The term "reserve active-status list" means a single list for the Army, Navy, Air Force, or Marine Corps, respectively, that contains the names of all officers of that armed force except warrant officers who are in an active status in a reserve component and are not on an active-duty list.[58]

Duty Status

Active Duty

The term "active duty" means full-time duty in the active military service of the United States.[59] It includes full-time training duty, annual training duty, and attendance, while in the active military service, at a school designated as a service school by law or by the Secretary of the military department concerned. Such term does not include full-time National Guard duty.[60]

Active Duty for a Period of More than 30 Days

The term "active duty for a period of more than 30 days" means active duty under a call or order that does not specify a period of 30 days or less.[61]

Active Service

The term "active service" means service on active duty or full-time National Guard duty.[62]

Active Status

The term "active status" means the status of a member of reserve component who is not in the inactive Army National Guard or inactive Air National Guard, on an inactive status list, or in the Retired Reserve.[63]

Other Duty Status Definitions

Federal statutes define other duty statuses: *"full-time National Guard duty,"*[64] *"active Guard and Reserve Duty,"*[65] and *"inactiveduty training."*[66]

Discharge from the Miliary: Classification and Status

The servicemember usually leaves the United States military service at the time of his or her *discharge* or release from military service. At that time, the servicemember's status changes, and his or her eligibility for various benefits and services may change.

Concept of "Veteran"

Not all discharged service members are considered "veterans" for the purposes of Veterans Administration benefits and programs. It should also be considered that services and benefits provided to a servicemember during his or her military service may not be available after his or her discharge.

In order to be eligible for most VA benefits, it is necessary for the discharged servicemember to be classified as a "veteran," or in some circumstances, the survivor or the dependent of a veteran. It should also be considered that available benefits may vary for "veterans" and for fully retired members of the armed services.

Definition of "Veteran"

Within the context of the VA, a "veteran" is defined as a "person who served in the active military, naval, or air service, and who was discharged or released therefrom under conditions other than dishonorable."[67] The VA largely bases its determination of veteran status upon military department service records.[68]

In addition to the member's service records, other factors affect his or her classification as a "veteran," and may affect future benefits. These include *discharge criteria,*[69] a requirement of "*active military, naval or air service*,"[70] whether the military service was during *time of war*,[71] and the *length of duty requirement.*[72]

After it has been proven that the discharged servicemember meets these criteria, he or she is considered to be a "veteran" who may be eligible for certain benefits relating to health care, education, and other services provided by the VA.

End Notes

[1] Dana Priest and Anne Hull, "Soldiers Face Neglect, Frustration at Army's Top Medical Facility," *Washington Post*, February 18, 2007.

[2] Among other discrepancies, several news reports mistakenly referred to soldiers at WRAMC as "veterans." For example, on February 20, 2007, *The Seattle Times* reprinted the second article in *The Washington Post* series, describing conditions at Mologne House on the WRAMC campus, under the headline "Injured Vets Now Battle for Benefits." See the first of two text boxes in this chapter for a definition of "veteran."

[3] In the DOD, 11% of disability evaluations involve personnel injured in war, while 89% involve servicemembers transitioning to disability retirement. See the testimony of Gordon R. England, Deputy Secretary of Defense, before a joint hearing of the Senate Committees on Armed Forces and Veterans' Affairs on the DOD and VA disability rating systems and the transition of servicemembers from the DOD to veteran status, April 12, 2007, at [http://armed-services. In the VA, 54% of all claims are claims reopened for worsening of chronic conditions. See the testimony of Ronald R. Aument, Deputy Under Secretary for Benefits, Department of Veterans Affairs, U.S. Congress, House Committee on Veterans Affairs, Hearing on the Impact of OEF/OIF on the VA Claims Process, Statement, March 13, 2007, at [http://www.va.gov/OCA/testimony/hvac/sdama/0703 1 3RA.asp].

[4] Government Accountability Office (GAO), "Modernizing Federal Disability Programs," in *High Risk Series: An Update,* GAO-07-3 10, p. 83, January 31, 2007.

[5] Each individual condition must, independently of the others, result in unfitness for duty.

[6] For more information on eligibility, see CRS Report RL33113, *Veterans Affairs: Basic Eligibility for Disability Benefit Programs*, by Douglas Reid Weimer.

[7] For more information on the disability process, see CRS Report RL33323, *Veterans Affairs: Benefits for Service-Connected Disabilities*, by Douglas Reid Weimer.

[8] A veteran can receive a 0% rating for a service-connected disability.

[9] This section was prepared by Scott Szymendera, Analyst in Disability Policy, Domestic Social Policy Division, CRS.

[10] For more information on the SSDI and SSI programs, see CRS Report RL32279, *Primer on Disability Benefits: Social Security Disability Insurance (SSDI) and Supplemental Security Income (SSI)*, by Scott Szymendera.

[11] For 2008, the monthly federal SSI benefit is $637 for an individual and $956 for a couple; 44 states and the District of Columbia offer a state supplement to some SSI benefits.

[12] This section was prepared by Edward Rappaport, a former (retired) staff member of the Domestic Social Policy Division, CRS. For questions on Workers Compensation, please contact Scott Szymendera, Analyst in Disability Policy, Domestic Social Policy Division, CRS.

[13] Workers compensation payments are tax-exempt.

[14] Maximal medical improvement is the greatest degree of cure likely to be achieved with further medical services.

[15] Reville, Robert T. et al., *An Evaluation of California's Permanent Disability Rating System*, Appendix A, Santa Monica CA, RAND Corp, Institute for Civil Justice, 2005, at [http://www.rand.org/pubs/monographs/2005/RAND_MG258.pdf].

[16] Five states (California, Hawaii, New Jersey, New York, Rhode Island) and Puerto Rico have Temporary Disability Insurance (TDI) programs that provide limited non work-related disability benefits. In most cases, these benefits cover up to a half-year or year of disability.

[17] Tenuta, Joachim J., "From the Battlefields to the States: The Road to Recovery. The Role of Landstuhl Regional Medical Center in US Military Casualty Care," *Journal of the American Academy of Orthopedic Surgeons*, vol. 14, (2006), S45-S47.

[18] See, for example, Army regulation 40-400, "Medical Services: Patient Administration." Reserve component personnel who have an illness or injury that prevents their deployment or return to duty with their unit are placed on "medical holdover" status.

[19] Department of Defense Directive 61 30.3 , *Physical Standards for Appointment, Enlistment and Induction*, May 2, 1994.

[20] Department of Defense Directive 1332.18, *Separation or Retirement for Physical Disability*, November 4, 1996 (certified current as of December 1, 2003), at [http://www. dtic.mil/whs/directives 3321 8p.pdf].

[21] GAO, *Military Disability System: Improved Oversight Needed to Ensure Consistent and Timely Outcomes for Reserve and Active Duty Service Members*, GAO-06-362, March 31, 2006.

[22] See CRS Report RS22366, *Military Support to the Severely Disabled: Overview of Service Programs*, by Charles A. Henning.

[23] See CRS Report RL33449, *Military Retirement, Concurrent Receipt, and Related Major Legislative Issues*, by Charles A. Henning.

[24] Ibid.

[25] DOD Instruction 1332.38, *Physical Disability Evaluation*, July 10, 2006.

[26] GAO, *Military Disability System: Improved Oversight Needed to Ensure Consistent and Timely Outcomes for Reserve and Active Duty Service Members*, GAO-06-362, March 31, 2006.

[27] U.S. Army, "Army Inspector General Details Findings on Soldier Disability System," press release with link to full report, March 12, 2007, at [http://www.army.mil/news/jumparchive/newsreleases/].

[28] A veteran (former servicemember) has received a DD 214 (Certificate of Release or Discharge from Active Duty) form.

[29] See CRS Report RL33985, *Veterans' Benefits: Issues in the 110th Congress*, by Carol D. Davis, Shannon S. Loane, Meredith Peterson, Christine Scott, Charmaine Mercer, Libby Perl, and Douglas Reid Weimer.

[30] Lower-income wartime veterans who are elderly or have a nonservice-connected disability may apply for a VA pension. The pension benefits are offset by income from other sources.

[31] For more detail on the VA disability process, see CRS Report RL33323, *Veterans Affairs: Benefits for Service-Connected Disabilities*, by Douglas Reid Weimer.

[32] For information on the appeal process, see CRS Report RL33704, *Veterans Affairs: The Appeal Process for Veterans' Claims*, by Douglas Reid Weimer.

[33] Department of Veterans Affairs, Office of Inspector General, Review of State Variances in VA Disability Compensation Payments, Report No. 05-00765-137, May 19, 2005.

[34] Government Accountability Office, *VA Disability Benefits, Routine Monitoring of Disability Decisions Could Improve Consistency*, GAO-06-120T, October 20, 2005.

[35] In addition to having VA claims counselors at major MTFs to assist severely injured servicemembers going through the DOD disability evaluation process and transitioning out of military service, the VA operates a Benefits Delivery at Discharge (BDD)program. Under the BDD program, which is available at certain military installations around the world, the VA begins processing servicemembers' claims for benefits prior to separation from the military. See the statement of Daniel. L. Cooper, Under Secretary for Benefits, Department of Veterans Affairs, before the Senate Committee on Veterans' Affairs, hearing on VA Claims Adjudication Process, March 7, 2007.

[36] U.S. Congress, House Committee on Veterans Affairs, Hearing on the Impact of OEF/OIF on the VA Claims Process, Statement of Ronald R. Aument, Deputy Under Secretary for Benefits, Department of Veterans Affairs, March 13, 2007, at [http://www.va.gov/OCA/testimony/hvac/sdama/070313RA.asp]. The number of

disability claims reflects total claims for all disability-related benefits, and not just claims for disability compensation.

[37] Currently, each of the services specifies its own training requirements.

[38] The National Defense Authorization Act for FY2004, P.L. 108-136, 38 U.S.C. § 1101 note. See [http://www.vetscommission.org/index.asp].

[39] Statement of Lieutenant General James Terry Scott, USA (Ret.), Chairman, Veterans' Disability Benefits Commission, before a joint hearing of the Senate Committees on Armed Forces and Veterans' Affairs on the DOD and VA disability rating systems and the transition of servicemembers from the DOD to veteran status, April 12, 2007, at [http://armed-services 2-07. pdf .

[40] VDBC full report, pp. 378-395, and executive summary, pp. 12-15. One commissioner's separate views on four of the Commission's recommendations are published as Appendix L in the full report.

[41] See [http://www.ha.osd.mil/DHB/default.cfm]. Secretary Gates also established a DOD web site to provide a centralized location for news articles pertaining to health care problems at WRAMC. See [http://www.defenselink.mil/home/features/2007/walter_reed/].

[42] Independent Review Group on Rehabilitative Care and Administrative Processes at Walter Reed Army Medical Center and National Naval Medical Center, *Rebuilding the Trust*, April 2007, at [http://www.ha.osd.mil/dhb/recommendations/2007/IRG-Report-Final.pdf].

[43] Ibid., pp. 28-34.

[44] Baker III, Fred W., "Gates Puts Punch Behind Fixing Wounded Warrior Care," *American Forces Press Service*, May 2, 2007, at [http://www.defenselink.mil/news/newsarticle.aspx? id=33033]. press release with link to full report, March 12, 2007, at [http://www.army.mil/news/ jumparchive/newsreleases/].

[45] U.S. Department of Veterans Affairs, "Task Force Report to the President on Returning Global War on Terror Heroes," April 2007, at [http://www1.va.gov/taskforce/].

[46] White House, "Executive Order: Establishing a Commission on Care for America's Returning Wounded Warriors and a Task Force on Returning Global War on Terror Heroes," press release, March 6, 2007.

[47] President's Commission on Care for America's Returning Wounded Warriors report, p. 28, chart.

[48] CRS has prepared a Congressional Distribution Memorandum that compares key recommendations of two Commissions discussed in this chapter. *See Comparison of Selected Recommendations of the President's Commission on Care for America's Returning Wounded Warriors and the Veterans' Disability Benefits Commission,* by Christine Scott and Sara A. Lister, November 15, 2007, that

[49] U.S. Army, "Army Inspector General Details Findings on Soldier Disability System," press release with link to full report, March 12, 2007, at [http://www.army.mil/news/jumparchive/newsreleases/].

[50] Appendix prepared by Douglas Reid Weimer, Legislative Attorney, American Law Division, CRS.

[51] 10 U.S.C. § 101(a)(4).

[52] Ibid., § 101(c).

[53] Ibid., § 101(c)(1).

[54] Ibid., § 101(c)(3).

[55] Ibid., § 101(c)(4).

[56] Ibid., § 101(c)(5).

[57] Ibid., § 101(c)(6).

[58] Ibid., § 101(c)(7).

[59] Ibid., § 101(d)(1).

[60] Full-time national guard duty is considered state service rather than federal service.

[61] 10 U.S.C. § 101(d)(2).

[62] Ibid., § 101(d)(3).

[63] Ibid., § 101(d)(4).

[64] Ibid., § 101(d)(5). See note 11.

[65] Ibid., § 101(d)(6).

[66] Ibid., § 101(d)(7).

[67] 38 U.S.C. § 101(2); 38 C.F.R. § 3.1(d).

[68] See CRS Report RL33 113, *Veterans Affairs: Basic Eligibility for Disability Benefit Programs*, at 2-3, by Douglas Reid Weimer.

[69] Ibid., at 3-4.

[70] Ibid., at 4-6. See 38 U.S.C. § 101(2); 38 C.F.R. § 3.1(d).

[71] Ibid., at 6-7. See 38 U.S.C. § 101 (6)-(1 1); 38 C.F.R. § 3.2.

[72] Ibid., at 7.

In: Veterans' Benefits and Care
Editor: Mathew H. Bradley

ISBN: 978-1-60692-500-3

Chapter 7

VETERANS AFFAIRS: BASIC ELIGIBILITY FOR DISABILITY BENEFIT PROGRAMS

Douglas Reid Weimer

SUMMARY

A broad range of benefits is offered to American veterans and to certain members of their families by the United States Department of Veterans Affairs (VA). Among these benefits are various types of financial benefits and assistance — which include disability compensation and pensions.

The VA administers two disability programs. These programs pay monthly cash benefits to disabled veterans. *Disability compensation* provides a monthly benefit if the veteran is disabled as a result of his/her military service. Disability compensation relates specifically to a disability which directly resulted from military service. A *disability pension* is paid to a wartime veteran if the veteran has limited income, is no longer able to work, or is age 65 or older. The pension is not related to a service-connected injury or medical condition. Award of the pension takes into consideration the material needs of the veteran (i.e., it is a "needs-based" pension).

There is no deadline or time limit for applying for disability benefits. A veteran cannot simultaneously receive both disability compensation and a disability pension. There are certain basic criteria which must be met in order to be eligible to receive either of these benefits.

This chapter examines the eligibility criteria and the fundamentals of the VA-administered disability benefit programs and related issues.

INTRODUCTION

The United States Department of Veterans Affairs (VA)[1] offers a broad range of benefits to American veterans and to certain members of their families.[2] Among the benefits which are extended to veterans are: various types of health care and related services, such as nursing homes, clinics, and medical centers;[3] various types of financial benefits, including disability compensation and pensions; education, vocational training, and related career assistance; home financing;[4] life insurance; burial benefits;[5] and benefits for certain family survivors. This chapter focuses upon the basic eligibility/entitlement requirements for disability benefits.[6]

The VA administers two disability programs. Both of these programs pay monthly cash benefits to disabled veterans. *Disability compensation* provides a monthly benefit if the veteran is at least 10% disabled[7] as a result of his/her military service. A *disability pension* is paid to a wartime veteran with limited income, who is no longer able to work, or is age 65 or older. The pension is not related to a service-connected injury or medical condition, and takes into consideration the material needs of the veteran (i.e., it is a "needs-based" pension).[8] There is no deadline or time limit for applying for disability benefits. A veteran cannot simultaneously receive both disability compensation and a disability pension. There are certain basic criteria which must be met in order to be eligible to receive either of these benefits. These eligibility criteria and the fundamentals of the disability benefit programs are examined below.

THE BASIC "TWO STEP" CLAIMS DECISION PROCESS

In its evaluation of disability claims, as well as in its determination of eligibility for other VA benefits, the VA utilizes a two-step process in its initial review. First, the claimant must demonstrate that he/she is *eligible* for the VA benefit. That is, the claimant must prove that he/she is a bona fide veteran and verify certain related matters (discussed below). In this sense, the eligibility relates to the veteran's general qualification(s) for the benefit(s). Second, the veteran must prove *entitlement* to the particular benefit being sought. After it has been determined that the veteran is eligible and that he/she is entitled, the VA will then provide the appropriate benefit.

Step One: Eligibility Criteria

Definition of "Veteran"

In order to be eligible for most VA benefits, it is necessary for the claimant to be a veteran, or in some circumstances, the survivor or the dependent of a veteran. Within the context of the VA, a "veteran" is defined as a "person who served in the active military, naval, or air service, and who was discharged or released therefrom under conditions other than dishonorable."[9]

In evaluating the evidence to determine whether the applicant is a "veteran" within the context of VA benefits, the VA relies substantially upon military department service records. Generally speaking, the VA findings must be in accord with the information contained in the applicant's service records.[10]

If a claimant submits an original service department record, the VA may accept it as evidence of service and/or character of discharge.[11] The VA may accept a copy issued by the service department with the certification that it is a true document. The VA may also accept a copy submitted by an accredited agent, attorney, or service representative with special training, who certifies that it is a copy of an original service document or a copy of a copy of such a document.[12] In addition to meeting these criteria, the document needs to contain data regarding the length, time, and character of the service, and the VA must believe that the document is genuine and accurate.[13] The VA is bound by the information that the service documents contain.[14] If the claimant does not provide the requisite documentation or other evidence, or the submitted documentation does not meet the requirements, the VA must seek to verify service directly from the appropriate military service department.[15]

Discharge Criteria

The statutory definition of "veteran" requires that the individual has been discharged or released from military service "under conditions other than dishonorable."[16] There are currently five types of discharges: 1) honorable discharge (HD); 2) discharge under honorable conditions (UHC), or general discharge (GD); 3) discharge under other than honorable conditions (UOTHC), or undesirable discharge (UD); 4) bad conduct discharge (BCD); and 5) dishonorable discharge (DD).[17]

The language of the statute does not precisely match the current categories of the discharges, and the VA often makes a case-by-case determination, as discussed below. In most cases, the VA considers honorable discharges and discharges under honorable conditions to fall within the "conditions other than dishonorable" category, and will usually qualify the claimant as a veteran under the first step of the eligibility test. Usually, honorable and general discharges qualify a veteran for most benefits.

A bad conduct discharge from a special court-martial and other discharges made under other than honorable conditions may or may not allow the claimant to be considered a veteran.[18] In such circumstances, the VA will determine the issue of the character of the service by making a special "character of service determination," based on the facts in each claimant's case. After considering the service record, the VA will decide whether the veteran was separated from service under "dishonorable conditions" or under "other than dishonorable conditions." The "character of service determination" is the VA's review of the entire period of the claimant's enlistment(s) to determine the quality of the service and to determine whether it is sufficient to deserve the award of veterans' benefits.[19] The issue of discharge is further complicated if a claimant has served more than one period of enlistment, and hence the claimant may have two or more different discharge categories. The VA will review the entire service record and make its determination.

The VA Federal Benefits guide offers the following on discharges:

> Dishonorable and bad conduct discharges issued by general courts-martial may bar VA benefits. Veterans in prison and parolees may be eligible for certain VA benefits. VA regional offices can clarify the eligibility of prisoners, parolees and individuals with multiple discharges issued under differing conditions. VA benefits will not be provided to any veteran or dependent wanted for an outstanding felony warrant.[20]

Certain exceptions exist to permit the award of VA benefits, even if the character of the discharge would ordinarily bar VA benefits. For example, if it is determined that the claimant was insane at the time of the offense leading up to the discharge, the claimant may be granted

VA benefits. There does not need to be a direct connection between the insanity and the misconduct.[21]

The Requirement of Active Service

It is required that an applicant have "active military, naval, or air service" in order for the applicant to be considered a veteran for VA benefits.[22] However, not all types of service are considered active military service for the determination of eligibility for VA benefits.[23]

The VA Federal Benefits guide makes the following general statement on the active service requirement:

> Eligibility for most VA benefits is based upon discharge from active military service under other than dishonorable conditions. Active service means full-time service, other than active duty for training, as a member of the Army, Navy, Air Force, Marine Corps, Coast Guard, or as a commissioned officer of the Public Health Service, the Environmental Science Services Administration or the National Oceanic and Atmospheric Administration, or its predecessor organization, the Coast and Geodectic [sic] Survey. Men and women veterans with similar service are entitled to the same VA benefits.[24]

Active service has been determined to include 1) active duty;[25] 2) a period of active duty for training during which the person was disabled or died from an injury or disease incurred or aggravated in the line of duty;[26] and 3) any period of inactive duty for training during which the person was disabled or died from an injury incurred or aggravated in the line of duty or from certain health conditions incurred during the training.[27]

Additional circumstances of service, and whether they are deemed to be active military service, are set out in VA statutes.[28] For example: if on authorized travel to and from the performance of active duty training or inactive duty for training, the person is disabled or dies while proceeding directly to or returning from such duty, the duty will be considered to be active duty for training or inactive duty for training.[29]

The determination of whether a claimant has met the "active service" requirement may not be a simple process. It is possible that the claimant and the VA may have to scrutinize the claimant's service record(s) to determine whether service fits into one of the many categories of active service, or whether an exception has been made for his/her service, so that it is considered to be active service for the purposes of veterans' benefits. In addition, a claimant may have more than one period of service, which may further complicate the determination.

Whether the Military Service was During Time of War

Whether or not a veteran has served during time of war may impact his/her potential VA benefits. All military service is classified as either wartime or peacetime service. Certain benefits are extended only to veterans with wartime service.[30]

Congress has set out the periods of "wartime" for the purposes of veterans' pensions and other benefits.[31] To be considered to have "served during wartime" by the VA, a veteran does not have to have served in an actual combat zone, but during the specified periods of war set out below. Those time periods not designated by Congress as "wartime" are considered to be "peacetime." A veteran may have served his/her duty part during wartime and part during peacetime. The veteran would meet the "wartime" criteria if the veteran served ninety consecutive days, at least one day of which occurred during a period designated as wartime.

Following is a list of those periods of "wartime" as so designated by Congress:[32]

- *Indian Wars* — January 1, 1817, through December 31, 1898[33]
- *Spanish-American War* — April 21, 1898, through July 4, 1 902[34]
- *Mexican Border War* — May 19, 1916, though April 5, 1917[35]
- *World War I* — April 6, 1917, through November 11, 1918; extended to April 1, 1920; by regulation extended to July 1, 1921, under certain specific conditions[36]
- *World War II* — December 7, 1941, through December 31, 1946, extended to July 25, 1947[37]
- *Korean Conflict* — June 27, 1950, through January 31, 1955[38]
- *Vietnam Era* — August 5, 1964, through May 7, 1975[39]
- *Persian Gulf War* — August 2, 1990, through a date to be prescribed by Presidential proclamation or law[40]

Service Requirements: Length of Duty

Prior to September 8, 1980, there was no minimum length of service necessary to vest most VA benefits. However, for an individual who enlisted after September 8, 1980, there are now certain minimum length of service requirements. The general requirement is either twenty-four months of continuous active duty or the "full period" for which the service person was called or ordered to active duty.[41] But, several significant exceptions exist to this general rule.

Service-connected compensation benefits are exempt from the minimum active duty requirements. A veteran with a disease or injury incurred during active service should almost always be able to receive service-connected compensation for his/her condition or disability.[42]

Other significant exceptions to the minimum service requirements include claims for VA insurance benefits;[43] hardship discharges;[44] and persons retired or separated from service because of a service-related disability.[45]

If the former service member does not fall into one of the two eligible categories (twenty-four months active duty or the "full period" of active duty), or fall within one of the statutory exceptions, then the veteran has not completed a minimum period of active duty and is "not eligible for any benefit under Title 38, United States Code or under any law administered by the Department of Veterans Affairs based on that period of active service."[46]

Impediments to VA Benefits: Willful Misconduct

If the VA determines that an injury or disease resulted from "willful misconduct" on the part of the claimant, such misconduct may serve as a bar for any disability benefits. Regulations define willful misconduct as "deliberate or intentional wrongdoing with knowledge of or wanton or reckless disregard of its probable consequences."[47] Such willful misconduct is an act that involves conscious wrongdoing or known prohibited action.[48]

Veterans whose health conditions or disabilities have come about as a result of willful misconduct may not receive compensation from either the non-service-connected pension plan[49] or the service-connected disability compensation program.[50] Likewise, vocational rehabilitation benefits and certain other benefits will be denied, as such benefits are based on a service-connected condition.[51] Customarily, the VA reviews all of the circumstances of each claimant's case to determine whether there was willful misconduct on the part of the claimant.

Alcohol Abuse

For the purpose of VA benefits, alcohol abuse has been defined as "the use of alcoholic beverages over time, or such excessive use at any one time, sufficient to cause disability to or death of the user."[52] Alcohol abuse is deemed to be "willful misconduct," even though the "simple drinking of alcoholic beverage is not of itself willful misconduct."[53]

Drug Abuse

The VA has defined drug abuse rather broadly. For the purposes of VA benefits, drug abuse has been defined as the use of an illegal drug, the use of a prescription drug illegally or illicitly obtained, the use of a drug for a purpose other than that for which it was medically intended, or the use of a drug (any substance other than alcohol) to enjoy its intoxicating effect.[54] Should the claimant's use of a drug coincide with any portion of this definition, then the claimant's use is considered drug abuse. Such resultant death or disability is then not considered to have occurred in the line of duty.[55]

Unusual situations may occur when the VA considers it not to be a case of willful misconduct when a drug is used for medical purposes or when during the use of drugs, addiction or habituation to drugs results from a service-connected disability.[56] Accordingly, if a claimant develops a medical problem because of the use of prescribed medications used as prescribed to respond to a service-connected problem, the resultant problem could be considered to be service-connected and not willful misconduct.

Venereal Disease

Under certain circumstances, the VA will consider the effects of venereal disease as not the result of willful misconduct. Thus, disabilities that result from venereal disease contracted during a period of military service may be compensable.[57] However, such compensation may be withheld if it is determined that the venereal disease predated military service and that the resultant medical problems were as a result of the progress of the disease.[58]

Step Two: Entitlement to Disability Benefits

Disability Benefit Programs

Once it has been determined that the claimant is *eligible* for veterans' benefits, then it must be determined whether the claimant is *entitled* to certain benefits. Again, there are two basic disability benefit programs for veterans: the disability compensation program and the pension program. The disability compensation program is service-connected and the pension program is non-service-connected.

Requirements for the Award of Service-Connected Disability Compensation

The award of service-connected disability compensation has several requirements. First, the fundamental eligibility requirements discussed above — service and discharge requirements — must be met. Then, for a veteran to be entitled to service-connected disability compensation, the veteran must prove three elements. These elements are: 1) a medical diagnosis of the current disability; 2) medical evidence, and in some instances lay evidence, of the in-service occurrence or worsening of an injury or disease; and 3) a link between the in-service-incident or the worsening of a disease or injury and the current disability.[59] If the VA is satisfied that these three elements are proved, then the VA determines the severity of the disability.[60] The VA assigns a percentage evaluation from 0% to 100% for the amount of disability that the VA determines that the veteran has sustained.[61]

After the VA determines the percentage of disability, the VA sets an effective date for the award of the disability compensation and payments begin to the veteran.[62] Should the VA deny disability benefits, or should the veteran disagree about the percentage determination, the veteran may appeal the decision(s) through a VA appeals process.

Requirements for the Award of a Non-Service-Connected Pension

Like the service-connected disability compensation, the fundamental eligibility requirements of discharge and active wartime service must be met prior to the award of a non-service-connected pension. Then, several additional criteria must be met. First, the veteran must have a limited income.[63] In addition, it must be determined that the veteran's net worth does not provide sufficient income to meet his/her needs, known as the "needs test."[64] Second, the veteran must be permanently and totally disabled or age 65 at the time of filing the pension application.[65] Finally, the disability of the veteran must not be attributable to the willful misconduct of the veteran.[66]

Procedurally, a veteran's application for pension benefits is reviewed by the VA regional office adjudicators. They will first determine the basic eligibility of the applicant for pension benefits. After this fundamental eligibility is established, the adjudicators will look at the claimant's income and net worth. If the claimant's income or net worth is a bar to the pension benefits, the claim will be denied without a determination of the claimed disability. If the income or net worth does not seem to serve as a bar to pension benefits, the pension claim is sent on to the rating board for a disability determination.[67]

The disability determination is undertaken on a case by case basis. Congress has provided some guidance in this process. A veteran is to be considered to be permanently and totally disabled if the veteran is in *any* of the following circumstances: 1) nursing home patient for long term care because of a disability; 2) disabled, as determined by the Commissioner of Social Security for the payment of Social Security benefits; 3) unemployable because of a disability which is reasonably certain to continue through the claimant's life; or 4) suffering from a) a disability adequate to render it impossible for the average person to be gainfully employed, if the disability is expected to continue for the life of the person; or b) a disease or disorder determined by the Secretary of Veterans Affairs to *per se* result in permanent and total disability.[68]

Special rules exist for claimants who are age 65 or older. A veteran, 65 or older, who applies for a pension is presumed to be permanently and totally disabled for pension purposes. Hence, a disability determination is not required for a veteran age 65 or older to be granted pension entitlement.[69]

After the disability status is determined,[70] pension benefits are paid to the claimant on a monthly basis. However, a determination adverse to the veteran may be appealed through appropriate VA channels.

End Notes

[1] The VA was established as an executive department by the Department of Veterans Affairs Act (P.L. 100-527, 102 Stat. 2635 [October 25, 1988]). The predecessor of the Department, the Veterans Administration, had been established as an independent agency under the President by Executive Order No. 5398 of July 21, 1930, in accordance with the act of July 3, 1930 (46 Stat. 1016), which authorized the President to consolidate and coordinate the U.S. Veterans Bureau, the Bureau of Pensions, and the National Home for Volunteer Soldiers. See [http://www.va.gov].

[2] See generally *Federal Benefits for Veterans and Dependents*, published by the Department of Veterans Affairs (2008 edition)(cited to afterward as "Federal Benefits"). See [http://www 1 .va.gov/opa/vadocs/current_benefits.asp] for the publication online.

[3] See CRS Report RL33993, *Veterans' Health Care Issues*, by Sidath Viranga Panangala.

[4] See CRS Report RS20533, *VA-Home Loan Guaranty Program: An Overview*, by Bruce E. Foote, updated by Meredith Peterson.

[5] See CRS Report RS2 1545, *Military Funeral Honors: Frequently Asked Questions*, by Mari-Jana "M-J" Oboroceanu, and CRS Report RL3 27 69, *Military Death Benefits: Status and Proposals*, by David F. Burrelli and Jennifer R. Corwell.

[6] Within the VA, the Veterans Benefits Administration (VBA) administers nonmedical benefits programs for veterans, and their dependents and survivors. These benefits include veterans' compensation and pensions, survivors' benefits, education and rehabilitation assistance, home loan benefits, certain burial benefits, and insurance coverage. See [http://www.vba.va.gov].

[7] The severity of a veteran's disability is evaluated by the VA and a determination is made as to what percentage of employment capacity is impaired. For example, a 10% disability (physical or psychological) is a relatively minor disability, whereas a 80% disability determination represents a significant impairment.

[8] Federal Benefits at 29.

[9] 38 U.S.C. § 101(2); 38 C.F.R. § 3.1(d).

[10] 38 C.F.R. § 3.203.

[11] 38 C.F.R. § 3.203(a)(1). See CRS Report RS21282, *Military Records and Unit Histories A Guide to Locating Sources*, by Julissa Gomez-Granger and Kim Walker Klarman.

[12] Id.

[13] 38 C.F.R. § 3.203(a)(2), (3).

[14] Venturella v. Gober, 10 Vet. App. 340, 34 1-342 (1997); Duro v. Derwinski, 2 Vet. App. 530, 532 (1992).

[15] Duro, 2 Vet. App. at 532.

[16] 18 U.S.C. § 101(2); 38 C.F.R. § 3.12(a).

[17] Barton F. Stichman et al., *Veteran Benefits Manual*, at § 2.2.1 (Cited to afterward as "Veterans Benefits Manual").

[18] Id.

[19] Id.

[20] Federal Benefits at vii.

[21] 38 U.S.C. § 5303(b).

[22] See note 9.

[23] For example, National Guard and Reserve duty are not considered active service unless an individual performing this duty was disabled or died from a disease or injury incurred or aggravated in the line of duty. (38 U.S.C. § 101(24); 38 C.F.R. § 3.6(a)).

[24] Federal Benefits at vii.

[25] Active duty is considered to include 1) Full-time service in the Army, Navy, Marine Corps, Air Force, or Coast Guard, other than active duty for training (38 U.S.C. § 101(21)(A); 38 C.F.R. § 3.6(b)(1)); 2) Full-time service as a commissioned officer in the Public Health Service (38 U.S.C. § 101(21)(B); 38 C.F.R. § 3.6(b)(2)); 3) Full-time service as a commissioned officer at the Coast and Geodetic Survey, Environmental Services Administration, or National Oceanic and Atmospheric Administration (38 U.S.C. § 101(21)(C); 38 C.F.R. § 3.6(b)(3)); 4) Service as a cadet at a military academy (38 U.S.C. § 101(21)(D); 38 C.F.R. § 3 .6(b)(4)); 5) Attendance by active-duty members at certain prep schools associated with military academies (38 C.F.R. § 3 .6(b)(5)); and 6) Authorized travel to or from such duty or service (38 U.S.C. § 101(21)(E); 38 C.F.R. § 3.6(b)(6)).

[26] Active duty for training is a tour of active duty that is used for training members of reserve and other components to fill the Armed Forces during time of war or national emergency. Active duty for training has been determined to mean: 1) full-time duty for training performed by Reservists (38 U.S.C. § 101(22)(A); 38 C.F.R. § 3.6(c)(1)); 2) full-time duty for training purposes as a commissioned officer in the Reserved Corps of the Public Health Service (38 U.S.C. § 101(22)(B); 38 C.F.R. § 3.6(c)(2)); 3) full-time training duty by members of the Air or Army National Guard of any state (38 U.S.C. § 101 (22)(C): 38 C.F.R. § 3 .6(c)(3)); 4) duty by

members of the Senior ROTC program on field training or a practice cruise (38 U.S.C. § 101 (22)(D); 38 C.F.R. § 3.6(c)(4)); and 5) authorized travel to and from duty for training (38 U.S.C. § 101(22)(E); 38 C.F.R. § 3.6(c)(6)).

[27] 38 U.S.C. § 101(24). Inactive duty for training has been defined to mean: 1) duty, other than full-time duty, for Reservists (38 U.S.C. § 101(23)(A); 38 C.F.R. § 3.6(d)(1)); 2) other duties authorized for Reservists performed on a voluntary basis (38 U.S.C. § 101(23)(B); 38 C.F.R. § 3.6(d)(2)); 3) training (other than active duty for training) by a member of, or applicant for membership in, Senior ROTC (38 U.S.C. § 101(23)(C); 38 C.F.R. § 3.6(d)(3)); and 4) for the members of the Air or Army National Guard of any state, such training means duty other than full-time duty (38 U.S.C. § 101(23); 38 C.F.R. § 3.6(d)(4)).

[28] 38 U.S.C. §§ 101, 106. See Federal Benefits at 2.

[29] 38 U.S.C. § 106(d); 38 C.F.R. § 3.6(e).

[30] For instance, only veterans having wartime service are eligible for non-service connected disability pension benefits (38 U.S.C. §1521(j)).

[31] 38 U.S.C. § 101 (6)-(1 1); 38 C.F.R. § 3.2.

[32] See Federal Benefits at 2.

[33] See 38 C.F.R. § 3.2(a).

[34] 38 U.S.C. § 101(6); 38 C.F.R. § 3.2(b).

[35] 38 U.S.C. § 101(30); 38 C.F.R.§ 3.2(h).

[36] 38 U.S.C. § 101(7); 38 C.F.R. § 3.2(c).

[37] 38 U.S.C. § 101(8); 38 C.F.R. § 3.2(d).

[38] 38 U.S.C. § 101(9); 38 C.F.R. § 3.2(e).

[39] 38 U.S.C. § 101(29); 38 C.F.R. § 3.2(f).

[40] 38 U.S.C. §§ 101(33), 1501(4); 38 C.F.R. §§ 3.2(I), 3.3(a)(3), 3.17, 3.54(a)(3)(viii). At the present time, no termination date has been established.

[41] 38 U.S.C. § 5303A(b); 38 C.F.R. § 3.12a(a)(1).

[42] 38 U.S.C. § 5303A(b)(3)(C); 38 C.F.R. § 3.12a(d)(4).

[43] 38 U.S.C. § 5303A(b)(3)(E); 38 C.F.R. § 3.12a(d)(5).

[44] 38 U.S.C. § 5303A(b)(3)(A); 38 C.F.R. § 3.12a(d)(1).

[45] 38 U.S.C. § 5303A(b)(3)(B); 38 C.F.R. § 3.12a(d)(2).

[46] 38 U.S.C. § 5303A(b)(1); 38 C.F.R. § 3.12a(b).

[47] 38 C.F.R. § 3.1(n)(1).

[48] Id.

[49] 38 U.S.C. § 1521(a); 38 C.F.R. § 3.301(b).

[50] 38 U.S.C. § 105(a); 38 C.F.R. § 3.301(a).

[51] 38 U.S.C. § 3102.

[52] 38 C.F.R. § 3.301(d).

[53] 38 C.F.R. § 3.301(c)(2).

[54] Id. § 3.301(d).

[55] Id.

[56] 38 C.F.R. § 3.301(c)(3).

[57] 38 C.F.R. § 3.301(c)(l).

[58] Id.

[59] Veteran Benefits Manual at § 3.1.5.

[60] Id.

[61] 38 U.S.C. § 1155; 38 C.F.R. pt. 4. See CRS Report RL33991, *Disability Evaluation of Military Servicemembers*, by Christine Scott, Sidath Viranga Panangala, Sarah A. Lister, and Charles A. Henning.

[62] Rates of disability compensation are set by statute. See 38 U.S.C. § 1114 for the rates of wartime disability compensation.

[63] 38 U.S.C. § 1521; 38 C.F.R. §§ 3.271-273.

[64] 38 U.S.C. § 1522; 38 U.S.C. § 3.274.

[65] 38 U.S.C. § 1521(a); 38 C.F.R. § 4.17.

[66] See discussion at pp. 8-9.

[67] Veterans Benefits Manual at § 6.1.2.

[68] 38 U.S.C. § 1502.

[69] 38 U.S.C. §1513.

[70] The monthly benefit is offset by any other income that the veteran may have.

In: Veterans' Benefits and Care
Editor: Mathew H. Bradley

ISBN: 978-1-60692-500-3

Chapter 8

VETERANS' BENEFITS: PENSION BENEFIT PROGRAMS

Carol D. Davis and Christine Scott

SUMMARY

The Department of Veterans Affairs (VA) administers several pension benefit programs for veterans as well as their surviving spouses and dependent children. The most current pension programs available (for those meeting the eligibility criteria on or after January 1, 1979) are the Improved Disability Pension for certain low-income veterans and the Improved Death Pension for certain low-income surviving spouses or children of veterans. There is also a special pension for Medal of Honor recipients. This chapter describes these programs, including the eligibility criteria and current benefit levels. This chapter will be updated as needed to reflect legislative activity and changes to benefits or eligibility requirements.

OVERVIEW

The Department of Veterans Affairs (VA) administers several pension programs for veterans and their surviving spouses and dependent children. There are two types of pension programs administered by the VA: (1) pension programs for veterans of specific periods of war; and (2) pension programs for certain low-income veterans. The pension programs for specific periods of war are for periods before World War I. They include pension programs for veterans, as well as their surviving spouses and dependent children, of certain periods of war such as the Civil War, the Indian Wars, and the Spanish- American War. The pension programs for certain low-income veterans include the Old Law Disability Pension, the Section 306 Disability Pension, and the Improved Disability Pension. The VA pension programs for certain low-income surviving spouses and dependent children of veterans include the Old Law Death Pension, the Section 306 Death Pension, and the Improved Death Pension.

In addition to the pension programs related to periods of service for certain low- income veterans and surviving spouses and dependent children, the VA administers a special pension program for Medal of Honor recipients.

This chapter will provide information on the most current pension programs — those programs for which a veteran, a surviving spouse, or a dependent child becomes eligible on or after January 1, 1979 — and on the special pension program for Medal of Honor recipients. The current pension program for veterans is the Improved Disability Pension, which is for certain low-income veterans. The current pension program for certain low- income surviving spouses and dependent children of veterans is the Improved Death Pension. Both pension programs were created by P.L. 95-588, the Veterans and Survivors Pension Improvement Act of 1978.

The Improved Disability Pension Benefit

The Improved Disability Pension provides a monthly benefit to certain low-income veterans. The monthly benefit is based on a maximum annual benefit, and the actual benefit received by the veteran reflects a reduction (from the maximum amount) of the veteran's "countable" income. This means that a veteran with countable income above the maximum benefit amount is not eligible for the pension.

Maximum Annual Benefit Amount

The maximum annual benefit amounts for the veterans' pension benefit are set in statute[1] and are based on the presence of a spouse or dependent child (or children) and the need for aid and attendance.[2] The annual benefit amounts are adjusted automatically by law[3] each year to reflect a cost-of-living adjustment (COLA) equal to the COLA for Social Security benefits. For example, beginning December 1, 2007, the maximum annual amount for the pension benefit is $11,181 for a veteran and $14,643 for a veteran with one dependent.[4] If two veterans are married to each other, the maximum annual amount is $14,643, the same as for a veteran with one dependent. The maximum annual benefit amount will be higher if the veteran is housebound or requires aid and attendance.[5]

Eligibility Criteria

To be eligible for the pension benefit, a veteran must meet eligibility criteria related to combat/period of service; income/net worth; and age or disability.

Combat/Period of Service

A veteran must meet military service requirements related to combat, or service during a period of war.[6] Specifically, a veteran must have been discharged from military service under conditions other than dishonorable and must have served in the active military:

- for at least 90 days during a period of war;[7]
- during a period of war and was released from service for a service- connected disability;
- for 90 or more consecutive days which began or ended during a period of war; or

- for a total of 90 days or more in two or more separate periods of service during one or more periods of war.

Income/Net Worth

As noted previously, the pension benefit for a veteran who meets the other eligibility requirements (combat/period of service and disability/age) is calculated by subtracting the veteran's annual countable income from the statutory annual maximum benefit. This means that a veteran with annual countable income above the annual maximum benefit amount will receive no pension benefit. A veteran with annual countable income below the annual maximum benefit amount will have his or her benefit reduced dollar for dollar by the amount of annual countable income. In addition, a veteran may not have a net worth, or estate, large enough that it would be reasonable for part of the estate to be used for the veteran's maintenance.[8]

Annual countable income includes income from nearly all sources. However, there are several specific sources of income that are *not included* in determining annual countable income:[9]

- donations from public welfare or private relief organizations;
- pension benefits administered by the VA;
- expenses paid by a veteran's spouse (or the veteran's surviving spouse or child) for the veteran's last illness, burial, or debts;
- amounts paid by the veteran for the last illness and burial of the veteran's spouse or child;
- amounts paid by a veteran's spouse for the last illness and burial of the veteran's child;
- insurance reimbursement for property casualty loss (up to the greater of fair market value or replacement value);
- profit from disposing of personal or real property (other than in the course of business);
- amounts in joint accounts the veteran acquires by the death of the other owner(s);
- amounts paid by the veteran, spouse, or child for unreimbursed medical expenses (limited to a maximum of 5% of the pension benefit); and
- amounts paid by a veteran or surviving spouse to pursue education, vocational rehabilitation, or training, including tuition, fees, books, and, if the veteran or surviving spouse needs aid and attendance, travel expenses above reasonable expenses for a nondisabled person.

Disability/Age

To be eligible for the pension benefit, the veteran must be totally disabled[10] due to non-service connected injuries or illnesses that are not a result of the veteran's willful misconduct.[11] However, to determine if a veteran is totally disabled, the Secretary of Veterans Affairs may combine the disability ratings for service-connected disabilities with the disability ratings for non-service connected disabilities. The restriction is that if the veteran's service-connected disabilities have contributed to making the veteran eligible for the pension benefit, the veteran will receive the greater of the pension benefit or the disability compensation benefit (for the service-connected disabilities). A veteran cannot receive both disability compensation and the pension benefit.

P.L. 107-103, the Veterans Education and Benefit Expansion Act of 2001, extended the pension benefit to veterans aged 65 or over, regardless of disability status (or disability rating), who meet the other pension requirements (combat/period and income/net worth).

Other

The pension benefit for a veteran convicted of a felony or misdemeanor will be stopped beginning 61 days after the veteran is imprisoned, and it will resume when the imprisonment ends. The veteran's pension benefit may be paid to the veteran's spouse or dependent children during the veteran's imprisonment.

To apply for the pension benefit, a veteran must complete and submit VA Form 21- 526, which is the application form for both disability compensation and the pension benefit. As part of the claims processing, the veteran will receive a disability rating, which may require a physical examination.

Interaction with Social Security and Supplemental Security Income (SSI)

Countable income for the veterans' pension benefit includes any Social Security benefits received. Therefore, the receipt of Social Security benefits can reduce or eliminate a veteran's pension benefit. Countable income does not include any Supplemental Security Income (SSI) payments received. However, because the SSI program includes veterans' benefits as unearned income in calculating the income limitations for SSI, a veteran's pension benefit could reduce the veteran's SSI benefit.[12]

The Improved Death Pension Benefit

The surviving spouse or dependent child of a veteran may be eligible for the Improved Death Pension Benefit if eligibility requirements with respect to the deceased veteran and surviving spouse or dependent child are met, along with an income requirement.

Deceased Veteran

The deceased veteran must have met the military service requirements for the Improved Disability Pension with respect to the veteran's discharge and period of service.[13] However, for the Improved Death Pension, an individual who has at least two years of honorable military service and who dies in military service but not in the line of duty is also considered a veteran.[14]

Surviving Spouse

The surviving spouse cannot be remarried and must have been married to the deceased veteran:[15]

- for at least one year (there is no minimum if the surviving spouse and veteran had a child), and
- must have been wed before December 14, 1944 for deceased veterans of the Mexican border period and World War I; before January 1, 1957 for deceased veterans of

World War II; before February 1, 1965 for deceased veterans of the Korean conflict; before May 8, 1985 for deceased veterans of the Vietnam era; or before January 1, 2001 for deceased veterans of the Persian Gulf War.

Surviving Children

Surviving children must be under age 18 (or under age 23 if in school) or must have become incapable of self-care before age 18.

Income

The countable income for a surviving spouse or child is calculated like that of a veteran for the Improved Disability Pension. However, for a surviving spouse with custody of a deceased veteran's child, part of the child's income that is available to the surviving spouse may be included in countable income.[16] For a veteran's surviving child, his or her current work income is excluded from countable income, if the income is not more than the income level at which a federal income tax return must be filed[17] *plus* postsecondary education or vocational rehabilitation or training expenses paid by the child.[18] In addition, for a surviving spouse or child, the proceeds from a life insurance policy on the veteran is excluded from countable income.[19]

Maximum Benefit Amount

The maximum annual benefit amounts for surviving spouses and dependent children, like those for veterans, are set in statute and are automatically increased to reflect the COLA for Social Security benefits. For example, effective December 1, 2007,[20] the maximum annual benefit amount for a surviving spouse without a dependent child is $7,498, and $9,815 for a surviving spouse with a dependent child (there is an incremental amount for each dependent child). Maximum annual benefit amounts are higher if the surviving spouse is housebound or requires aid and attendance.[21] For a surviving child, the maximum annual benefit amount is $1,909.

Medal of Honor Pension

A veteran who has been awarded a Medal of Honor is eligible for a monthly pension ($1,129 as of December 1, 2007).[22] Eligibility for the pension is based solely on receipt of the Medal of Honor, and receipt of the special pension (the Medal of Honor recipient must elect to receive the special pension) does not reduce any other benefits under U.S. law. A veteran who has received more than one Medal of Honor is, however, limited to receiving only one Medal of Honor pension benefit.[23]

End Notes

[1] 38 U.S.C. §1521(b)-§1521(g).

[2] Aid and attendance is provided when a veteran needs another person's help to perform activities of daily living, such as eating, dressing, or taking a shower.

[3] 38 U.S.C. §53 12.

[4] These figures reflect the cost-of-living adjustment (COLA) for Social Security benefits beginning January 2008. For more information on the Social Security COLA, see CRS Report 94-803, *Social Security: The Cost-of-Living Adjustment in January 2008*, by Gary Sidor.

[5] For more information on current rates, please see the Department of Veterans Affairs Website at [http://www.vba.va.gov/bln/2 1/Rates/pen0 1 .htm].

[6] 38 U.S.C. §1521(j).

[7] For information on periods of war, see CRS Report RS21405, *Periods of War*, by Barbara Salazar Torreon.

[8] 38 U.S.C. § 1522.

[9] 38 U.S.C. § 1503.

[10] The VA rates disability on a scale of 0-100 in 10% increments, with 100% being totally disabled. The rating is used for pensions and for disability compensation. For more information on disability evaluation by the VA, see the "VA Disability Evaluation" section of CRS Report RL3399 1, *Disability Evaluation of Military Servicemembers*, by Christine Scott, Sidath Viranga Panangala, Sarah A. Lister, and Charles A. Henning.

[11] 38 U.S.C. §1513 and 38 U.S.C. §1521.

[12] For more information on the SSI program, see CRS Report 94-486, *Supplemental Security Income (SSI): A Fact Sheet*, by Scott Szymendera, and CRS Report RS20294, *SSI Income and Resource Limits: A Fact Sheet*, by Scott Szymendera.

[13] 38 U.S.C. § 1541(a) and § 1542(a).

[14] 38 U.S.C. § 1541(h).

[15] 38 U.S.C. §1541(f).

[16] 38 U.S.C. § 1541(g).

[17] The income level at which a tax return must be filed (the filing requirement) is equal to the sum of the standard deduction and personal exemption amounts. For tax year 2008, the filing requirement for a single taxpayer is $8,950 for a taxpayer under age 65.

[18] 38 U.S.C. §1503(a)(10).

[19] 38 U.S.C. §1503(a)(11).

[20] These figures reflect the cost-of-living adjustment (COLA) for Social Security benefits beginning January 2008. For more information on the Social Security COLA, see CRS Report 94-803, *Social Security: The Cost-of-Living Adjustment in January 2008*, by Gary Sidor.

[21] For more information on current rates, please see the Department of Veterans Affairs Website at [http://www.vba.va.gov/bln/2 1/Rates/pen02.htm].

[22] The pension benefit was increased to $1,000 and a COLA was provided by P.L. 107-330, the Veterans Benefits Act of 2002.

[23] 38 U.S.C. §1562.

In: Veterans' Benefits and Care
Editor: Mathew H. Bradley

ISBN: 978-1-60692-500-3

Chapter 9

HEALTH CARE FOR DEPENDENTS AND SURVIVORS OF VETERANS

Sidath Viranga Panangala and Susan Janeczko

SUMMARY

The Civilian Health and Medical Program of the Department of Veterans Affairs (CHAMPVA) is primarily a fee-for-service program that provides reimbursement for most medical care for certain eligible dependents and survivors of veterans rated permanently and totally disabled from a service-connected condition. This chapter provides an overview of CHAMPVA and includes a series of questions and answers about the program. The report will be updated as legislative or programmatic changes warrant.

OVERVIEW

The Veterans Health Administration (VHA) of the Department of Veterans Affairs (VA) provides health care services to veterans who meet certain eligibility requirements. The VHA is primarily a direct service provider of primary care, specialized care, and related medical and social support services to veterans though an integrated health care system. In 1973, Congress established the Civilian Health and Medical Program of the Department of Veterans Affairs (CHAMPVA) as a means of providing health care services to dependents and survivors of certain veterans.[1] As stated in the House report accompanying P.L. 93-82:

> "The nation has long recognized that the widow and children of a veteran who dies of service-connected disease or injury or of a veteran who has a service-connected total disability are in a special category and deserving of substantial compensation and assistance in return for the sacrifice the family has made. This recognition has been shown in title 38 programs which provide for death compensation benefits, home loans, and educational assistance

benefits for wives, widows, and war orphans. Failure to provide for the medical care of such individuals is an oversight which should be corrected."[2]

CHAMPVA primarily is a fee-for-service program that provides reimbursement for most medical care for certain eligible dependents and survivors of veterans rated permanently and totally disabled from a service-connected condition.[3] CHAMPVA is a cost-sharing program that reimburses providers and facilities a determined allowable amount, minus patient co-pay and deductible. CHAMPVA was designed to provide medical care in a manner similar to the care provided to certain eligible beneficiaries under the Department of Defense (DOD) TRICARE program (see the description below). The number of beneficiaries enrolled in CHAMPVA has grown over the years. From FY2002 through the second quarter of FY2008, enrollment grew by 175% — from 112,403 to 308,700 beneficiaries (see **Figure 1**). The 2001 expansion of CHAMPVA eligibility to certain individuals aged 65 years and older has contributed to the increase in enrollment. Moreover, there has been an increase in enrollment of dependents and spouses of certain Vietnam-era veterans with service-connected disabilities. This increase in Vietnam-era CHAMPVA sponsorship has occurred as aging Vietnam-era veterans with service-connected disabilities experience a worsening of symptoms and a change in disability status. Once a veteran becomes VA-rated permanently and totally disabled for a service-connected disability, the veteran's spouse and dependents are then eligible to enroll in CHAMPVA.

Moreover, the number of unique CHAMPVA users has grown by 149% from FY2002 to FY2007 (see **Figure 2**). Unique users are enrollees who utilize a health benefit at least once in a fiscal year.

Funding for CHAMPVA is provided through the VHA's Medical Services account.[4] As shown in **Table 1**, spending for CHAMPVA grew from approximately $200 million in FY2002 to approximately $835 million in FY2008, a 311% increase over the seven- year period. Between FY2002 and FY2007, CHAMPVA expenditures increased by 251%, while the number of unique users increased by only 149% during the same period. These data imply an increased average cost per patient from approximately $2,495 per patient in FY2002 to $3,512 per patient in FY2007. A demographic shift in CHAMPVA enrollees from less expensive younger beneficiaries to more expensive aging beneficiaries, in addition to the general inflation of medical costs, has contributed to the increase in CHAMPVA expenditures.

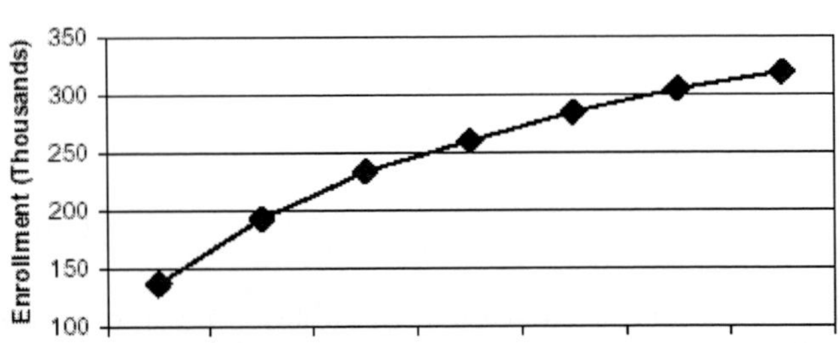

Source: Chart prepared by CRS, based on data from the Department of Veterans Affairs.
*Note: Projected enrollment; actual second quarter enrollment 308,700.

Figure 1. CHAMPVA-Enrolled Beneficiaries, FY2002-FY2008

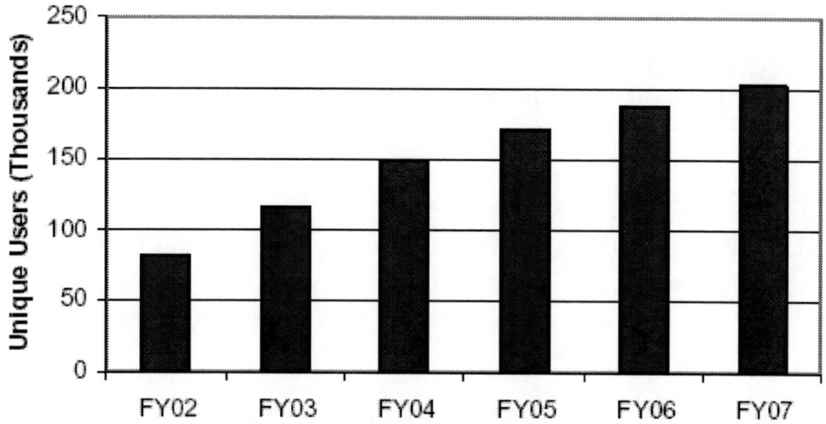

Source: Chart prepared by CRS, based on data from the Department of Veterans Affairs.

Figure 2. CHAMPVA Unique Users, FY2002-FY2007

Table 1. CHAMPVA Expenditures, FY2002-FY2008 (Dollars in millions)

	FY2002 Actual	FY2003 Actual	FY2004 Actual	FY2005 Actual	FY2006 Actual	FY2007 Actual	FY2008 Estimated
Expenditures	$203.1	$318.2	$454.5	$565.5	$656.9	$712.2	$834.8

Source: Table prepared by CRS, based on data from the U.S. Department of Veterans Affairs, *Congressional Budget Submissions (FY2004-09), Medical Programs*.

The next section provides answers to frequently asked questions about the program.

Questions and Answers[5]

Who Is Eligible to Receive CHAMPVA Benefits?

Eligibility for CHAMPVA requires inclusion in one of the following categories:[6]

- the individual is the spouse or child of a veteran who has been rated permanently and totally disabled for a service-connected disability;
- the individual is the surviving spouse or child of a veteran who died from a VA-rated service-connected disability;
- the individual is the surviving spouse or child of a veteran who was at the time of death rated permanently and totally disabled from a service-connected disability;
- or the individual is the surviving spouse or child of a military member who died on active duty, not due to misconduct (in most cases, these family members are eligible under TRICARE, not CHAMPVA).

What Happens if a CHAMPVA-Eligible Spouse Divorces or Remarries?

CHAMPVA eligibility is terminated by divorce or annulment of marriage to the qualifying veteran. CHAMPVA has specific eligibility rules for widows. When a

CHAMPVA-eligible widow remarries, eligibility is terminated if the marriage occurs before the age of 55. As of February 4, 2003, a CHAMPVA-eligible widow who remarries at age 55 or older remains eligible for CHAMPVA. If a CHAMPVA-eligible widow under the age of 55 remarries, and the remarriage is later terminated, the widow is again eligible for CHAMPVA.

When Does a Child Lose Eligibility?

In general, eligibility for CHAMPVA is lost when either a child (other than a helpless child)[7] turns 18, unless enrolled in an accredited school as a full-time student; a child, who has been a full-time student, turns 23 or loses full-time student status; a child marries; or a stepchild no longer lives in the household of the sponsor.

What Is the Difference Between CHAMPVA and TRICARE?

Before distinguishing between the two programs, it is important to make the distinction between a veteran and a military retiree. Title 38 of the United States Code defines a "veteran" as a person who has been discharged under conditions other than dishonorable from active military, naval, or air service.[8] All military retirees, by definition, are veterans. However, to be considered a "military retiree," an individual generally must have spent at least 20 years on active duty in the armed services. CHAMPVA is a comprehensive program run by the VA for eligible family members of veterans rated permanently and totally disabled for a service-connected disability or the family members of veterans who died from a VA-rated service-connected disability. The sponsoring veteran does not receive services through CHAMPVA, as he or she is eligible to receive services through the VA. Dependents of military retirees are not eligible for CHAMPVA, and must apply for benefits through TRICARE. TRICARE is a health care program run by the DOD for families of active duty military service members, families of service members who died while on active duty, and retired military service men, women, and their families, regardless of their disability status. TRICARE has no disability criteria required for eligibility.[9]

What Is the Relationship of CHAMPVA and Medicare?

Under section three of the Veterans' Survivors Benefits Improvement Act of 2001, referred to as CHAMPVA for Life (P.L. 107-14), CHAMPVA benefits were expanded to those over the age of 65 in the following circumstances. CHAMPVA is the secondary payer for beneficiaries with Medicare coverage.

- If a beneficiary turns 65 before June 5, 2001, and only receives Medicare Part A, the beneficiary is eligible for CHAMPVA without having to purchase Medicare Part B coverage.
- If a beneficiary turns 65 before June 5, 2001, and receives both Medicare Part A and Part B, the beneficiary must retain both parts to be eligible for continued CHAMPVA as secondary coverage.
- If a beneficiary turns 65 on or after June 5, 2001, the beneficiary must be enrolled in Medicare Parts A and B to be eligible for CHAMPVA.
- Enrollment in Medicare Part D is not required to become or remain eligible for CHAMPVA.

- Individuals aged 65 or older not entitled to Medicare Part A retain CHAMPVA eligibility.

What Happens if the Beneficiary Has Other Health Insurance?

By law, CHAMPVA is generally the secondary payer for beneficiaries having any other form of health insurance. The primary health insurance company is billed first, and then beneficiaries submit an explanation of benefits (EOB) for additional reimbursement by CHAMPVA. The exception is for beneficiaries with Medicaid, beneficiaries receiving care under the State Victims of Crime Compensation Program, or beneficiaries with a CHAMPVA supplementary insurance policy. In those cases, CHAMPVA is the first payer.[10]

What Medical Benefits Are Available to Eligible Beneficiaries?

The CHAMPVA program covers most health care services and supplies that are determined to be medically necessary, including inpatient and outpatient care, prescription drugs, mental health services, and skilled nursing care. By law, CHAMPVA is required to provide health care benefits that are similar to the DOD's TRICARE program. Chiropractic services, routine eye examinations, hearing aids, and most dental benefits are excluded from both the federal CHAMPVA and TRICARE programs.[11]

What Is the CHAMPVA Payment Structure?

CHAMPVA is a cost-sharing program that reimburses at rates comparable to the Medicare and TRICARE programs. CHAMPVA has an outpatient deductible of $50 per person and $100 per family per calender year. After the deductible is reached, CHAMPVA pays 75% of the allowable amount, and the beneficiary pays 25% of the total amount.[12] The patient typically pays the cost share at the time the service is provided, unless the beneficiary has another health insurance plan. In cases where a beneficiary has another form of health insurance, CHAMPVA is the secondary payer (with the exception of the circumstances outlined in question five), and pays the lesser of either 75% of the allowable amount after the deductible or the rest of the billed charges. There is a $3,000 cap on cost sharing per CHAMPVA-eligible family. There is also an exception to the payment scheme outlined here for instances in which medical services are rendered through VA facilities participating in the CHAMPVA In-house Treatment Initiative (CITI).[13]

What Is the CHAMPVA In-House Treatment Initiative (CITI)?

The CITI is a voluntary program for CHAMPVA beneficiaries that provides medical care through local VA facilities on a space-available basis. Beneficiaries receiving care at the VA through the CITI program are not required to pay a deductible or participate in cost sharing. No extra enrollment is necessary to participate in the CITI program; the beneficiary simply has to determine if the local VA is a participating facility. The majority of VA facilities are CITI participants. It is important to emphasize that care is delivered based on the availability of space. Beneficiaries on Medicare or who have an HMO plan as their primary insurance are not eligible for the CITI program.

How Are CHAMPVA ClaimsPprocessed?

All CHAMPVA claims are processed through the VA Health Administration Center (HAC) in Denver, Colorado. Claims can be submitted by either the provider or the beneficiary, with each case requiring a different set of forms. All claims must be filed within one year after the date of service. For inpatient care, the claim must be filed within one year of the discharge date, and all payments will be made to the hospital regardless of which party submits the billing. Claims submitted after the one-year deadline will be denied.

End Notes

[1] Veterans Health Care Expansion Act of 1973 (P.L. 93-82).

[2] U.S. Congress, Committee on Veterans' Affairs, *Veterans Health Care Expansion Act of 1973*, report to accompany H.R. 9048, 93rd Congress, first session, H.Rept. 93-3 68 (Washington: GPO, 1973).

[3] The term "service-connected" means, with respect to disability, that such disability was incurred or aggravated in the line of duty in the active military, naval, or air service. VA determines whether veterans have service-connected disabilities, and for those with such disabilities, assigns ratings from 0 to 100% based on the severity of the disability. Percentages are assigned in increments of 10%.

[4] For detailed information on VHA appropriations, see CRS Report RL34063, *Veterans' Medical Care: FY2008 Appropriations*, by Sidath Viranga Panangala.

[5] This part was drawn from: Department of Veterans Affairs Health Administration Center, *CHAMPVA 2006 Handbook,* November 2006, at [http://www.va.gov/hac/forbeneficiaries/ champva/handbook/chandbook.pdf] and [http://www.va.gov/hac], visited June 2, 2008.

[6] 38 U.S.C. § 1781; 38 C.F.R. § 17.270-17.278.

[7] A helpless child is established after a fact-based analysis completed by a VA Regional Office determines the child to be permanently incapable of self-support by the age of 18. See 38 C.F.R. § 3.356 and [http://www.va.gov/hac/forbeneficiaries/champva/handbook/chandbook.pdf].

[8] 38 U.S.C. § 101.

[9] For further information on TRICARE, see CRS Report RL33 537, *Military Medical Care: Questions and Answers*, by Richard A. Best Jr.; and the Department of Defense, *Evaluation of the TRICARE Program: FY2005 Report to the Congress*, March 1, 2005, pp. 63. For specific provisions, see [http://www.TRICARE.osd.mil]; relevant regulations are at 32 C.F.R. § 199.

[10] 38 C.F.R. § 17.275.

[11] 38 C.F.R. § 17.272.

[12] An allowable amount is the maximum payment that is authorized by the VA for a covered medial service or supply.

[13] 38 C.F.R. § 17.274.

In: Veterans' Benefits and Care
Editor: Mathew H. Bradley

ISBN: 978-1-60692-500-3

Chapter 10

"WOUNDED WARRIOR" AND VETERANS PROVISIONS IN THE FY2008 NATIONAL DEFENSE AUTHORIZATION ACT

Sarah A. Lister, Sidath Viranga Panangala and Christine Scott

SUMMARY

This chapter summarizes provisions in Division A, Titles XVI and XVII, of the National Defense Authorization Act for Fiscal Year 2008, P.L. 110-181, signed by the President on January 28, 2008. Titles XVI and XVII address matters related to the care and treatment of servicemembers and former servicemembers (i.e., veterans) who were wounded, or who contracted an illness, while serving on active duty. These individuals are widely referred to as "wounded warriors."

Provisions in the act reflect congressional concern about the quality and availability of medical, mental health, and dental care services for servicemembers returning from active duty in Iraq and Afghanistan, and the difficulties that some of theseindividuals haveexperiencedin their transition from military service to veteran status. The provisions vary in scope. Some of them alter specific aspects of existing services or benefits programs in either the Department of Defense (DOD) or the Department of Veterans Affairs (VA). Others call for comprehensive and long-term redesign of programs or systems in one or both of the departments. Congress and others have determined that certain programs and systems that involve both departments are particularly problematic in providing continuity and quality of care and services to wounded warriors. Among the problems addressed in the act are the efficient maintenance and transfer of servicemembers' health and benefits records between the departments, and the separate evaluations of disability by each department. Efforts to address these and other transition problems were already underway in both departments, partly in response to the recommendations of several DOD and independent commissions and task forces. The act codifies various mandates for these activities, including deadlines.

This chapter does not attempt to analyze provisions in the act, but provides brief outlines of the matters addressed.

LEGISLATIVE HISTORY AND OVERVIEW

The FY2008 National Defense Authorization bill, H.R. 1585, was adopted by the House on December 12, and by the Senate on December 14, 2007. On December 28, the White House announced that the President would "pocket veto" the bill, a procedure that would preclude efforts by Congress to override the veto. The President objected to a provision of the bill that would allow lawsuits in U.S. courts against the current Iraqi government for damages resulting from acts of the Saddam Hussein regime. On January 16, 2008, the House passed H.R. 4986, a version of H.R. 1585 that was modified to allow the President to waive application to Iraq of the provision that he had cited as grounds for his veto.[1] H.R. 4986 was subsequently passed by the Senate and signed by the President on January 28, 2008, becoming P.L. 110-181, the National Defense Authorization Act for Fiscal Year 2008.

Division A of the act provides Department of Defense authorizations. Within Division A, Titles XVI ("Wounded WarriorMatters") and XVII ("Veterans Matters") address matters related to the care and treatment of injured or ill servicemembers. These individuals are widely referred to as "wounded warriors." Provisions in the act reflect congressional concern about the quality and availability of medical, mental health, and dentalcare services for servicemembers returning from active dutyinIraq and Afghanistan, and thedifficulties that some of these individuals have experienced in their transition from military service to veteran status. The provisions vary in scope. Some of them alter specific aspects of existing services or benefits programs in either the Department of Defense (DOD) or the Department of Veterans Affairs (VA). Others call for comprehensive and long-term assessment and/or redesign of programs or systems in one or both of the departments. This chapter does not attempt to analyze each of the provisions in the act, but provides brief outlines of the matters addressed.[2]

ABBREVIATIONS AND ACRONYMS

Unless otherwise noted, references in this chapter to activities of "DOD" (including mentions in Title XVI) or "VA" (including mentions in Title XVII) are activities to be carried out by the Secretary of the stated department. The following acronyms and abbreviations are used:

MTF: military treatment facility
OEF: Operation Enduring Freedom
OIF: Operation Iraqi Freedom
PDES: the DOD's Physical Disability Evaluation System
PTSD: post-traumatic stress disorder
TBI: traumatic brain injury
TDRL: Temporary Disability Retired List
TSGLI: Traumatic Servicemembers' Group Life Insurance
VASRD: Veterans Administration Schedule for Rating Disabilities
WRAMC: Walter Reed Army Medical Center

TITLE XVI: WOUNDED WARRIOR MATTERS

Section 1601 is the short title.

Sec. 1602. General Definitions

This section provides a number of definitions for terms used in the act. Selected definitions are provided below.

The term "medical care" includes mental health care. The term "outpatient status," with respect to a recovering servicemember, means the status of a recovering servicemember assigned to a military medical treatment facility (MTF) as an outpatient, or to a unit established for the purpose of providing command and control of members of the Armed Forces receiving medical care as outpatients. The term "recovering servicemember" means a member of the Armed Forces, including a member of the National Guard or a Reserve, who is undergoing medical treatment, recuperation, or therapy and is in an outpatient status while recovering from a serious injury or illness related to the member's military service. The term "serious injury or illness," in the case of a member of the Armed Forces, means an injury or illness incurred by the member in the line of duty while on active duty in the Armed Forces that may render the member medically unfit to perform the duties of the member's office, grade, rank, or rating.

Sec. 1603. Gender-Specific Needs

Requires the Secretaries of Defense and Veterans Affairs to take into account and address fully any unique gender-specific needs of recovering servicemembers and veterans when developing and implementing a comprehensive policy on improvements to their care, management, and transition.

Subtitle A: Care, Management, and Transition Policy

At the core of this subtitle is a joint requirement of the Secretaries of DOD and VA to develop a comprehensive policy on the care and management of covered servicemembers, to address medical care and case management, medical and disability evaluation, return to duty when appropriate, and transition from DOD to VA.

Sec. 1611. Comprehensive Care and Transition Policy

Requires DOD and VA, not later than July 1, 2008, and updated at least annually, to develop and implement a comprehensive policy on the care and management of covered servicemembers. The Secretaries are to consult with heads of other relevant federal departments and agencies, and to consider the recommendations of a number of listed studies, reviews, reports, and evaluations. The policy shall address care and management, medical and disabilityevaluation, return to duty when appropriate, and transition from DOD to VA.

Requires the development, in policy, of uniform standards, among the military departments and with the VA, for the training and skills of health care professionals, recovery care coordinators, medical care case managers, and non-medical care managers for recovering servicemembers. Requires the development of *comprehensive recovery plans*, and the assignment of a *Recovery Care Coordinator,* for each recovering servicemember. Special attention is to be paid to recognizing early warning signs of post-traumatic stress disorder (PTSD) and suicide, and managing these conditions. The policy is to address several additional aspects of access to health care and other assistance, including waiting times, patient tracking, family support, and others.

Sec. 1612. Medical and Disability Evaluations

Requires DOD to develop uniform standards and procedures for disability evaluations of recovering servicemembers across military departments. Requires the Secretaries of DOD and VA to report to Congress on the feasibility and advisability of combining the two departments' disability evaluation systems.[3]

Sec. 1613. Return to Active Duty

Requires DOD to establish standards for determinations by the military departments on the return of recovering servicemembers to active duty.

Sec. 1614. Transition from DOD to VA Care

By July 1, 2008, DOD and the VA are jointly to develop and implement detailed procedures and standards for servicemembers in their transition from health care and treatment provided by DOD to health care, treatment, and rehabilitation provided by the VA. Procedures and standards are to address, among other things, patient tracking, enrollment for benefits, and training and deployment of personnel.

Sec. 1615. Reports

Requires the Secretaries of DOD and VA jointly to report to Congress on the status of certain requirements in Section 1611, namely the policy to improve the care, management, and transition of recovering service-members; the review of current policies and procedures; and the review of the recommendations of a number of studies, reviews, reports, and evaluations listed in Section 1611. Requires the Comptroller General, within six months of enactment and annually through 2010, to report to Congress regarding implementation of the policy required in Section 1611. Requires the Secretary of Defense, not later than February 1, 2009, to report to Congress on the number of instances between October 7, 2001, and September 30, 2006, in which a disability rating assigned to a member of the Armed Forces by an informal DOD physical evaluation board was reduced upon appeal, and the reasons for such reduction.

Sec. 1616. Wounded Warrior Resource Center

Requires the Secretary of Defense to establish a wounded warrior resource center to provide wounded warriors, their families, and their primary caregivers with a single point of contact for assistance with reporting deficiencies in covered military facilities, obtaining health care services, receiving benefits information, and any other difficulties encountered while supporting wounded warriors. (See also the reporting requirement in Section 1648.)

Sec. 1617. Congressional Notification of Combat Wounded

Requires DOD to notify appropriate congressional offices of hospitalization of servicemembers evacuated from a theater of combat. Consent of the servicemember is required.

Sec. 1618. Comprehensive TBI/PTSD Plan

Requires the Secretaries of DOD and VA to conduct joint planning for the prevention, diagnosis, mitigation, treatment, and rehabilitation of, and research on, traumatic brain injury (TBI), PTSD, and other mental health conditions in members of the Armed Forces, including planning for the seamless transition of such members to veteran status. Twelve required planning elements are specified, including designation of a lead agent to develop and coordinate the plan, development of screening protocols, and other matters. The required plan shall include a program whereby all servicemembers who incur TBI or PTSD while on active duty receive the highest quality, evidence-based treatment and rehabilitation.

Subtitle B: Centers of Excellence

This subtitle requires the Secretary of Defense to establish three centers of excellence, addressing TBI, PTSD, and military eye injuries, respectively. In establishing each center, the Secretary is to collaborate with the Department of Veterans Affairs, institutions of higher education, and other appropriate public and private entities, including international entities. The TBI and PTSD Centers are required, among other things, to implement the comprehensive TBI/PTSD plan developed pursuant to Section 1618 of this act. The Center of Excellence for Military Eye Injuries is required, amongother things, to implement a comprehensive plan and strategy for a DOD "Military Eye Injury Registry" regarding the diagnosis, treatment, and follow up of significant eye injuries (defined) incurred by a servicemember while on active duty. The Secretary of Defense is required, within 180 days of enactment, and annually thereafter, to report to Congress regarding each center, its activities, and its progress in discharging its responsibilities.

Subtitle C: Health Care Matters

Sec. 1631. Medical Care and Other Benefits

Former servicemembers with serious injuries or illnesses may receive medical and dental care from DOD if care is not "reasonably available" from the VA. DOD is not authorized to provide such care after December 31, 2012, if such care had not been provided to a former servicemember prior to that date.

Sec. 1632. Reimbursement of Travel Expenses

Requires the Secretaries of the military services to establish outreach programs to ensure that retired servicemembers with a combat-related disability receive travel reimbursements for which they are eligible, for specialty care, services, or supplies related to a combat-related disability.

Sec. 1633. Respite Care and Other Extended Care Benefits

Requires the Secretary of Defense to make servicemembers who incur a serious injury or illness on active duty eligible for the respite care and aid and personal attendant benefits comparable to those currently provided in the Tricare Extended Care Health Option. Requires the Secretary to prescribe in regulations the individuals who shall be considered as the primary caregivers of the servicemember, and the definition of serious injury or illness.

Sec. 1634. Reports

Requires the Secretary of Defense, within 90 days of enactment, to report to Congress regarding the implementation of provisions in the FY2007 Defense authorization relating to a longitudinal study on TBI incurred by servicemembers in Operation Enduring Freedom (OEF) and Operation Iraqi Freedom (OIF), and pilot projects on early diagnosis and treatment of PTSD and other mental health conditions. Requires the Secretary, not later than March 1, 2008, and each year thereafter through 2013, to report to Congress regarding funding for the preceding year for activities relating to the improved diagnosis, treatment, and rehabilitation of servicemembers with TBI or PTSD.

Sec. 1635. Interoperable Electronic Health Information

Requires DOD and VA jointly to develop and implement a system of electronic health records that allows for full interoperability of personal health care information between the two departments. Establishes an interagency program office to act as a single point of accountability for the departments, and to implement, not later than September 30, 2009, the required system of records. Establishes leadership, membership, staffing, funding, reporting requirements, and other matters regarding the office. The system of records shall be developed in coordination with the Office of the National Coordinator for Health Information Technology, in the Department of Health and Human Services.

The office shall develop, and prepare for deployment, a joint electronic health record to be used by both departments in the provision of medical care and treatment to members of the Armed Forcesand veterans, in compliance with applicable federal interoperability standards, implementation specifications, and certification criteria (including for the reporting of quality measures). Requires the Secretaries of Defense and Veterans Affairs, within 30 days of enactment, to establish a schedule and benchmarks for implementing the required interoperable system of records. Authorizes the Secretaries to conduct pilot projects to assess the technical feasibility of various approaches, consistent with privacy regulations promulgated pursuant to the Health Insurance Portability and Accountability Act of 1996 (42 U.S.C. 1320d-2 note). Requires the Comptroller General, within six months of enactment and every six months thereafter until completion of implementation, to report to Congress regarding progress in implementing the required system of records.

Sec. 1636. Enhanced DOD Personnel Authorities

Authorizes the Secretary of Defense, until September 30, 2010, to exercise authorities for the appointment and pay of health care personnel that are currently available to the Secretary of Veterans Affairs for the purposes of recruitment, employment, and retention of civilian health care professionals.[4] Requires the Secretaries of the military services to each develop and implement a strategy to disseminate, among appropriate personnel of the military departments, information about authorities and best practices for the recruitment of medical and health professionals.

Sec. 1637. Continuation of Transitional Health Benefits

Authorizes DOD to provide transitional medical and dental care benefits to servicemembers with service-connected medical conditions beyond the existing 180-day transition period. The care is for service-connected conditions only.

Subtitle D: Disability Matters

Sec. 1641. Presumption of Sound Condition

Servicemembers with a disability are presumed to have suffered such disability in connection with military service if they had been on active duty for six months or more, and if the disability was not noted at the time of entrance into active duty.

Sec. 1642. DOD Determinations of Disability

Requires the Secretaries of the military services to use the VASRD to the extent feasible in making a determination of disability of a member of the armed services. The Secretaries may not deviate from the schedule or any such interpretation of the schedule, unless they use alternate criteria that the Secretaries of DOD and VA jointly may prescribe for purposes of this subsection, if using such criteria will result in a determination of a greater percentage of disability than would be otherwise determined by using the schedule. In rating the disability of servicemembers, the Secretaries shall consider all medical conditions, whether individually or collectively, that render the servicemember unfit to perform the duties of his or her office, grade, rank, or rating.

Sec. 1643. Review of Separations Less than 30% Disabled

Requires the Secretary of Defense to establish a "Physical Disability Board of Review" to review the disability determinations of covered individuals by Physical Evaluation Boards (PEBs). *Covered individuals* are members and former members of the Armed Forces who, during the period beginning on September 11, 2001, and ending on December 31, 2009 (1) are separated from the Armed Forces because of unfitness for duty due to a medical condition with a disability rating of 20% disabled or less, and (2) are found to be not eligible for retirement. Upon the request of a covered individual, or a survivingspouse, nextof kin, or legal representative, or upon its own motion, the review board is to review the findings and decisions of the PEB with respect to such individuals and make appropriate recommendations with respect to the disability ratings of servicemembers and former servicemembers.

Sec. 1644. Disability Evaluation Pilot Programs

Authorizes the Secretary of Defense, in consultation with VA, to carry out pilot programs with respect to the DOD disability evaluation system, in order to reduce processing times, identify statutory or administrative improvements, and improve consistency in evaluations, among other things. Pilot programs must be completed within one year of their commencement. Requires the Secretary of Defense to provide periodic reports to Congress regarding the implementation of pilot programs. Authorized pilot programs are as follows:

- Disability determinations by DOD using VA-assigned disability ratings: Upon a determination by the DOD (the Secretary of the relevant service branch) that the servicemember is unfit for duty, the VA may conduct an evaluation of the member for physical disability and assign the member a rating of disability, using the VASRD, based on all medical conditions that render the member unfit for duty, and DOD may make the determination of disability regarding the member using the rating of disability assigned by the VA.
- Disability determinations using joint DOD/VA-assigned disability ratings: Upon a determination by the DOD (the Secretary of the relevant service branch) that the member is unfit for duty, the relevant Secretary may: provide for the joint DOD/VA evaluation of the member for disability, including theassignment of a rating, using the VASRD, based on all medical conditions (whether individually or collectively) that render the member unfit for duty, and make the determination of disability regarding the member using the rating assigned in this manner.
- Authorizes DOD to establish an electronic information clearinghouse regarding disability, for use by participating servicemembers.

Sec. 1645. Reports on Army Plan Regarding Disability Evaluation

Requires the Secretary of Defense to report on the implementation of corrective measures by DOD with respect to the Physical Disability Evaluation System (PDES) in response to recommendations in the following reports: (1) the report of the Inspector General of the Army on the PDES of March 6, 2007; (2) the report of the Independent Review Group on Rehabilitation Care and Administrative Processes at Walter Reed Army Medical Center (WRAMC) and National Naval Medical Center; and (3) the report of the Department of Veterans Affairs Task Force on Returning Global War on Terror Heroes.

Each report shall include current information on the total number of cases, and the number of cases involving combat disabled servicemembers, pending resolution before the Medical and Physical Disability Evaluation Boards of the Army, including information on the number of members of the Army who have been in a medical hold or holdover status for more than each of 100, 200, and 300 days. In addition, each report shall include current information on the status of the implementation of modifications to disability evaluation processes of the DOD in response to recommendations in the reports listed in the previous paragraph. The Secretary shall, within 24 hours, post each report required by this section on a publicly available DOD Internet website.

Sec. 1646. Disability Severance Pay

Changes the maximum number of years of service for computing disability severance pay from 12 years to 19 years, and discontinues the deduction (offset) of disability severance pay from disability compensation from the VA. (Previously, a veteran's disability compensation from the VA was fully offset for the amount of disability severance pay).

Sec. 1647. Assessments of the TDRL

Requires the Secretary of Defense to report to Congress regarding (1) a statistical history, since January 1, 2000, of the numbers of servicemembers who are returned to dutyor separated following a tenure on the temporary disability retired list (TDRL) and, in the case of members who were separated, how many were granted disability separation or retirement, and their disability ratings; (2) the results of certain required assessments regarding the utility of the TDRL, and its current and future implementation; and (3) such recommendations for the modification or improvement of the TDRL as the Secretary considers appropriate in response to the assessments.

Sec. 1648. Standards and Reports for MTFs

Requires the Secretary of Defense to establish standards for MTFs, and deadlines for compliance, in regard to appearance, maintenance and operations, compliance with the Americans with Disabilities Act of 1990, and such other matters relating to the appearance, size, operation, and maintenance of facilities as the Secretary considers appropriate.

Sec. 1649. Reports on WRAMC

Requires the Secretary of Defense to report regularly to Congress, beginning in February 2008, on the implementation of the Army Medical Action Plan to correct deficiencies identified in the condition of facilities and patient administration at WRAMC.[5]

Sec. 1650. Required Certifications Regarding WRAMC

In implementing the decision to close WRAMC, the Secretary of Defense shall submit to Congress a certification that (1) a transition plan has been developed, and resources have been committed, to ensure that patient care services, medical operations, and facilities are sustained at the highest possible level at WRAMC until replacement facilities are staffed and ready to assume at least the same level of care; (2) the closure of WRAMC will not result in a net loss of capacity in the major medical centers in the National Capitol Region in terms of total bed capacity or staffed bed capacity; and (3) the capacity of medical hold and outpatient lodging facilities operating at WRAMC as of the date of the certification will be available in sufficient quantities at designated replacement facilities by the date of the closure of WRAMC.

Sec. 1651. Compensation and Benefits Handbook

Requires the Secretary of Defense to develop and maintain, in handbook and electronic form, a comprehensive description of the compensation and other benefits to which a member of the Armed Forces, and the family of such member, would be entitled upon separation or retirement as a result of a serious injury or illness. The handbook will be available to servicemembers and next of kin, and its electronic form will be updated at least annually.

Subtitle E: Studies and Reports

Sec. 1661. Study on Readjustment Needs

Requires DOD, in consultation with the National Academy of Sciences, to prepare a study on the physical and mental health of servicemembers who deployed to combat operations in Iraq and Afghanistan.

Sec. 1662. Access to Adequate Outpatient Residential Facilities

Facilities occupied by recovering servicemembers shall be inspected semiannually for the first two years after enactment, and annually thereafter.

Sec. 1663. Study and Report on Support Services

Requires the Secretary of Defense to conduct a study of the provision of support services for families of recovering servicemembers, and to report to Congress on the findings of such study within 180 days of enactment.

Sec. 1664. Report on TBI Classifications

Requires the Secretaries of DOD and VA, within 90 days of enactment, jointly to submit to Congress a report describing the changes undertaken within the two departments to ensure that TBI victims receive a medical designation that clearly identifies TBI as a specific disease condition, rather than a generic classification (such as "organic psychiatric disorder").

Sec. 1665. Program Evaluation

Requires the DOD to conduct an evaluation of specific aspects of the Polytrauma Liaison Officer/Non-Commissioned Officer program, which is the program operated by each of the military departments and the VA for the purpose of (1) assisting in the seamless transition of servicemembers from DOD to VA health care systems, and (2) expediting the flow of information and communication between MTFs and VA Polytrauma Centers. DOD shall report to Congress on the findings of such evaluation, and any recommendations, within 90 days of enactment.

Subtitle F: Other Matters

Sec. 1671. Prohibition on Transfer of Resources from Medical Care

Prohibits the Secretary of Defense and the Secretaries of the military departments from transferring funds or personnel from medical care functions to administrative functions within DOD in order to comply with the new administrative requirements imposed or the amendments made by this title.

Sec. 1672. Medical Care for Families

Authorizes medical care at MTFs, on a space-available basis, for family members of a recovering servicemember who are on invitational orders or receiving per diem payments while caring for the servicemember.

Sec. 1673. Deployment Assessments of Cognitive Function

Requires DOD to incorporate an assessment of PTSD in its pre- and post-deployment medical examination of servicemembers deployed overseas. To support this requirement and a preexisting requirement regarding TBI, DOD is required to a develop a protocol for the pre-deployment assessment and documentation of cognitive function, including memory. DOD is required to conduct relevant pilot programs, and to report to Congress on their implementation. Also, DOD is required to ensure the quality of such pre-and post-deployment assessments, and to prescribe in regulations minimal health standards for deployment regarding TBI.

Sec. 1674. Guaranteed Funding for WRAMC

Requires that funding of WRAMC for a given fiscal year shall not be less than the FY2006 amount, until the Secretary of Defense submits to Congress a plan for the provision of health care for military beneficiaries and their dependents in the National Capital Region. Such plan shall, at a minimum, include (1) the manner in which patients, staff, bed capacity, and functions will move from WRAMC to expanded facilities; (2) a timeline and milestones for such moves; (3) projected budgets, including budget transfers, for MTFs within the region; (4) the management or disposition of MTF properties within the region; and (5) staffing projections for the region. After submission of such plan, the Secretary shall certify to Congress on a quarterly basis that patients, staff, bed capacity, functions, or parts of functions at WRAMC have not been moved or disestablished until the expanded facilities elsewhere in the region are completed, equipped, and staffed with sufficient capacity to accept and provide, at a minimum, the same level of and access to care that patients received at WRAMC during FY2006.

Sec. 1675. Use of Federal Leave Transfer Program

Eliminates, for federal civilian employees who sustained a combat-related disability for which they are undergoing medical treatment, the requirement that they exhaust annual and sick leave before any transferred (donated) annual leave may be used. This provision is in effect only while the servicemember is receiving medical treatment for the combat-related disability, and only for a maximum of five years from the beginning of treatment. This provision is effective upon enactment.

Sec. 1676. Moratorium on Contractor Conversions at MTFs.6

Requires the Secretary of Defense to meet certain criteria before the announcement or conduct of an OMB Circular A-76 study pursuant to 10 U.S.C. 2461 (regarding public-private competition required before conversion to contractor performance) for any study carried out at an MTF. These criteria include certifying to Congress that appropriate steps have been taken to ensure that neither the quality of military medical care nor the availability of qualified personnel will be adversely affected by the competition process, or by the conversion to performance by a contractor; reporting to Congress within 180 days of enactment on certain data regarding each public-private competition; and performing an assessment of whether other types of business reform or reengineering methods might in the future achieve anyanticipated or budgeted savings rather than through a public-private competition.[7]

TITLE XVII: VETERANS MATTERS

Title XVII includes several provisions that have an impact on programs administered by the VA. A majority of these provisions are focused on improving health care services for those with TBI. Following is a summary of each of these provisions.

Sec. 1701. Sense of Congress

Expresses the sense of Congress, recognizing that VA is a leader in the field of TBI care, and also acknowledges that DOD and VA have made efforts to provide a smooth transition of medical care and rehabilitative services to servicemembers as they transition from the DOD health care system to that of the VA. However, it is the sense of Congress that more can be done to assist veterans and their families in the continuum of the rehabilitation, recovery, and reintegration of wounded or injured servicemembers and veterans into their communities.

Sec. 1702. TBI Rehabilitation and Reintegration Plans

Amends 38 U.S.C., Chapter 17, and adds a new section. It requires the VA Secretary to develop an individualized plan for rehabilitation and reintegration into the community for each veteran or servicemember who receives inpatient or outpatient care at the VA for TBI. This plan must be provided in writing to each veteran or servicemember before such individual is discharged from inpatient care at a VA medical facility, or as soon as practicable following a diagnosis of TBI by the VA. It requires that each individualized plan for rehabilitation include (1) rehabilitation objectives for improving the physical, cognitive, and vocational functioning of a veteran or servicemember with a TBI in order that such individual regain independence and reintegrate into the community; (2) access, as needed, to all appropriate rehabilitative components of the TBI continuum of care; (3) a description of specific rehabilitative treatments and other services, to include the type, frequency, duration, and location of such treatments and services; (4) the name of the designated case manager responsible for the implementation of the individualized plan; and (5) the dates on which the effectiveness of the plan will be reviewed.

Requires the VA Secretary to develop the individualized plan based on a comprehensive assessment of the physical, cognitive, vocational, neuropsychological and social impairments of the veteran or servicemember. The assessment must also take into consideration the family education and family support needs of such individual after discharge from inpatient care. The assessment will be performed by a team of individuals, with relevant expertise as stipulated in this section.

Requires the VA Secretary to assign a case manager for each veteran or servicemember with a TBI. The case manager will be responsible for the implementation of the individualized plan, and the coordination of care. The Secretary must ensure that such case manager has specific expertise, either through experience, education, or training, in the care required by the individual to whom such case manager is assigned.

Requires the VA Secretary, to the maximum extent practicable, to involve the family members or legal guardian of the veteran or servicemember with a TBI in developing the individualized plan. It also requires the Secretary to collaborate with a state protection and advocacy system if the veteran or servicemember covered by such plan requests such collaboration, or, in the event that the individual is incapacitated, the family or guardian of the servicemember or veteran requests collaboration. In the event that the servicemember is still on active duty, the VA must collaborate with DOD in developing the individualized plan for rehabilitation and reintegration.

Requires the VA Secretary to periodically review the effectiveness of each individualized plan and refine it as appropriate after such review. Moreover, the Secretary is required to review the individualized plan at the request of the veteran with a TBI or in the case of a veteran or servicemember who is incapacitated, at the request of the guardian or designee of the veteran.

Sec. 1703. Use of Non-VA Facilities for TBI

Amends 38 U.S.C., Chapter 17, and adds a new section. It authorizes the VA, at its discretion, to provide hospital care and medical services through appropriate public or private entities to veterans and servicemembers who receive TBI care from the VA. Such care in non-VA facilities may be authorized if the VA is unable to provide care at the frequency or duration prescribed in the individualized plan, for rehabilitation and reintegration.

Sec. 1704. TBI Research, Education, and Clinical Care

Amends 38 U.S.C., Chapter 17, Subchapter II. Requires the VA to conduct research on mild to severe forms of TBI; visually related neurological conditions; means of improving the diagnosis, rehabilitative treatment, and prevention of TBI; and dual diagnosis of PTSD and TBI, among other conditions. Requires the VA to collaborate on this research with the Defense and Veterans Brain Injury Center (DVBIC) and other relevant programs of the federal government. Requires the Secretary to conduct educational programs on recognizing and diagnosing mild and moderate cases of TBI. Moreover, this section requires the VA to establish a TBI registry to be known as the "Traumatic Brain Injury Veterans Health Registry." When possible, the VA Secretary must notify each individual listed in the registry of significant developments in research on the health consequences of military service in OIF and OEF theaters of operations.

Sec. 1705. TBI Pilot Program on Assisted-living Services

This section requires the VA Secretary to implement, within 90 days of enactment, a five-year pilot program to assess the effectiveness of providing assisted-living services to eligible veterans to enhance the rehabilitation, quality of life, and community integration of such veterans. The pilot program must be carried out in locations selected by the Secretary.

However, at least one program must be located in a Veterans Integrated Service Network (VISN) that has a VA polytrauma center. Other locations must be in areas that contain high concentrations of veterans with TBI. The Secretary must also give special consideration to rural areas when selecting program locations.

Authorizes the Secretary to enter into agreements for the provision of assisted living services with a provider participating in Medicaid (42 U.S.C. 1396 et seq.). Suchassistedliving facilities must meet standards prescribed by the Secretary for the purposes of the pilot program. Requires the Secretary to continue to provide case management services for veterans participating in the pilot program. Requires the Secretary to submit a report on the pilot program to the House and Senate Veterans' Affairs Committees not less than 60 days after the completion of the pilot program. The report must include information about the program, utility of the program, and recommendations regarding the extension or expansion of the program.

Sec. 1706. Provision of Age-appropriate Nursing Home Care

Amends 38 U.S.C. 1710A and adds a new provision that requires the Secretary to provide age-appropriate nursing home care.

Sec. 1707. Extension of Period of Eligibility

This section extends from two to five years the period of automatic eligibility for VA health care, for veterans who served in a combat theater of operations and are discharged or released five years before the date of enactment of this Act. For those veterans who served in a combat theater of operations after November 11, 1998, but more than five years before the date of enactment of this act, and have not enrolled in the VA health care system, the period of automatic eligibility will be three years.

Sec. 1708. Mental Health Service-connection

Amends 38 U.S.C. 1702 that pertains to presumption of service-connection, and inserts the term "mental illness" instead of "psychosis." Requires the Secretary to provide a veteran who served in a period of war after the Persian Gulf War, or in combat against a hostile force during a period of hostilities after November 11, 1998, a preliminary mental health evaluation as soon as practicable, but not later than 30 days after a request for such evaluation.

Sec. 1709. Modification Regarding Outpatient Dental Services

Amends 38 U.S.C. 1712 and extends from 90 days to 180 days after discharge or release, the eligibility for outpatient dental treatment for a veteran with service-connected dental conditions or disabilities who served on active duty.

Sec. 1710. Clarification Regarding Outreach Services

Amends 38 U.S.C. 6301 to include National Guard and Reserve components among those who are eligible for VA outreach services. Defines the term "outreach" as the act or process of reaching out in a systematic manner proactively to provide information, services, and benefits counseling to veterans, and to the spouses, children, and parents of veterans who may be eligible to receive benefits under the laws administered by the Secretary, to ensure that such individuals are fully informed about, and assisted in applying for, any benefits.

Sec. 1711. Designation of Fiduciary or Trustee

Amends 38 U.S.C. 1980A, and provides for the designation of a fiduciary or trustee for benefits under the Traumatic Servicemembers' Group Life Insurance (TSGLI) for servicemembers who are medically incapacitated.[8]

End Notes

[1] For more information, see CRS Report RL33999, *Defense: FY2008 Authorization and Appropriations*, by Pat Towell, Stephen Daggett, and Amy Belasco.

[2] For more information on the authorities and programs discussed in this summary, see CRS Reports regarding "Military Personnel and Compensation" and "Health Care for Military Personnel and Veterans" at [http://apps.crs.gov/cli/level_2.aspx? PRDS_CLI_ITEM_ ID=3], and regarding "Veterans' Benefits" at [http://apps.crs.gov/cli/level_2. aspx?PRDS_ CLI_ ITEM_ID=13].

[3] For more information regarding the DOD and VA disability evaluation processes, see CRS Report RL33991, *Disability Evaluation of Military Servicemembers*, by Christine Scott and Sidath Viranga Panangala (Domestic Social Policy Division) and Charles A. Henning (Foreign Affairs, Defense, and Trade Division).

[4] Pursuant to 38 U.S.C., Chapter 74, VA has special authorities for recruiting and retaining certain categories of health professionals. These authorities include providing advance payments, recruitment or relocation bonuses, retention allowances, and pay adjustments based on market rates and performance.

[5] The Army Medical Action Plan was developed as a result of critical media scrutiny of soldier care at WRAMC and other Army medical facilities, and is a comprehensive Armywide plan to improve aspects of medical care and support for injured servicemembers. For more information, see testimony of Brigadier General Sheila Baxter, hearing regarding "Mental Health Concerns of Veterans," U.S. Senate, Committee on Veterans Affairs, 11th Cong., 1st Sess., August 17, 2007.

[6] This information provided by Valerie Bailey Grasso, Foreign Affairs, Defense, and Trade Division.

[7] For more information, see CRS Report RL34140, *Walter Reed Army Medical Center (WRAMC) and Office of Management and Budget (OMB) Circular A-76: Implications for the Future*, by Valerie Bailey Grasso.

[8] Traumatic Servicemembers' Group Life Insurance is a traumatic injury protection rider under Servicemembers' Group Life Insurance (SGLI) that provides for a payment to members of the armed services covered by SGLI who sustain a traumatic injury that results in certain severe losses.

In: Veterans' Benefits and Care
Editor: Mathew H. Bradley

ISBN: 978-1-60692-500-3

Chapter 11

SUICIDE PREVENTION AMONG VETERANS

Ramya Sundaraman, Sidath Viranga Panangala and Sarah A. Lister

SUMMARY

Numerous news stories in the popular print and electronic media have documented suicides among servicemembers and veterans returningfrom Operation Iraqi Freedom (OIF) and Operation Enduring Freedom (OEF). In the United States, there are more than 30,000 suicides annually. Suicides among veterans are included in this number, but it is not known in what proportion. There is no nationwide system for surveillance of suicide specifically among veterans. Recent data show that about 20% of suicide deaths nationwide could be among veterans. It is not known what proportion of these deaths are among OIF/OEF veterans.

Veterans have a number of risk factors that increase their chance of attempting suicide. These risk factors include combat exposure, post-traumatic stress disorder (PTSD) and other mental health problems, traumatic brain injury (TBI), poor social support structures, and access to lethal means.

Several bills addressing suicide in veterans have been introduced in the 110th Congress. On November 5, 2007, the Joshua Omvig Veterans Suicide Prevention Act (P.L. 110-110) was signed into law, requiring the Department of Veterans Affairs (VA) to establish a comprehensive program for suicide prevention among veterans. More recently, the Veterans Suicide Study Act (S. 2899) was introduced. This bill would require the VA to conduct a study, and report to Congress, regarding suicides among veterans since 1997.

The VA has carried out a number of suicide prevention initiatives, including establishing a national suicide prevention hotline for veterans, conducting awareness events at VA medical centers, and screening and assessing veterans for suicide risk.

This chapter discusses data sources and systems that can provide information about suicides in the general population and among veterans, and known risk and protective factors associated with suicide in each group. It also discusses suicide prevention efforts by the VA.

It does not discuss Department of Defense (DOD) activities, or VA's treatment of risk factors for suicide, such as depression, PTSD, and substance abuse.

INTRODUCTION

Considerable public attention has been drawn toward the mental health care needs of veterans, especially those returning from combat in Iraq and Afghanistan. Numerous news stories in the popular print and electronic media have documented suicides among servicemembers and veterans returning from Operation Iraqi Freedom (OIF) and Operation Enduring Freedom (OEF).[1] Some veterans advocacy groups have filed a class-action lawsuit claiming that the Department of Veterans Affairs (VA) is not providing adequate and timely access to mental health care, and that this has led to an "epidemic of suicides."[2]

However, most often the data cited in these press reports do not differentiate between suicides among veterans and active duty servicemembers.[3] It is important to make this distinction, because two separate health care systems — at the VA and the Department of Defense (DOD), respectively — are responsible for providing mental health care to these two distinct populations. This chapter explains the difficulties in determining the incidence of suicide among veterans, summarizes what is known about suicides in the general population and among veterans, and discusses known risk and protective factors associated with suicide in each group. It also discusses recent congressionalaction toaddress suicide among veterans, and suicide prevention efforts by the VA. The report does not discuss DOD activities, or VA's treatment of risk factors for suicide, such as depression, post-traumatic stress disorder (PTSD), and substance abuse.

DATA AND DATA SYSTEMS FOR TRACKING SUICIDE

Suicide is the act of intentionally ending one's life,attempted suicideis an effort that does not have a fatal outcome, and suicidal ideation is thinking about or wanting to end one's life. Because completed (versus attempted) suicide results in death, national statistics on suicide come from death certificate data.[4] These data are collected by state and territorial health officials, under their authority, and are voluntarily reported to the Centers for Disease Control and Prevention's (CDC's) National Vital Statistics System. The CDC analyzes the data and publishes information on numbers and rates of death, and important trends, in the United States.[5] The CDC also publishes a U.S. standard death certificate, which states and territories can modify. Most U.S. deaths are not investigated by government officials. Possible suicides may be investigated, however, pursuant to state and territorial authorities. To the extent that a death is recognized as a suicide, the standard death certificate provides the means to report suicide as the manner of death, but it has limited options for noting other information that may be relevant to the suicide.

In 2003, CDC launched the National Violent Death Reporting System (NVDRS), an active surveillance system that provides detailed information about the circumstances of violent deaths, including suicide.[6] The NVDRS augments death certificate data by linking it to death investigation reports filed by coroners, medical examiners, and law enforcement officials. These added layers of information allow the NVDRS to identify suicide risk factors, such as depression; to gather additional information, such as toxicology results; and to more reliably capture information that could have been, but was not, completed on the standard death certificate. At this time, the NVDRS is not in operation nationwide, but only in 17 states, and NVDRS data might not be generalizable to the entire U.S. population. Also, because protocols for death investigation vary from one state to the next, NVDRS data might not be comparable between those states in which it is in operation. CDC's goal is to expand the system to all 50 states, all U.S. territories, and the District of Columbia, and to continue efforts to standardize data collection and analysis across states.

At this time, there is no nationwide system for surveillance (i.e., tracking) of suicide among all veterans. As with all suicides in civilian jurisdiction, suicides among veterans may be investigated, and the death certificates completed, by state and territorial authorities. Unless a veteran's suicide occurs in a VA facility, opportunities for the VA to become aware of the incident may be limited. Three approaches are being used to track the incidence of suicide among veterans, though each of them has serious shortcomings.

First, CDC's standard death certificate allows officials to note if a decedent *has ever served*[7] in the U.S. Armed Forces. However, the fact that a decedent is a veteran is not always known when the certificate is completed. Although suicides among veterans are a part of total national suicide statistics, it is not known what proportion of that total is made up of veterans.

Second, VA data may be linked to CDC's vital statistics data through the National Death Index (NDI). This CDC data system allows authorized researchers to link national death data to other data systems, identifying the fact that an individual had died of suicide, and that a death certificate has been filed.[8] This would allow the VA to identify suicide deaths among its enrollees. (Subsequent research steps are cumbersome. For example, researchers typically must contact state officials to access the actual death certificates.) The NDI is not an ongoing data linkage that would constitute surveillance for suicide. It can be used, however, to support special studies by linking specific data sets. For example, researchers from the VA and the University of Michigan conducted a study in which they linked data from VA's National Registry for Depression (NARDEP) to the NDI, allowing VA to match its patient registry to certified suicide deaths even when the decedent's veteran status had not been noted on the death certificate.[9] However, because only about one-third of veterans receive their health care from the VA, using VA health systems data for linkage would not capture the complete experience of suicide among veterans.

Third, the NVDRS resolves many of the problems discussed above. Through ongoing active surveillance, NVDRS substantially improves the likelihood that a suicide victim's veteran status will be captured, and it provides additional useful information about suicide incidents. But NVDRS is in operation in only 17 states. Though CDC intends it to become a nationwide system, expansion would depend on appropriations. Congress first provided funding for NVDRS in FY2002 and has expressed support for the program in annual appropriations report language. The program has not received a specified appropriation in recent years, but rather is funded through CDC's budget for intentional injury prevention and control.

SUICIDE IN THE U.S. GENERAL POPULATION

There are *risk factors* that increase the likelihood that someone will attempt suicide, and *protective factors* that decrease that likelihood. This section provides some context for suicide among veterans by discussing the incidence, and risk and protective factors, for suicide in the U.S. general population.[10]

Incidence of Suicide

Suicide is a serious public health problem in the United States. According to CDC, there were more than 32,000 suicide deaths in the United States in 2004, making it the 11th leading cause of death that year. On average, there are four suicides among males for each one among females. Use of firearms is the most common method of suicide among males, while poisoning is the most common method among females. Suicide is the second leading cause of death among 25-34 year olds, and the third leading cause of death among 15-24 year olds. Although suicide is a leading cause of death in younger adults, the *rate* of suicide (number of suicides within the age group per 100,000 resident population in the age group) is actuallyhighest in individuals aged 45 or older. **Table 1** presents suicide rates across age groups in the United States for 2004, as published by CDC. It is important to note that except in the youngest age group, these rates may, and probably do, include suicides among veterans, though in proportions that are not known.

There are no official national statistics on attempted suicide (i.e., attempts that were not fatal), but it is generally estimated that there are 25 attempts for each death by suicide. Also, it is reported that there are three suicide attempts among females for every one among males.

Risk and Protective Factors

No single cause or factor leads to suicide. It is a "final common outcome with multiple potential antecedents, precipitants, and underlying causes."[11] A number of factors are known to increase or decrease the likelihood that an individual will attempt suicide. Factors that increase this likelihood are called *risk factors*. Risk factors exist at multiple levels, involving individual, family, community, and societal factors. Conversely, factors that decrease a person's inclination to attempt suicide are called *protective factors*, which also exist at multiple levels. It is important to note that none of these factors in isolation is known to cause or prevent suicide.

The single best predictor of an increased risk of suicide is a history of a prior suicide attempt. Other risk factors for suicide in the general population include certain mental illnesses such as depression, alcohol and substance abuse, history of trauma or abuse, family history of suicide, job or financial stress, the stigma associated with seeking mental health care, barriers to health care access, and easy access to lethal means. Protective factors include strong family or community connections; accessible and effective clinical care; skills in problem solving,conflict resolution, and nonviolent handling of disputes; and cultural and religious beliefs that discourage suicide.[12]

Table 1. U.S. Death Rates for Suicide, by Age, 2004

Age Group	5-14 years	15-24 years	25-44 years	45-64 years	65 years and over	All age groups[a]
Suicide rate	0.7	10.3	13.9	15.4	14.3	10.9

Source: CDC, death rates for suicide, according to sex, race, Hispanic origin, and age: selected years, 1950-2004, "Health, United States, 2007," Table 46, at [http://www.cdc.gov/nchs/data/hus/hus07.pdf].

Notes: CDC does not calculate rates based on small numbers of suicides among those younger than five years of age, as such rates are not statistically reliable. In the source above, CDC also published rates for sub-intervals of the age intervals presented here (e.g., for those aged 25-34 years and 35-44 years).

a. This rate is age-adjusted, calculated using the year 2000 standard population.

SUICIDE AMONG VETERANS

In the absence of national surveillance for suicide among veterans, information is limited to the findings of special epidemiological studies and surveys. These vary considerably in their design and in the sub-population of veterans studied, and they often yield conflicting results.

It is tempting to makecomparisons between these studies, and with information about suicide in the general population. Such comparisons are often made, but they are not necessarily valid. Among other things, data about suicides in the general population includes suicides among veterans. Information about suicide in groups that exclude veterans is scant, as is information about the extent to which data for veterans may skew the data for the general population, if at all. An additional problem in interpreting the findings of these special studies is that they are often conducted on populations of veterans who are receiving treatment for suicide risk factors. On the one hand, this makes it difficult to determine whether study findings reflect the effects of risk factors, or the effects of interventions. On the other hand, it indicates that efforts to develop systematic surveillance of suicide among veterans may, with careful attention to design, also provide the means to evaluate the effectiveness of prevention and treatment programs. This section discusses the findings of some key studies of suicide among veterans.

Incidence of Suicide

The true incidence of suicide among veterans is not known. This section discusses information from two recent published studies that yield a partial picture of the burden of suicide in this group.

In 2005, the NVDRS identified 1,821 suicidesamongformer or current military personnel, comprising 20% of all suicides, in the 16 states in which the system was operational that year.[13] CDC's published findings about these 1,821 decedents include the following:

- 1,765 (96.9%) were male.

- 1,415 (77.7%) were 45 years of age or older.
- The most common method used was firearms (67.9%), followed by poisoning (12.7%), and hanging/strangulation/suffocation (11.5%).
- 47.2% were married, 25.0% were divorced, 13.0% were widowed, and 14.0% were never married.[14]

Researchers from the VA and the University of Michigan conducted a cohort study of 807,694 veterans who were diagnosed with depression in the VA health system, and registered in the VA's National Registry for Depression (NARDEP), between 1999 and 2004.[15] During the study period, 1,683 (0.21%) of the veterans in this high-risk group committed suicide. The researchers calculated a rate of 88.25 suicides per 100,000 person-years in this group, seven to eight times higher than the rate in the general population for the same time period. They noted that this rate was similar, though, to a more relevant comparison, namely, to suicides among those in the general population who were depressed.[16] They also found the rate among the group of veterans studied to be highest among those who were younger than 45 years of age, in contrast with the age trend in the general population.

In December 2007, VA testified that it had identified 144 known suicides among OIF/OEF veterans from the time the conflicts began through the end of 2005, and that this number translated into a rate that is not statistically different from the rate for age, sex, and race matched individuals from the general population. These data have not been published.[17]

Risk and Protective Factors

While there have been a number of studies to identify risk and protective factors for suicide in the general population, few studies have looked at factors specific to veterans. In the general population, suicide risk factors include male gender; older age; diminished psycho-social support (e.g., homelessness or unmarried status); availability and knowledge of firearms; and the co-existence of medical and psychiatric conditions. This profile describes a large portion of the veteran patient population, making suicide risk management particularly challenging in the VA health care system.[18] A study that screened 703 patients from a general medical outpatient clinic at a VA hospital found that 7.3% of the patients had suicidal ideation.[19] Younger and white patients were found to be at increased risk. The risk was higher in patients with self-described fair or poor mental health, a history of mental health treatment, and fair or poor perceived physical health. When major depression was controlled for, anxiety and substance abuse disorders continued to show an association with suicidal ideation.

CDC's NVDRS data identified the following associated circumstances among a group of 1,622 former or current military personnel who died by suicide in 2005:[20]

- Although almost half of them (47.2%) were depressed at the time of death, only about a fourth (26.7%) were receiving mental health treatment.
- 17.2% had an alcohol problem, and 7.7% had a problem with other substances.
- 24.5% had a problem with an intimate partner.
- 38.4% had a physical health problem.
- 28.0% had experienced an acute crisis during the prior two weeks.

- 33.9% had left a suicide note, 13.3% had made a previous suicide attempt, and 29.0% had disclosed their intent to commit suicide with enough time for someone to have intervened.

The VA/University of Michigan study of suicide among veterans with depression found that having a service-connected disability was associated with a lower risk of suicide in this group.[21] The authors suggest that greater access to VA health facilities and regular compensation payments may explain the protective effect.

The Effects of PTSD, TBI, and Depression on Suicide Risk

This section describes three suicide risk factors that are common among veterans: Post-traumatic Stress Disorder (PTSD), Traumatic Brain Injury (TBI), and depression. PTSD and TBI are common consequences of war, with distinct symptoms, treatment modalities, and long-term effects. PTSD has been recognized in various forms throughout military history. It is an anxiety disorder, with symptoms of varying severity, that can occur following experiences, such as military combat, in which grave physical injury occurred or was threatened. People who suffer from PTSD often relive the experience through nightmares and flashbacks, have difficulty sleeping, and feel detached or estranged. TBI occurs when a sudden physical trauma causes damage to the brain. Improvised explosive devices (IEDs), which have been used extensively in the current conflict in Iraq, can cause TBI, sometimes in the absence of obvious external signs of injury. Symptoms of TBI can be mild, moderate, or severe, depending on the extent of the brain injury. When symptoms of TBI or PTSD are mild, they may go undiagnosed, or be confused with conditions with similar symptoms, such as other mental illnesses, including depression, or substance use disorders. Either PTSD or TBI may co-occur with depression or substance abuse. Finally, some veterans have both a TBI and PTSD.

In April 2008, the RAND Corporation published a study of mental health problems in servicemembers and veterans.[22] From their review of the literature, the authors found that in the general population, depression, PTSD, and TBI are each independent risk factors for suicide. More limited information from studies of servicemembers or veterans generally shows the same effect of these three risk factors in specific groups that were studied. This information also typically shows trends comparable to those in the general population with respect to other risk factors for suicide, though the demonstrated effects of interactions of these factors with depression, PTSD and TBI may differ. For example, studies have found that while males are at greater risk of death from suicide than are females, the effects that depression, PTSD and TBI have on increasing this risk is greater in females. Among the general population, substance abuse, prior nonfatal suicide attempts, severity of PTSD symptoms, and certain types of TBI are more predictive for suicide, and may signal areas of greater suicide risk among military and veterans populations as well. Researchers also found that combat exposure increases the risk of suicide, as well as the likelihood of PTSD, which itself also increases the risk of suicide.

The VA/University of Michigan study of suicide among veterans with depression found that PTSD was associated with a lower risk of suicide in this Zivin et al., study of depression and suicide in group.[23] The authors suggest that this unexpected finding may reflect the effect of treatment for PTSD, rather than a protective effect of PTSD itself.

CONGRESSIONAL ACTION

In the 109th Congress, two measures (H.R. 5771 and S. 3808) were introduced regarding the prevention of suicide among veterans. However, these bills did not see further legislative action.

In the 110th Congress, the Joshua Omvig Veterans Suicide Prevention Act (H.R. 327) was introduced in the House, and a companion version (S. 479) was introduced in the Senate.[24] The House passed H.R. 327 on March 21, 2007, and the Senate passed the House measure with an amendment on September 27. The bill was signed into law (P.L. 110-110) on November 5, 2007.[25] The act, among other things, requires the VA to establish a comprehensive program for suicide prevention among veterans. In carrying out this comprehensive program, the VA must designate a suicide prevention counselor at each VA medical facility. Each counselor is required to work with local emergency rooms, police departments, mental health organizations, and veterans service organizations to engage in outreach to veterans. The act also requires the VA to provide for research on best practices for suicide prevention among veterans, and requires the VA Secretary to provide for outreach and education for veterans and their families, with special emphasis on providing information to veterans of OIF and OEF. The act requires VA to provide for the availability of 24-hour mental health care for veterans and to establish a 24-hour hotline for veterans to call if needed.

Also in the 110th Congress, the National Defense Authorization Act for Fiscal Year 2008 (P.L. 110-181) requires the Secretaries of DOD and VA to develop a comprehensive care and transition policy for servicemembers who are recovering from serious injuries or illnesses related to their military service, and to specifically address the risk of suicide among these individuals in developing the required policy.[26]

More recently, the Veterans Suicide Study Act (S. 2899) was introduced. This measure would require the VA to study and report to Congress regarding suicides that have occurred among veterans since 1997. In carrying out this study, the VA Secretary would have to coordinate with the Secretary of Defense, Veterans Service Organizations, the CDC, and state public health offices and veterans agencies.

VA'S SUICIDE PREVENTION EFFORTS[27]

In response to legislation and congressional oversight, the VA has initiated several suicide prevention activities. Following is a summary of major activities.

Mental Health Strategic Plan

In 2004, the VA developed the Mental Health Strategic Plan (MHSP), which aimed to present a new approach to mental health care, to focus on recovery rather than pathology, and to integrate mental health care into overall health carefor veteran patients. This five-year action plan, with more than 200 initiatives, includes timetables and responsible offices identified for each action item. A number of these action items are specifically aimed at the prevention of suicide. In 2006, following a request by the House Committee on Veterans Affairs, the VA's Inspector General (IG) undertook an assessment of VA's progress in implementing the MHSP initiatives for suicide prevention, and provided recommendations.[28] The IG's findings revealed that MHSP initiatives pertaining to 24-hour crisis availability, outreach, referral, and development of methods for tracking veterans at risk have been implemented in multiple facilities, but not yet systemwide. Initiatives focused on the development of methods for screening, assessment of veterans at risk, emerging best practice treatment interventions, education of VA health providers, and an electronic suicide prevention database have been piloted or are in the process of being piloted at selected facilities.

Mental Health Research

VA's Mental Illness Research, Education and Clinical Center (MIRECC) at Denver, Colorado, and the Center of Excellence in Mental Health and PTSD at Canandaigua, New York, have been specifically focusing on research related to suicide prevention. According to the VA, ongoing studies at these centers are studying suicide risk factors, validation of suicide ideation screening instruments, quality of mental health care and its relationship to suicide prevention, and risk factors for suicide as it relates to depression.

Suicide Awareness

In April 2007, VA held its first Suicide Prevention Awareness Day at all VA medical centers (VAMCs). The program included recognizing risk factors for suicide, and proper protocols for responding to crisis situations. VA held its second Suicide Prevention Awareness Day in September 2007. The program consisted of required training for all staff on general principles of suicide prevention, and the use of the national VA Suicide Prevention Hotline (see below).

VA has also appointed Suicide Prevention Coordinators who are located at each VA medical center. They were appointed in response to P.L. 110-110, which required VA to appoint suicide prevention counselors in each VA medical facility. The primary function of these coordinators is to support the identification of patients at high risk for suicide, and to ensure that their monitoring and care are intensified. Furthermore, they are involved in training and education, both within the VA and in the community. All the coordinators are licensed mental health professionals.

Screening

A screening program aims to identify individuals who have mental or emotional problems that increase their risk for suicide.[29] VA has implemented a policy to screen all OEF/OIF veterans for depression, PTSD, and alcohol abuse upon their initial visit to VA medical centers or clinics. Furthermore, screening for depression and alcohol abuse is required on an annual basis for all veterans, and screening for PTSD is required annually for the first five years after enrollment, and every five years thereafter. Veterans who screen positive for one of these conditions are required to receive a follow-up clinical evaluation that considers both the condition(s) related to the positive screen, and the risk of suicide. When this process confirms the presence of a mental disorder or suicide risk, veterans are offered mental health treatment. When there is a referral or request for mental health services, veterans must receive an initial evaluation within 24 hours. If this evaluation identifies an urgent need, treatment is to be provided immediately. Otherwise, veterans must receive a full diagnostic and treatmentplanning evaluation and the initiation of care within two weeks.

In addition, the DOD administers a post-deployment health reassessment (PDHRA) 90-180 days after a servicemembember's return from deployment, to identify health concerns, with an emphasis placed on screening for mental health conditions that may have emerged since returning home. Information gathered during this assessment helps DOD identify servicemembers who require referrals for further evaluation.[30] The Government Accountability Office (GAO) has stated that DOD shares information gathered through the PDHRA with the VA. According to GAO, "VA officials obtain PDHRA information about servicemembers referred to VA and individual servicemembers' [PDHRA] when they access VA health care. Each month, VA receives a report that provides monthly and cumulative totals of servicemembers referred, including servicemembers referred to VA facilities."[31] However, it is unclear at this time if VA uses this information to specifically screen those who may be potentially at risk of suicide.

Suicide Prevention Hotline

The VA has also partnered with the Lifeline Program, a grantee of the Substance Abuse and Mental Health Services Administration (SAMHSA), of the Department of Health and Human Services (HHS), to develop a VA suicide prevention hotline. Those who call 1-800-273-TALK are asked to press "1" if they are a veteran, or are calling about a veteran.[32] When they do so, they are connected directly to VA's hotline call center, where they speak to a VA mental health professional with real-time access to the veteran's medical records. The responders at the VA suicide prevention hotline have received American Association of Suicidology (AAS) credentialing and certification.

In emergencies, the hotline contacts local emergency resources such as police or ambulance services to ensure an immediate response. In other cases, after providing support and counseling, the hotline transfers care to the suicide prevention coordinator at the nearest VAMC for follow-up care.

From October 7 to November 10, 2007, 1,636 veterans and 311 family members or friends called the VA suicide prevention hotline. These calls led to 363 referrals to suicide prevention coordinators and 93 rescues involving emergency services.[33]

Funding for Suicide Prevention

According to VA estimates, in FY2008, spending for the suicide prevention program will include $970,000 to establish the suicide prevention hotline; $1.97 million for the Center of Excellence in Canandaigua, New York; $2.20 million for the Mental Illness Research, Education and Clinical Center in Denver, Colorado; $90,000 for the Serious Mental Illness Research, Education and Clinical Center for monitoring of suicide rates and risk factors; and $14.32 million for Suicide Prevention Coordinators.[34]

Conclusion

There has been considerable recent interest in the burden of suicide among veterans, in particular those who have recently returned from military service in Operation Iraqi Freedom and Operation Enduring Freedom. This interest has thrown a spotlight on the fact that there is not, at this time, a system of surveillance for suicide among veterans.

Despite recent interest in comparing suicide rates between veterans and the general population, this may not be the most useful comparison. In numerous ways that affect their suicide risk, veterans are not like the general population. Also, the VA has an interest in decreasing the burden of suicide among veterans, whether this burden exceeds that of the general population or not. What may be more meaningful, and more important to achieve, is the establishment of data systems that support a more robust and reliable understanding of suicide among veterans. The ideal systems would describe a clear baseline, and provide a means to track changes going forward with respect to such things as risk and protective factors, and the effects of treatment — in order to know which interventions work, and where to target them.

End Notes

[1] Ken Fuson and Jennifer Jacobs, "Iowans Lauded for Anti-suicide Efforts," *The Des Moines Register,* January 26, 2008; Dana Priest, "Soldier Suicides at Record Level," *Washington Post,* January 31, 2008, Page A01; "Soldier, After Bipolar Treatment and Suicide Attempts, Sent Back to War Zone," *Editor & Publisher,* February 11, 2008; "Suicide Epidemic Among Veterans — A CBS News Investigation Uncovers a Suicide Rate for Veterans Twice That of Other Americans," aired November 13, 2007. OEF, which began in October 2001, conducts combat operations in Afghanistan and other locations. OIF, which began in March 2003, conducts combat operations in Iraq and other locations.

[2] *Veterans for Common Sense and Veterans United for Truth, Inc., v. James B. Peake, Secretary of Veterans Affairs, et al.*, Plaintiffs Trial Brief, Case No. C-07-3758-SC, filed April 17, 2008.

[3] Within the context of the VA, a veteran is defined as a "person who served in the active military, naval, or air service, and who was discharged or released therefrom under conditions other than dishonorable." [38 U.S.C. § 101(2); 38 C.F.R. § 3.1(d)]. The VA largely bases its determination of veteran status upon military department service records.

[4] In reference to fatal suicides, the public health community prefers to use the term "completed," rather than "committed" or "successful," to recognize the frequent association of suicide with mental illness, and reduce the accompanying stigma.

[5] For more information, see Centers for Disease Control and Prevention (CDC), Mortality Data from the National Vital Statistics System, at [http://www.cdc.gov/nchs/deaths.htm], visited May 2, 2008.

[6] See CDC, National Violent Death Reporting System, at [http://www.cdc.gov/ncipc/ profiles/nvdrs/default.htm].

[7] This definition captures current and former U.S. military servicemembers.

[8] See CDC, National Death Index, at [http://www.cdc.gov/nchs/ndi.htm].

[9] Zivin et al., "Suicide Mortality among Individuals Receiving Treatment for Depression in the Veterans Affairs Health System: Associations with Patient and Treatment Setting Characteristics," *American Journal of Public Health*, Vol. 97, No. 12, pp. 2193-8, December 2007, hereafter referred to as Zivin et al., study of depression and suicide in veterans.

[10] Unless otherwise noted, information in this section is drawn from CDC: "Suicide, Facts at a Glance," Summer 2007, and "Understanding Suicide, Fact Sheet," 2006, at [http://www.cdc.gov/ncipc/dvp/suicide/]; and "Surveillance for Violent Deaths — National Violent Death Reporting System, 16 States, 2005," *MMWR,* vol. 57(SS03), April 11, 2008, hereafter referred to as NVDRS 2005 report, at [http://www.cdc.gov/mmwr/preview/ mmwrhtml/ss5703a1.htm].

[11] Testimony of Michael Shepherd, M.D, Office of Healthcare Inspections, Office of Inspector General, Department of Veterans Affairs, in U.S. Congress, House Committee on Veterans' Affairs, hearing on *Stopping Suicides: Mental Health Challenges Within the Department of Veterans Affairs,* December 12, 2007.

[12] Suicide Prevention Resource Center, "Risk and Protective Factors for Suicide," at [http://www.sprc.org/library/srisk.pdf], visited April 30, 2008.

[13] NVDRS 2005 report. The definition "current and former military personnel" is likely to include both current military personnel and veterans, but the publication does not provide information about each group separately, or about whether such separate information is available.

[14] The remaining small number of decedents were "married but separated," "single, not otherwise specified," or their marital status was not known. These findings were not cross-tabulated by age.

[15] Zivin et al., study of depression and suicide in veterans. The authors used CDC's National Death Index to link NARDEP registrants with death certificate data, in order to identify registrants who had died, and determine that they died of suicide, during the study period.

[16] The authors cited only one study on which to base this comparison, though, which likely reflects the limited availability of studies in groups that are meaningful for comparison. It is not clear whether the comparison group included or excluded veterans.

[17] Testimony of Ira Katz, M.D., Ph.D., Deputy Chief Patient Care Services Officer, Office of Mental Health, Veterans Health Administration, Department of Veterans Affairs in U.S. Congress, House Committee on Veterans' Affairs, *Stopping Suicides: Mental Health Challenges Within the U.S. Department of Veterans Affairs,* hearings, 110th Cong., 1st sess., December 12, 2007.

[18] Lambert et al., "Suicide RiskFactors among Veterans: Risk Management in the Changing Culture of the Department of Veterans Affairs," *Journal of Mental Health Administration*, Vol. 24, No. 3, pp. 350-8, Summer 1997.

[19] Lish et al., "Suicide Screening in a Primary Care Setting at a Veterans Affairs Medical Center," *Psychosomatics*, Vol. 37, No. 5, pp. 413-24, 1996.

[20] NVDRS 2005 report. This group is a subset of the 1,821 former or current military personnel whose suicides were recorded in NVDRS in 2005, for whom these additional types of information were collected.

[21] Zivin et al., study of depression and suicide in veterans.

[22] Tanelian and Jaycox, "Invisible Wounds of War," RAND, 2008, at [http://rand.org/pubs/ monographs/2008/RAND_MG720.1.pdf], visited April 28, 2008. group.

[23] Zivin et al., study of depression and suicide in veterans.

[24] The Joshua Omvig Veterans Suicide Prevention Act is named for a veteran who completed suicide on December 22, 2005.

[25] Codified at 38 U.S.C.§ 1720F. For a detailed legislative history of P.L. 110-110, see H.Rept. 110-55 and S.Rept. 110-132.

[26] See CRS Report RL34371, *"Wounded Warrior" and Veterans Provisions in the FY2008 National Defense Authorization Act*, by Sarah A. Lister, Sidath Viranga Panangala, and Christine Scott.

[27] Drawn from the Department of Veterans Affairs, Report to Congress, *P.L. 110-110, Comprehensive Program for Suicide Prevention Among Veterans*, February 2008.

[28] Department of Veterans Affairs, Office of Inspector General, "Implementing VHA's Mental Health Strategic Plan Initiatives for Suicide Prevention," Report No. 06-03706-126, 2007.

[29] For more information on screening tools and their effectiveness, see CRS Report RS22647, *Screening for Youth Suicide Prevention*, by Ramya Sundararaman.

[30] The PDHRA (DD Form 2900) includes questions about feeling down, depressed, or hopeless, the occurrence of nightmares, relationship issues with family and friends, and increased alcohol use.

[31] U.S. Government Accountability Office (GAO), *DOD's Post-Deployment Health Reassessment,* GAO-08-181R, January 25, 2008, p.7.

[32] VA is using the national suicide prevention hotline to provide this service to veterans.

[33] Testimony of Ira Katz, M.D., Ph.D., Deputy Chief Patient Care Services Officer, Office of Mental Health, Veterans Health Administration, Department of Veterans Affairs in U.S. Congress, House Committee on Veterans' Affairs, *Stopping Suicides: Mental Health Challenges Within the U.S. Department of Veterans Affairs,* hearings, 110th Cong., 1st sess., December 12, 2007.

[34] Department of Veterans Affairs, Report to Congress, *P.L. 110-110, Comprehensive Program for Suicide Prevention Among Veterans*, p. 7, February 2008.

In: Veterans' Benefits and Care
Editor: Mathew H. Bradley

ISBN: 978-1-60692-500-3

Chapter 12

VETERANS AFFAIRS: HISTORICAL BUDGET AUTHORITY, FISCAL YEARS 1940 THROUGH 2007

Christine Scott

SUMMARY

Budget authority — the amount of money a federal department or agency can spend or obligate to spend by law — for veterans' benefits and services has increased significantly since FY1 940. In FY1 940, the budget authority for veterans' benefits and services was $561.1 million, and in FY2007 the budget authority was $82. 0 billion, or *146 times* the FY1940 budget authority. In constant 2007 dollars (i.e., inflation-adjusted), the FY2007 budget authority is *9.9 times* the FY1 940 budget authority. The increases over time have reflected the impact of increases in the number of veterans as the result of wars and other conflicts, the aging of the veteran population, and changes in benefits and services provided for veterans. This chapter provides information on the historical budget authority of the Department of Veterans Affairs (formerly the Veterans Administration) for FY1 940 through FY2007. Budget authority is presented in both current dollars and constant 2007 dollars (i.e., inflation-adjusted).

INTRODUCTION

Because of the annual budget and appropriation process in Congress and the current conflicts involving U.S. servicemembers overseas, there is a strong interest in the levels of spending by the federal government for veterans' benefits and services[1] among members of Congress and the public. For this chapter, veterans' benefits and services include direct spending on veterans (such as disability compensation or health care) and indirect spending (such as administration and construction of facilities). This chapter provides information on the historical budget authority for veterans' benefits and services for FY1940 through

FY2007. Budget authority is presented in both current dollars and constant 2007 dollars (i.e., inflation-adjusted).

Budget Authority for Veterans' Programs FY1940 - FY2007

The budget authority[2] for veterans' benefits and services over the FY1 940 - FY2007 period has generally shown a steady increase. As can be seen in **Table 1** and **Figure 1**, the FY2007 budget authority in current dollars was *146 times* the FY1940 budget authority, reflecting an average annual growth rate for the period of 7.7%.[3] In constant 2007 dollars (i.e., inflation-adjusted), the FY2007 budget authority is *9.9 times* the FY1 940 budget authority and reflects a 3.4% average annual growth rate over the period.[4]

World War II

A large number of Americans, 16.1 million,[5] served in the military in World War II (WWII, December 7, 1941, through December 31, 1946), making WWII the largest conflict to date in terms of the number of servicemembers. Because the servicemembers volunteered (or were drafted) for "the duration," a large number of servicemembers were released in a relatively short period of time at the end of the war.

Before the end of the war, the Servicemen's Readjustment Act (P.L. 346 of the 78th Congress), commonly known as the GI Bill, was signed into law in 1944, providing a major change in benefits for veterans. The GI Bill introduced education and training benefits that enabled millions of servicemembers who may have otherwise been unable to attend college or training schools to receive a college education or specific job skills training. In addition, the housing loan guarantee benefits provided by the GI Bill enabled WWII veterans to purchase homes for their families.

As shown in **Table 1**, the combination of the large number of veterans being released in a short period of time and the change in benefits resulted in the budget authority for veterans increasing from $561.1 million before the war in FY1 940 to a peak in the postwar period in FY1 947 of $8.4 billion.

In current dollars, the FY1947 budget authority was *14.9 times* the pre-war budget authority for veterans. In constant 2007 dollars, the FY1 947 budget authority for veterans was $80.8 billion, or *9.8 times* the pre-war budget authority for veterans.

The Vietnam Era

The Vietnam era (February 28, 1961 through May 7, 1975) was significantly longer than WWII, with a total of 8.7 million Americans who served in the military during the period. Until the end of 1972, a military draft was in place (the last drafted servicemembers began service in 1973), and drafted servicemembers were released through the period at the end of their military obligation. Also, while benefit changes or expansions were made during the period, no new large benefit programs were started during the period (unlike the WWII period). As a result of the regular release of servicemembers from the military over the period and the relatively stable levels of veterans' benefits and services, the large peak in budget authority at the end of WWII was not repeated at the end of the Vietnam era.

There was however a smaller peak in budget authority for the FY1975-FY1976 period that reflected an increase in the number of veterans at the end of the Vietnam conflict. While the current dollar budget authority for FY1975 and FY1976 was 2.0 and 2.3 times the FY1947 budget authority, in constant 2007 dollars (after adjusting for inflation) the budget authority for FY1975 and FY1976 was below that of FY1947. This reflects in large part the differences between the two conflicts in terms of the timing for release of servicemembers and veterans benefits and services (compared to the pre-conflict period).

Current Conflicts

During the current conflicts, Operation Enduring Freedom (OEF, which began October 2001) and Operation Iraqi Freedom (OIF, which began March 2003), there is no military draft in place. Servicemembers generally leave at the end of their obligation, or at retirement. The somewhat steady increase in budget authority for veterans' benefits and administration each year since the late 1 990s may reflect the impact of the aging of the veteran population more than the impact of the returning OEF/OIF veterans. In FY1999, of the 87,384 veterans who began receiving disability compensation that year, 19.2% were over age 55. By FY2006, of the 162,805 veterans who began receiving disability compensation that year, 41.5% were over age 55.[6]

Over time, the increases in the budget authority for veterans' benefits and services have reflected the impact of increases in the number of veterans as the result of wars and other conflicts, the aging of the veteran population, and changes in the benefits and services provided for veterans. The most dramatic impact of the combination of an increase in the number of veterans and changes in veterans' benefits can be seen in the period shortly after World War II.

Table 1. Historical Budget Authority for the Department of Veterans Affairs (VA) in Current and Constant (2007) Dollars, FY1 940-FY2007 (dollars in millions)

Fiscal Year	Current Dollars	Constant (2007) Dollars
1940	$561.1	$8,244.3
1941	582.0	8,441.1
1942	611.0	8,046.8
1943	608.6	7,380.5
1944	947.8	11,168.7
1945	1,517.2	17,510.3
1946	4,780.6	53,813.3
1947	8,354.4	80,823.6
1948	6,972.7	61,449.1
1949	5,961.8	50,778.7
1950	6,611.1	57,319.6
1951	5,831.6	47,644.2
1952	4,409.3	34,447.3
1953	4,157.2	32,011.3
1954	4,199.7	32,068.2

Table 1. (Continued)

Fiscal Year	Current Dollars	Constant (2007) Dollars
1955	4,232.4	32,478.5
1956	4,706.9	35,951.6
1957	4,792.1	35,587.7
1958	4,985.0	35,842.9
1959	5,070.7	35,955.5
1960	5,153.4	36,013.3
1961	5,424.2	37,438.5
1962	4,946.5	33,791.0
1963	5,333.1	35,993.0
1964	5,425.2	36,120.3
1965	5,641.1	37,086.8
1966	6,002.6	38,628.4
1967	6,438.0	40,161.3
1968	6,707.1	40,496.6
1969	7,408.6	42,652.2
1970	8,473.3	46,059.5
1971	9,909.4	51,221.7
1972	10,935.8	54,569.4
1973	12,391.3	59,437.3
1974	$13,540.8	$59,634.2
1975	16,304.0	64,640.6
1976	19,300.0	71,459.4
1977	18,572.9	63,935.2
1978	18,515.0	59,543.3
1979	19,901.4	58,012.9
1980	20,551.8	52,745.4
1981	22,455.2	51,876.1
1982	24,205.4	52,076.7
1983	24,607.0	51,145.6
1984	25,634.4	51,178.6
1985	26,387.0	50,808.2
1986	26,230.4	49,296.9
1987	26,605.4	48,611.4
1988	28,242.0	49,558.4
1989	29,344.9	49,155.4
1990	29,778.1	47,510.5
1991	32,525.0	49,401.2
1992	33,157.6	48,888.4
1993	35,154.7	50,306.9
1994	36,780.1	51,286.4
1995	37,466.1	50,816.6
1996	38,634.9	50,976.6

Table 1. (Continued)

Fiscal Year	Current Dollars	Constant (2007) Dollars
1997	40,054.4	51,476.8
1998	41,686.6	52,713.8
1999	43,137.8	53,521.7
2000	44,818.9	53,895.1
2001	48,665.2	56,694.2
2002	53,495.0	61,400.7
2003	59,673.1	66,920.7
2004	63,824.8	69,952.9
2005	69,436.4	73,681.3
2006	73,736.8	75,466.0
2007	82,013.8	82,013.8

Source: Table prepared by the Congressional Research Service (CRS) using data provided by the Department of Veterans Affairs, Office of the Budget, General Administration & Coordination Service.

Note: Budget authority shown in constant (2007) dollars was calculated using the Consumer Price Index All Urban Consumers (CPI-U) published by Bureau of Labor Statistics.

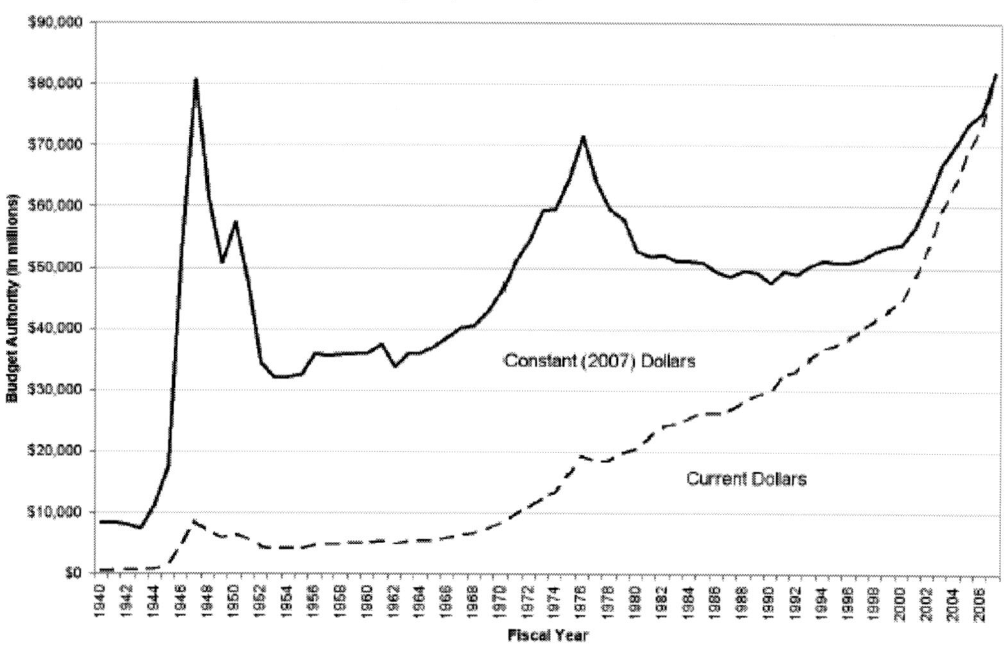

Source: Table prepared by the Congressional Research Service (CRS) using data provided by the Department of Veterans Affairs, Office of the Budget, General Administration & Coordination Service.

Note: Budget authority shown in constant (2007) dollars was calculated using the Consumer Price Index All Urban Consumers (CPI-U) published by Bureau of Labor Statistics.

Figure 1. Historical Budget Authority for the Department of Veterans Affairs (VA) in Current and Constant (2007) Dollars, FY1 940 - FY2007

End Notes

[1] For information on FY2008 appropriations for veterans' benefits and services, see CRS Report RL34038, *Military Construction, Veterans Affairs, and Related Agencies: FY2008 Appropriations*, by Daniel H. Else, Christine Scott, and Sidath Viranga Panangala.

[2] Budget authority is the amount of money the federal department or agency can spend or obligate to spend by law. Budget authority has several forms, including appropriations; authority to borrow; contract authority; and authority to spend from offsetting collections. For more information see CRS Report 98-721, *Introduction to the Federal Budget Process*, by Robert Keith.

[3] The federal fiscal year changed between 1976 and 1977. For fiscal years 1940 through 1976, the federal fiscal year was July through June. For fiscal years 1977 and later, the federal fiscal year was October through September. The adjustment quarter in 1976 is not shown in the figures used in this chapter.

[4] For this chapter, constant dollar budget authority figures were calculated using the current dollar budget authority data provided by the Department of Veterans Affairs and the Consumer Price Index for All Urban Consumers (CPI-U) published by the Bureau of Labor Statistics.

[5] For information on the number of military personnel serving in American war and military operations, see CRS Report RL32492, *American War and Military Operation Casualties: Lists and Statistics*, by Hannah Fischer, Kim Klarman, and Mari-Jana "M-J" Oboroceanu.

[6] Department of Veterans Affairs, Annual Benefits Report, various years, available at [http://www.vba.va.gov/reports/index.htm].

In: Veterans' Benefits and Care
Editor: Mathew H. Bradley

ISBN: 978-1-60692-500-3

Chapter 13

VA HEALTH CARE: FACILITIES HAVE TAKEN ACTION TO PROVIDE LANGUAGE ACCESS SERVICES AND CULTURALLY APPROPRIATE CARE TO A DIVERSE VETERAN POPULATION

United States Government Accountability Office

WHY GAO DID THIS STUDY

The Department of Veterans Affairs (VA) faces challenges in bridging language and cultural barriers as it seeks to provide quality health care services to an increasingly diverse veteran population in terms of race, ethnicity, sex, and age. To meet the needs of veterans with limited English proficiency (LEP), VA issued an LEP Directive that provides guidance for medical centers in assessing language needs and, if needed, developing language access services designed to ensure effective communication between English-speaking providers and those with LEP. In addition, VA is also challenged to deliver health care services in ways that are culturally appropriate—that is, respectful of and responsive to the cultural values of a diverse veteran population. In light of these challenges, GAO was asked to discuss the (1) actions VA has taken to implement its LEP Directive and the status of veterans' utilization of language access services, and (2) efforts VA has made to provide culturally appropriate health care services.

GAO reviewed VA's policies and the LEP Directive, interviewed VA officials and reviewed efforts by 6 VA medical centers and 10 other VA facilities to implement VA's LEP Directive and to provide culturally appropriate health care services. GAO also reviewed documents from 17 other VA medical centers related to implementation of the LEP Directive.

To view the full product, including the scope and methodology, click on GAO-08-535. For more information, contact Randall B. Williamson, (202) 512-7114, williamsonr@ gao. gov.

WHAT GAO FOUND

VA reported that as of June 2007, all of its medical centers had taken action to implement the guidance in VA's LEP Directive. Specifically, medical center officials told VA that they had assessed the language needs of their veteran service populations, and, if necessary, developed language assistance policies and offered language access services, including providing translated materials and interpretation services. The VA medical centers GAO reviewed provided translated materials to meet the various language needs of their veteran service populations and offered interpretation services as well. For example, VA medical centers maintained a list of bilingual medical center staff who can provide interpretation services during a clinical encounter between a provider and a veteran with LEP. In addition, five of the six VA medical centers GAO reviewed can access telephone interpretation services that are provided through a contract to help ensure that medical staff can communicate with veterans and their families with LEP. According to officials at medical centers GAO reviewed, utilization of language access services is low. However, VA officials told GAO that they expect the demand for language access services to grow as the increasingly diverse military servicemember population transitions to veteran status.

VA medical centers are addressing the need for culturally appropriate health care services through staff training and tailoring health care services. Medical centers provide training for medical center staff to facilitate the delivery of culturally appropriate health care services including an annual mandatory training on the health care needs of veterans in various age groups. VA medical centers and other VA facilities GAO reviewed have implemented a variety of measures to meet the needs of their culturally diverse veteran populations. For example, three VA facilities GAO reviewed offer spiritual services, such as the use of medicine men and traditional healing rituals, in order to meet the needs of Native American veterans. Also, VA has minority veterans program coordinators at each medical center to identify barriers to health care for minorities and advise medical center officials in developing services to make health care more accessible and culturally appropriate for minority veteran populations. VA medical centers GAO reviewed have also initiated outreach efforts to promote the availability of culturally appropriate care.

In commenting on a draft of this chapter, VA stated that it agreed with the information presented as it pertained to VA.

MOTIVOS DE ESTE ESTUDIO DE LA GAO

El Departamento de Asuntos de los Veteranos (VA) se enfrenta a retos en su empeño por sobrepasar barreras culturales y de lenguaje para proporcionar buenos servicios de atención de salud a una población de veteranos que es cada vez más diversa en cuanto a raza, origen étnico, sexo y edad. A fin de satisfacer las necesidades de los veteranos que tienen conocimiento limitado de inglés (LEP, por sus siglas en inglés), el VA emitió una Directiva LEP para guiar a los centros médicos en su evaluación de la necesidad de servicios lingüísticos y, cuando era necesario, establecerlos con el fin de asegurar la comunicación eficaz entre los proveedores anglófonos y los que tienen LEP. Además, el VA también se enfrenta al reto de prestar servicios de atención de salud en formas que sean culturalmente aceptables; es decir, que respeten los valores culturales de una población diversa de veteranos y sean sensibles a esos valores. En vista de estos retos, se pidió a la GAO que analize (1) las medidas que el VA ha tomado para aplicar su Directiva LEP y el estado relativo de la utilización de los servicios lingüísticos por parte de los veteranos y (2) los esfuerzos que el VA ha realizado para proporcionar servicios de atención de salud culturalmente aceptables.

La GAO examinó las políticas del VA y la Directiva LEP, entrevistó a funcionarios del VA y examinó los empeños de 6 centros médicos y 10 establecimientos más del VA dirigidos a la aplicación de la Directiva LEP del VA y a la prestación de servicios de atención de salud culturalmente aceptables.

Para ver el informe completo, su ámbito y metodología, pulse en GAO-08-535. Para más información, llame a Randall B. Williamson, (202) 512-7144, williamsonr@gao.gov.

Conclusiones de la GAO

El VA informó que en junio de 2007, todos sus centros médicos habían tomado medidas para aplicar lo estipulado en la Directiva LEP del VA. En concreto, los funcionarios de los centros médicos informaron al VA que habían evaluado las necesidades lingüísticas de sus poblaciones de veteranos y que, cuando era necesario, habían elaborado políticas de asistencia lingüística y ofrecido servicios lingüísticos, lo que incluía información traducida y servicios de interpretación. Los centros médicos del VA que la GAO examinó proporcionaron información traducida para satisfacer las diferentes necesidades lingüísticas de los veteranos a los que atienden, y también ofrecieron servicios de interpretación. Por ejemplo, los centros médicos del VA tenían una lista de su personal bilingüe que podía interpretar durante una consulta clínica entre un proveedor y un veterano con LEP. Además, cinco de los seis centros médicos del VA que la GAO examinó tienen acceso a servicios de interpretación telefónica proporcionados por contrato, lo cual ayuda a garantizar que el personal médico pueda comunicarse con los veteranos y sus familiares que tienen LEP. Según los funcionarios en los centros médicos que la GAO examinó, los servicios lingüísticos se utilizan poco. Sin embargo, los funcionarios del VA informaron a la GAO que ellos anticipan un aumento en la demanda de servicios lingüísticos en vista de la diversidad cada vez mayor de los militares que pasan a ser veteranos.

Con manera de abordar la necesidad de atención de salud culturalmente aceptable, los centros médicos del VA ofrecen capacitación de personal y adaptan sus servicios de atención de salud. Los centros médicos capacitan a su personal para facilitar la prestación de servicios de atención de salud culturalmente aceptables, lo cual incluye capacitación anual obligatoria sobre las necesidades de atención de salud de los veteranos en diferentes grupos de edad. Los centros médicos del VA y otras instalaciones que la GAO examinó han puesto en marcha una serie de medidas para responder a las necesidades de sus poblaciones de veteranos culturalmente diversas. Por ejemplo, tres instalaciones del VA que la GAO examinó ofrecen servicios espirituales, como curanderos y rituales tradicionales de curación, para satisfacer las necesidades de los veteranos que sean indios nativos de los EEUU. Así mismo, en cada centro médico el VA tiene coordinadores de programas para los veteranos que forman parte de grupos de minoría. Estos coordinadores identifican los obstáculos que se interponen a la atención de salud de las minorías, y asesoran a los funcionarios de los centros médicos en la elaboración de servicios para que la atención de salud sea más accesible y culturalmente aceptable para los veteranos que forman parte de grupos de minoría. Los centros médicos del VA que la GAO examinó también han iniciado actividades de divulgación para promover la disponibilidad de atención de salud culturalmente aceptable.

El VA, al comentar sobre una versión preliminar de este informe, afirmó que estaba de acuerdo con la información relativa al VA que se presenta.

ABBREVIATIONS

CBOC	community-based outpatient clinic
CMV	Center for Minority Veterans
DOJ	Department of Justice
EEO	Equal Employment Opportunity
EO	executive order
HHS	Department of Health and Human Services
LEP	limited English proficiency
NDAA	National Defense Authorization Act
VA	Department of Veterans Affairs
VHA	Veterans Health Administration
VISN	Veterans Integrated Service Network

May 28, 2008

The Honorable Michael H. Michaud
Chairman
Subcommittee on Health
Committee on Veterans' Affairs

House of Representatives
The Honorable John T. Salazar
House of Representatives

The Honorable Hilda L. Solis
House of Representatives

The veteran population served by the Department of Veterans Affairs (VA) will become more diverse in terms of race, ethnicity, sex, and age. VA data show that racial and ethnic minorities account for about 20 percent of the veteran population and that about 7 percent of veterans are women.[1] We reported in 2005 that racial and ethnic minorities accounted for about 33 percent of servicemembers in the military; about 16 percent of servicemembers were women.[2] Based on the higher diversity among servicemembers in the military compared to veterans, VA officials anticipate that the veteran population eligible to receive health care services from VA will become more diverse as current members of the military are discharged or released from active duty and transition to veteran status. In addition to racial and ethnic diversity, VA has seen an increase in the number of younger Operation Enduring Freedom and Operation Iraqi Freedom veterans using VA health care services and officials expect this number to continue to grow.

As its veteran population becomes more diverse, VA faces challenges in bridging language and cultural barriers as it seeks to provide quality health care services to its veteran population. For example, a study commissioned by the California Endowment and the Robert Wood Johnson Foundation found that to help meet the needs of a diverse patient population, health care institutions, such as VA medical facilities, should provide language access services.[3] Language access services are designed to ensure effective communication between English speakers and those with limited English proficiency (LEP). This may include providing translated versions of informational brochures or consent forms and making staff available who can interpret providers' instructions for patients or their family members with LEP. Several studies have found that the implementation of language access services in health care settings can increase access to care, quality of care, and health outcomes.[4]

Research suggests that providing culturally appropriate health care services is an integral part of quality health care, and that cultural factors can have a significant influence on the delivery of health care services and can compromise access for culturally diverse populations.[5] At the federal level, HHS has published a set of standards for medical facilities that state that health care services should be delivered in ways that are culturally appropriate—that is, respectful of and responsive to the cultural values of a diverse population.[6] This can mean, for example, recognizing the role of the extended family in medical decisions for a particular ethnic group and including these individuals in discussions of a patient's medical care and treatment. According to HHS's standards, providing culturally appropriate services to culturally diverse patients has the potential to improve access to care, quality of care, and ultimately, health outcomes. Prior to the enactment of the National Defense Authorization Act (NDAA) for Fiscal Year 2008, there was no specific statutory requirement for VA to provide culturally appropriate care. However, several provisions in the 2008 NDAA require the consideration of the gender-, ethnic group-, or age-specific needs of veterans, including a direction to provide age-appropriate nursing home care.[7]

To meet the needs of persons with LEP, the President issued an executive order[8] in August 2000 that required all federal agencies to develop and implement a system by which persons with LEP can have meaningful access to the services provided by the agency. The order also instructs federal agencies to work to ensure that recipients of federal financial assistance provide meaningful access to their LEP applicants and beneficiaries. According to the order, each agency must develop a plan that outlines the steps the agency will take to ensure that persons with LEP have meaningful access to the programs and services it provides.[9] In response to this order, in January 2002, VA issued a directive of its own—referred to in this chapter as the LEP Directive[10] —to assist VA programs, including its medical centers, in providing appropriate language access services for veterans with LEP. The LEP directive provides guidance to medical centers and other facilities within VA to help them comply with EO 13166; medical centers and other facilities that do not adopt all of the specific practices outlined in the directive are not necessarily out of compliance with the executive order as long as medical center officials take reasonable steps to assess and meet the language needs of the veteran service population. Additionally, because the diversity of the veteran service population varies across VA medical centers, some medical centers may not have a need to take all the actions identified in VA's LEP Directive.

In light of the increasing diversity of the veteran population in terms of race, ethnicity, sex, and age, you asked for information about the steps VA has taken to provide language access services for veterans and its efforts to deliver health care services in ways that are culturally appropriate for veterans' diverse cultural values. This chapter discusses the (1) actions VA has taken to implement its LEP Directive and the status of veterans' utilization of available language access services, and (2) efforts VA has made to provide culturally appropriate health care services. We did not assess VA's compliance with EO 13166 and instead describe actions taken under VA's LEP Directive in response to EO 13166.

To describe the actions VA has taken to implement its LEP Directive as well as veterans' utilization of available language access services and the efforts VA has made to provide culturally appropriate health care services, we reviewed an executive order, federal guidance, and VA policy and procedures. We also selected five Veterans Integrated Service Networks (VISN) to review.[11] We selected these five VISNs based on the number of racial and ethnic minority veterans living in each VISN and geographic variation.[12] Within these five VISNs we selected a judgmental sample of 16 VA facilities, including six VA medical centers, five community-based outpatient clinics (CBOC), and five Vet Centers, to include in our review.[13] From our sample of VA facilities, we conducted site visits to medical centers and associated CBOCs, and Vet Centers, located in Chicago, Illinois; Durham, North Carolina; and Los Angeles, California. For the remainder of VA facilities in our sample, we conducted in-depth telephone interviews with medical center, CBOC, and Vet Center officials in Bath, New York; Prescott, Arizona; and Richmond, Virginia.[14] We conducted in-depth interviews with VA officials and staff from each of the 16 VA facilities to learn about actions taken at their facility to provide language access services for veterans with LEP, the utilization of these services, and the efforts the facility has made to provide culturally appropriate health care services. At the six VA medical centers we reviewed in depth, we examined documents related to efforts by the centers to assess the language needs of their service population and, if necessary, provide language access services. In addition, we interviewed officials in each of the five VISNs we selected for review. The information we collected from the six medical centers and five VISNs we reviewed is not generalizable to all VISNs and VA medical centers.

Additionally, in order to obtain information on the steps VA has taken through its medical centers to provide language access services under its LEP Directive, we selected a random sample of 20 VA medical centers and requested copies of language needs assessments conducted by medical center officials and language assistance policies.[15] We received documentation from 17 of the 20 medical centers. We conducted follow-up with the three medical centers that did not provide documentation but did not receive the requested materials from them. We did not evaluate the quality of the language needs assessments or language access policies provided by the 17 medical centers or from the 6 medical centers we visited or reviewed in depth. The information we collected from our sample of 17 medical centers is not generalizable to all VA medical centers. In addition to interviews we conducted with VA officials, we also interviewed officials from the Department of Justice (DOJ), as well as experts in the field of language access services and the provision of culturally competent health care services.[16] We conducted this performance audit from February 2007 through March 2008, in accordance with generally accepted government auditing standards. Those standards require that we plan and perform the audit to obtain sufficient, appropriate evidence to provide a reasonable basis for our findings and conclusions based on our audit objectives. We believe that the evidence obtained provides a reasonable basis for our findings based on our audit objectives.

RESULTS IN BRIEF

As of June 2007, all VA medical centers had taken actions to implement VA's LEP Directive, according to VA. Specifically, all medical centers had assessed the language needs of their veteran service populations, and if necessary developed language assistance policies, and offered language access services. These language access services mainly involve providing translated materials and interpretation services. In addition, we found that all VA medical centers have computer software that generates medical treatment consent forms in Spanish and additional software that allows VA staff to access patient education materials in languages other than English. Medical centers offered interpretation services as well. For example, the six medical centers we reviewed maintained a list of bilingual medical center staff who volunteered to provide interpretation services during a clinical encounter between a provider and a veteran with LEP. In addition, five of the six medical centers included in our in-depth review can access telephone interpretation services that are provided through a contract to ensure that medical staff can communicate with veterans with LEP and their families. VA medical center officials reported to us that current utilization of language access services is low. However, VA officials told us that they expect the demand for language access services to grow as the increasingly diverse military servicemember population transitions to veteran status.

We found that the six VA medical centers we reviewed in depth are addressing the need for culturally appropriate health care services through staff training and tailoring health care services. The six medical centers we reviewed provided training for medical center staff to facilitate the delivery of culturally appropriate health care services, including a mandatory training on the health care needs of veterans in various age groups. We found that VA medical centers and other VA facilities we reviewed in depth implemented a variety of measures to meet the needs of their culturally diverse veteran populations. For example, some locations offered spiritual services to meet the needs of Native American veterans, including the use of medicine men and traditional healing rituals. Another offered a counseling group exclusively for African American veterans; another offered counseling groups specifically for women veterans. Also, minority veterans program coordinators at all VA medical centers are charged with identifying barriers to health care for minorities and advising medical center officials in developing services to make health care more accessible and culturally appropriate for minority veteran populations. Some VA medical centers have also initiated outreach efforts to promote the availability of culturally appropriate care. For example, at two VA medical centers we reviewed in depth, staff told us that they worked closely with military and National Guard bases located near the medical center to increase the awareness of VA health benefits among younger veterans and their families. According to VA officials, these outreach efforts helped younger veterans understand that VA serves veterans of all ages and from all military conflicts.

In commenting on a draft of this chapter, VA stated that it agreed with the information presented as it pertained to VA.

BACKGROUND

EO 13166, *Improving Access to Services for Persons with Limited English Proficiency*, requires that all federal agencies take reasonable steps to ensure meaningful access to their programs and services for people with LEP. DOJ has issued guidance that spells out four factors agencies need to consider in determining whether they are taking reasonable steps in this regard: (1) the number or proportion of LEP persons in the eligible service population; (2) the frequency with which LEP individuals come in contact with the program; (3) the importance the services provided by the program; and (4) the resources available.[17] Reasonable steps to ensure meaningful access could include developing language access services and guidance for implementing these services. The EO required that each federal agency create a plan outlining steps it will take consistent with DOJ guidance to ensure meaningful access to its services by LEP individuals. The EO did not require DOJ to evaluate the plans or to monitor the implementation of these plans.

In 2002, in response to EO 13166, VA created and implemented VHA Directive 2002-006. It provided a framework for VA medical centers to assess and determine if there was a need to develop language assistance policies and language access services. The medical centers retain flexibility to determine exactly how they will comply with the EO, but they must do so in accordance with the four factors as outlined by DOJ and reiterated in the LEP Directive. In February 2007, VA issued VHA Directive 2007-009, which renewed VA's guidance on language assistance policies.[18] In its LEP Directive, VA outlined the steps that constitute an effective language assistance program at its medical centers, including an assessment of the language needs of the veteran population served and identification of the non-English languages encountered by medical center staff. If a VA medical center identifies a specific language need among its veteran service population, VA's LEP Directive also indicated that the medical center should develop and implement a language assistance policy to ensure meaningful communication. According to the directive, the policy should describe how the medical center plans to provide language access services and ensure that all veterans receive meaningful access to VA health care services, regardless of the veterans' level of English proficiency. VA's LEP Directive also provided medical centers with examples of ways to provide language access services—including, translating written materials,[19] hiring bilingual staff, and contracting with interpreter services.

VA's Equal Employment Opportunity (EEO) office is responsible for overseeing the implementation of VA's LEP Directive. As such, this office conducted surveys of VA medical centers to assess whether medical center officials were following the steps outlined in the LEP Directive, such as conducting an assessment of language needs, or otherwise taking reasonable steps to provide language access services for veterans being served. VA's Center for Minority Veterans (CMV)[20] is also involved in helping medical centers meet the language and cultural needs of the veteran population. CMV is responsible for ensuring that eligible minority veterans receive VA benefits and services.

Culturally appropriate health care is care that is respectful of and responsive to the cultural needs of patients. According to HHS, providing culturally appropriate services to culturally diverse patients has the potential to improve access to care, quality of care, and ultimately, health outcomes. HHS has published a set of standards[21] for all medical facilities regarding the delivery of culturally appropriate care. Other national organizations also recognize the importance of culturally appropriate care and have established standards or recommendations for its provision. For example, the Joint Commission has standards related to culturally appropriate health care that must be met by hospitals, including VA medical centers, to receive accreditation.[22]

VA Medical Centers Are Implementing VA's LEP Directive; However, Utilization of Language Access Services Is Low

VA medical centers are implementing VA's LEP Directive in terms of assessing the language needs of its veteran service population, and, if necessary, developing language assistance policies. VA medical centers and facilities have offered language access services that include providing translated materials and interpretation services to meet the needs of veterans with LEP. VA medical center officials reported a low utilization of these language access services. However, VA and medical center officials told us that they expect the demand for language access services to grow as the increasingly diverse servicemember population transitions to veteran status.

VA Medical Centers Have Implemented the LEP Directive

VA stated that by June 2007 all of its medical centers had taken actions to implement the guidance in VA's LEP Directive. According to VA, all of its medical centers have assessed the language needs of its veteran service population, and, as necessary, developed language assistance policies. Our visits to three VA medical centers and in-depth telephone interviews with staff at three VA medical centers provided a more detailed account of the variety of language access services being offered at VA medical centers.

VA first surveyed each of VA's medical center directors in December 2005 to assess if medical centers were following the guidance in VA's LEP Directive.[23] The survey contained 10 "yes" or "no" questions to gauge the extent of medical centers' efforts to implement the LEP Directive. The questions ranged from issues such as overall language assistance policies to efforts to provide language access services. If a "no" response was provided for any question, the medical center directors completing the survey were instructed to indicate a tentative date by which they would take action to address the item. VA required medical center directors and VISN directors to ensure that the responses for individual medical centers were completed. However, VA did not require that VISN or medical center directors provide documentation to support their "yes" responses to the survey.

The results of the 2005 survey showed that 65 percent of VA medical centers had assessed the language needs of their veteran service population and that 60 percent of the centers had developed a language assistance policy.[24] While completing the survey, VA medical center directors reported information about other medical center efforts to meet the needs of LEP veterans, including efforts to translate documents and hire bilingual interpreters. For example, 87 percent of VA medical center directors reported establishing a list of staff available for interpretation services and that 24 percent of VA medical centers had translated written documents into languages other than English.

After conducting its initial survey, VA took several steps to help medical centers improve their efforts to implement the LEP Directive, according to a VA official. VA staff made follow-up calls to VA officials from the medical centers that did not respond to the survey or that were identified by the survey as not conducting efforts consistent with the LEP Directive.[25] During these follow-up efforts, VA staff offered guidance to medical center officials on conducting language needs assessments and developing language assistance policies in ways that were consistent with the LEP Directive. According to officials we interviewed at two VA medical centers, the guidance was helpful in their facilities' assessment of language needs among their service population and development of language assistance policies.

According to VA, the follow-up efforts proved successful, as all medical centers reported that they had assessed the language needs of their veteran service population, and, as necessary, developed language assistance policies. In July 2007, VA reported that as a result of its follow-up efforts, all of VA's medical centers, in accordance with the LEP Directive, had assessed the language needs of their veteran service population and developed language assistance policies as needed. VA concluded that because of the progress and efforts made by its medical centers to implement the LEP Directive, VA would not conduct any additional evaluations of medical center implementation of the LEP Directive. Instead, VA said it would rely on the medical centers to monitor their own LEP language access needs and programs.

VA Medical Centers and Facilities Offer a Variety of Language Access Services for Veterans with LEP

VA medical centers and other VA facilities have access to a variety of translation services. At the national level, VA has translated its widely distributed benefits publication into Spanish and makes information from this publication available in Spanish on its Web site.[26] All VA medical centers have computer software that offers medical treatment consent forms in Spanish and additional software that allows VA staff to access patient education materials in several languages other than English, such as Spanish and Korean.[27]

The VA medical centers and facilities included in our in-depth review also provide translated materials to meet the various language needs of their veteran service populations. We found that all six medical centers in our in-depth review translate written materials on their own. For example, staff at one medical center we interviewed told us that they translated educational materials on traumatic brain injuries into Spanish. However, staff at the medical centers reported that they primarily rely on publicly available translated documents rather than translating written materials on their own because of the cost of independently translating documents. The sources of these publicly available materials range from other federal agencies to results of an Internet search. For example, according to VA officials, patient educators at some medical centers use patient education materials on a range of topics including heart disease and diabetes that have been translated into Spanish by HHS's Food and Drug Administration. VA medical center staff can also use materials translated by staff at other medical centers. For example, staff at one medical facility we reviewed reported that the VA medical center located in San Juan, Puerto Rico, has shared patient education materials they have translated into Spanish with other VA medical centers. Medical center staff we interviewed also reported using professional groups within VA, such as EEO managers or patient educators, to identify and share existing translated materials. However, these groups are limited in their membership and, as such, might not be aware of all translated materials available at VA medical centers. Additionally, VA medical facilities included in our review generally offer translated materials specific to the services they provide, when needed. For example, one Vet Center we reviewed translated a pamphlet on post-traumatic stress disorder into Spanish for its largely Hispanic veteran service population.

As part of language access services, VA medical centers we reviewed in depth provide language interpretation services to help address the language needs of veterans with LEP. Staff we interviewed at all six medical centers we reviewed had the ability to provide interpretation services to veterans with LEP and were doing so in several different ways. For example, staff members at all six of these medical centers maintained a list of bilingual medical center staff who volunteered to provide interpretation services during a clinical encounter between a provider and a veteran with LEP. Medical center staff primarily used people from this list to provide needed interpretation services. In addition, staff at five of the six VA medical centers had contract telephone interpretation services available as a means to help effectively communicate with veterans and their families with LEP. Moreover, two of the three medical centers we visited advertised within the medical center, in languages other than English, the availability of language interpretation services to veterans and their families with LEP. In these medical centers, we observed signs posted near entrances and elevators that advertised, in multiple languages, free language interpretation services for veterans and their family members.

In addition to efforts made by VA's medical centers to provide language access services, some of VA's Vet Centers have also made efforts to provide language access services to ensure that veterans with LEP have meaningful access to counseling and other services. Vet Centers provide language access services to veterans' family members with LEP to ensure that they are able to participate in counseling sessions, such as marital and family counseling. For example, at one Vet Center we visited, the entire staff was bilingual to help accommodate the needs of its mostly Hispanic veteran service population. In cases where bilingual staff were not available, four of the five Vet Centers where we conducted interviews had agreements with the local VA medical center to access its list of bilingual staff available for interpretation services.

VA Medical Center Officials Report Low Utilization of Language Access Services; However, Officials Expect the Demand for These Services to Grow

Officials at the VA medical centers and facilities included in our in-depth review reported that veterans seldom use VA's language access services. For example, officials and staff we interviewed from five of the six medical centers in our review stated that their facility had a contract in place for telephone interpretation services but only one medical center reported ever utilizing these services. Staff at the medical center that reported utilizing the interpretation service stated that the use was infrequent. Moreover, staff we interviewed at the six VA medical centers we reviewed reported that most veterans speak English and staff at one medical center reported that veterans prefer to receive written materials in English. Staff at one medical center told us that they stopped routinely offering translated materials after veterans—for whom English was not their primary language—stated their preference for materials in English. However, translated documents were made available upon request. Despite the low utilization of interpretation services, such as the use of a contracted telephone interpretation service, officials at all six medical centers in our in-depth review reported using bilingual staff to serve as volunteer interpreters when needed.[28] In addition, in our review of 17 other medical centers' language needs assessments, officials from one medical center volunteered utilizing telephone interpretation services four times in the 2 years prior to our request in July 2007, while another medical center volunteered in its assessment that veterans at the facility never used the facility's contracted telephone interpretation service.

VA medical center officials told us that they expect the demand for language access services to grow as the increasingly diverse servicemember population transitions to veteran status. The servicemember population is more diverse—in terms of race, and ethnicity—than the current veteran population.[29] VA officials we interviewed projected that the increased diversity of the military servicemember population will directly translate to an increased level of diversity in the veteran population as these servicemembers end their military careers and become veterans who may be eligible for VA health care services. Staff from several VA facilities told us that they have recently witnessed demographic changes in their service population. For example, two Vet Centers we visited told us that they have experienced an increase in the number of veterans and family members needing language access services in Spanish to facilitate marital and family counseling sessions.

VA Medical Centers Are Addressing the Need for Culturally Appropriate Health Care Services through Staff Training and Tailoring Health Care Services

In an effort to address the cultural differences represented in its veteran service population, VA medical centers have conducted training programs to increase staff awareness about cultural diversity and the need for culturally appropriate health care services. Additionally, VA medical centers and facilities tailored a variety of health care services to different segments of the veteran population and promoted the availability of culturally appropriate health care services by targeting outreach efforts to different segments of the veteran population.

VA Medical Centers Provided Training to Staff to Increase Awareness about the Need for Culturally Appropriate Health Care Services

VA medical centers have provided a variety of training programs for staff to both raise cultural awareness and to assist medical center staff in providing culturally appropriate health care services. According to VA medical center officials we interviewed, medical center staff are required to annually complete one mandatory VA-developed training course on the health care needs of veterans of various age groups.[30] The six VA medical centers we reviewed have offered training to help staff understand cultural diversity as well as appreciate the need for culturally appropriate health care. These training efforts included locally-developed training on diversity given to new staff during orientation and on-line diversity training that is available to all staff. One of the six medical centers we reviewed in depth also developed training to help staff better understand what it was like for a veteran in general to serve in the military, as well as what it was like for a veteran who served during a particular military service era, such as the Vietnam War. The training materials also provided information on the types of medical diagnoses that may be related to a veteran's service, such as exposure to environmental hazards. Additionally, individual medical centers developed programs designed to increase awareness of veteran diversity and different cultural practices. For example, four VA medical centers we reviewed reported using celebrations and events in conjunction with heritage months (e.g., African American Heritage Month and Women's History Month) as educational opportunities to increase medical center staff awareness of veteran cultures and diversity. Programs included speakers, cultural fairs, and presentations open to staff and veterans at the individual VA medical centers.

VA Medical Centers and Facilities Have Provided Health Care Services Tailored to Meet the Needs of a Culturally Diverse Veteran Population

VA medical centers and facilities have provided numerous health care services designed to meet the needs of the culturally diverse veteran population that differs in terms of race, ethnicity, sex, as well as age. According to VA officials, these services have varied across VA medical centers, CBOCs, and Vet Centers, depending on the needs of the veteran populations served. During our in-depth review of 16 VA medical centers and facilities, officials identified a number of health care services that are provided in a culturally appropriate manner:

- Two medical centers and one Vet Center offer spiritual services, which include the use of medicine men and traditional healing rituals, in order to meet the needs of Native American veterans.
- Three medical centers and one CBOC have increased the use of modern technology, such as text-messaging appointment reminders, to communicate more effectively with younger veterans, who are typically accustomed to such means of communication.
- One Vet Center offered a counseling group exclusively for African American veterans and one Vet Center offered counseling groups for women veterans.

According to staff we interviewed, services tailored to different segments of the population are often designed using information gained from specific veteran requests, veteran focus groups, or through recommendations of special-emphasis population groups.[31]

To facilitate the delivery of culturally appropriate health care services, all VA medical centers have a minority veterans program coordinator.[32] The role of the minority veterans program coordinator is to identify barriers to health care and advise medical center officials in developing services to make health care more accessible and culturally appropriate for minority veteran populations. Minority veterans program coordinators also work directly with minority veterans in an effort to facilitate access to and use of VA health care services.

To promote the availability of culturally appropriate care, the six VA medical centers included in our in-depth review have implemented a variety of targeted outreach efforts to different veteran populations. For example, officials at two of the six medical centers we reviewed reported working closely with military and National Guard bases located near the medical center to increase awareness of VA health benefits among younger veterans and their families. According to VA staff, these outreach efforts helped younger veterans understand that VA was not just "their grandfather's VA" and that VA medical centers serve veterans from all military conflicts. At one medical center, officials we interviewed reported outreach efforts to help Hispanic, younger, and female veterans recognize when they might need medical services, for example treatment for post- traumatic stress disorder or depression. These outreach efforts included participating in community health fairs and ceremonies held to welcome home servicemembers from the combat theaters. VA staff said they tailored these efforts to different communities, and staff at one medical center reported including materials in Spanish.

GAO's Mission

The Government Accountability Office, the audit, evaluation, and investigative arm of Congress, exists to support Congress in meeting its constitutional responsibilities and to help improve the performance and accountability of the federal government for the American people. GAO examines the use of public funds; evaluates federal programs and policies; and provides analyses, recommendations, and other assistance to help Congress make informed oversight, policy, and funding decisions. GAO's commitment to good government is reflected in its core values of accountability, integrity, and reliability.

End Notes

[1] See Department of Veterans Affairs, *VA Benefits & Health Care Utilization* (Washington, D.C., 2007), and Department of Veterans Affairs, *Women Veterans: Past, Present and Future* (Washington, D.C., May 2005). VA data from 2007 show that about 80 percent of veterans are white, non-Hispanic; 11 percent are African American; 6 percent are Hispanic; and 4 percent are other racial groups.

[2] See GAO, *Military Personnel: Reporting Additional Servicemember Demographics Could Enhance Congressional Oversight*, GAO-05-952 (Washington, D.C.: Sept. 22, 2005). We reported that 67 percent of military servicemembers were white, non-Hispanic; 9 percent were Hispanic, 17 percent were African American; and 3 percent were Asian American/Pacific Islander.

[3] See Grantmakers in Health, *In the Right Words: Addressing Language and Culture in Providing Care* (San Francisco, Calif., August 2003).

[4] See Department of Health and Human Services (HHS), *A Patient-Centered Guide to Implementing Language Access Services in Healthcare Organizations* (Washington, D.C., September 2005); B. D. Smedley, A. Y. Stith, and A. R. Nelson, *Unequal Treatment: Confronting Racial and Ethnic Disparities in Health Care,* Institute of Medicine Report (Washington, D.C., 2003); Grantmakers in Health, *In the Right Words*; and Edward L. Martinez, Steve Hitov, and Mara Youdelman, *Language Access in Health Care Statement of Principles: Explanatory Guide* (Washington, D.C., October 2006, reissued November 2007).

[5] See Institute of Medicine, *Speaking of Health: Assessing Health Communication Strategies for Diverse Populations* (Washington, D.C., 2002), and The Henry J. Kaiser Family Foundation, *Compendium of Cultural Competence Initiatives in Health Care* (Washington, D.C., and Menlo Park, Calif., 2003).

[6] HHS, Office of Minority Health, *National Standards for Culturally and Linguistically Appropriate Services in Health Care* (Washington, D.C., 2001).

[7] See, for example, Pub. L. No. 110-181, §§ 1603, 1661, 1706, 122 Stat. 3.

[8] Exec. Order (EO) No. 13166, *Improving Access to Services for Persons with Limited English Proficiency*, 65 Fed. Reg. 50121 (Aug. 11, 2000).

[9] EO 13166 further states that these plans are to be consistent with the standards set forth in the Department of Justice (DOJ) guidance that was issued at the same time as the EO. See 65 Fed. Reg. 50123 (Aug. 16, 2000). The steps outlined in the plans are required to be consistent with, and not unduly burdensome to, the fundamental mission of the agency. DOJ serves as the central repository for materials related to implementation of EO 13166, including agency plans.

[10] In this chapter, the term "LEP Directive" refers to Veterans Health Administration (VHA) Directive 2002-006, *Limited English Proficiency (LEP) Title VI Prohibition Against National Origin Discrimination in Federally-Conducted Programs and Activities and in Federal Financial Assisted Programs*, renewed as VHA Directive 2007-009, unless otherwise noted.

[11] VA organizes its medical facilities into 21 regional networks, called Veterans Integrated Service Networks (VISN). For this chapter, we focus exclusively on health care services provided by VA in its medical centers, community-based outpatient clinics (CBOC), and Vet Centers, which are federally-conducted programs. The scope of this chapter does not include recipients of financial assistance from VA.

[12] There is geographic variation in this group of VISNs: VISN 2 includes upstate New York; VISN 6 includes Richmond, Virginia, and Raleigh-Durham, North Carolina; VISN 12 includes Chicago, Illinois; VISN 18 includes northern Arizona; and VISN 22 includes the greater Los Angeles, California, area. There is also variation in the racial and ethnic composition of veteran service populations in each VISN. For example, VISN 22 has significant Hispanic, African American, Asian/Pacific Islander, and Native American populations whereas the majority of veterans served in VISN 12 is Caucasian with smaller percentages of African American veterans.

[13] VA's health care system includes different types of health care facilities, including medical centers and community-based outpatient clinics (CBOC). VA medical centers offer services that range from primary care to complex specialty care, such as cardiac or spinal cord injury. VA's CBOCs are an extension of VA medical centers and mainly provide primary care services. VA also operates Vet Centers, which offer counseling services, including psychological counseling and psychotherapy, to combat veterans and their family members. Vet Centers are the only VA medical facilities authorized to provide services to family members. Vet Centers operate outside of the VISN structure but coordinate veterans' services and outreach with nearby VA medical centers.

[14] Specifically, we conducted site visits to Jesse Brown VA Medical Center, Auburn Gresham CBOC, and Chicago Vet Center in Illinois; Durham VA Medical Center, Raleigh CBOC, and Raleigh Vet Center in North Carolina; and West Los Angeles VA Medical Center, East Los Angeles CBOC, and East Los Angeles Vet Center in California. We conducted in-depth interviews with officials from Bath VA Medical Center, Rochester CBOC, and Rochester Vet Center in New York; Prescott VA Medical Center, Anthem CBOC, and Prescott Vet Center in Arizona; and Hunter Holmes McGuire Medical Center in Virginia. We conducted interviews with officials from the medical center in Richmond, Virginia, because the medical center operates one of four VA polytrauma centers that provide care to active duty servicemembers as well as veterans. We did not interview CBOC or Vet Center officials from the Richmond area.

[15] This sample did not include the six medical centers that we visited or reviewed in depth.

[16] We interviewed experts in the field including staff from HHS's Office of Minority Health; the National Health Law Program; and the National Center for Cultural Competence.

[17] See 65 Fed. Reg. 50123 (Aug. 16, 2000). EO 13166 indicated that the agency plans for their own programs should be consistent with this DOJ guidance.

[18] VHA Directive 2002-006 expired in January 2007. The current VHA Directive 2007-009, which contains the same guidance as the 2002 directive, expires in February 2012.

[19] VA's LEP Directive prescribes standards for written translations that, if implemented by medical centers, would constitute a "safe harbor" for the center. That is, VA will consider those facilities that adopt the LEP Directive's standards to be in compliance with EO 13166. For example, if a medical facility has a population of at least 3,000 veterans with LEP who speak the same primary language that facility will be considered in compliance with the EO if it provides translated written materials including vital documents in that primary language.

[20] The Veterans Benefits Improvement Act of 1994 required VA to create the CMV, which is organizationally aligned to VA's Office of the Secretary. See Pub. L. No. 103-446, § 509, 108 Stat. 4645, 4665-66 (codified as amended at 38 U.S.C. § 317). As required by law, CMV's primary emphasis is on minority veterans,

specifically veterans in the following groups: Pacific Islander, Asian American, African American, Hispanic/Latino, and Native American, including American Indian, Alaska Native, and Native Hawaiian.

[21] HHS , Office of Minority Health, *National Standards for Culturally and Linguistically Appropriate Services in Health Care* (Washington, D.C., 2001).

[22] The Joint Commission, previously known as the Joint Commission on Accreditation of Healthcare Organizations, is a not-for-profit organization that evaluates and accredits health care organizations throughout the United States to help assure the quality of care provided to patients. Accreditation is an assessment process by which an organization's performance is measured against certain standards defined by industry experts. VA requires its medical centers to obtain and maintain accreditation from the Joint Commission.

[23] VA initiated its survey in response to a November 2005 letter from members of Congress to VA's Secretary, which requested that VA monitor the implementation of VA's LEP Directive to help ensure that medical center's actions were consistent with the steps outlined in the directive.

[24] This survey showed that four of the medical centers we reviewed in depth assessed the language needs of their veteran service population and that three of the medical centers we reviewed in depth developed a language assistance policy.

[25] Staff from VA's EEO office conducted the follow-up calls to VA medical centers.

[26] Department of Veterans Affairs, *Federal Benefits for Veterans and Dependents* (Washington, D.C., 2008). This publication is available in Spanish at http://www.va.gov/opa/vadocs/fedbensp.pdf (accessed May 27, 2008).

[27] The iMed Consent application allows VA medical center staff to create medical consent forms in Spanish. Similarly, the KRAMES-on-Demand program allows medical center staff to provide patient education materials in several languages other than English. KRAMESon-demand provides all its education materials and drug information sheets in English and Spanish. Additionally, education materials covering 10 critical health topics are available in 10 languages: English, Spanish, Armenian, Chinese, Farsi, Hmong, Korean, Russian, Tagalog, and Vietnamese.

[28] According to VA medical center staff we interviewed, the use of volunteer staff interpreters is often not reported to medical center officials and as a result may be undercounted.

[29] See GAO-05-952 and Department of Veterans Affairs, *VA Benefits & Health Utilization* (Washington, D.C., 2007).

[30] Training of medical center staff on the health care needs of various age groups is an accreditation requirement from The Joint Commission. VA established a Cultural Competency Taskforce to identify and provide resources and training materials to medical centers to help facilitate the delivery of culturally appropriate health care. The taskforce is reviewing training modules on culturally appropriate health care in an effort to find a module that can be distributed to all VA medical centers for use in their efforts to provide culturally appropriate health care to veterans. The taskforce began work in spring 2006.

[31] Special-emphasis population groups are advocacy groups comprised of VA staff and focus on understanding the needs and promoting awareness of certain groups including Native Americans, Asian Pacific/Islanders, African Americans, Hispanics, women, and people with disabilities.

[32] Minority veterans program coordinators have been placed at each VA medical center by CMV as part of its systemwide effort to improve services for minority veterans.

In: Veterans' Benefits and Care
Editor: Mathew H. Bradley

ISBN: 978-1-60692-500-3

Chapter 14

A BRIEF OVERVIEW OF THE POST-9/11 VETERANS EDUCATIONAL ASSISTANCE ACT OF 2008

Shannon S. Loane

SUMMARY

The Post-9/11 Veterans Educational Assistance Act of 2008, enacted as Title V of P.L. 110-252 on June 30, 2008, provides enhanced educational benefits for veterans and servicemembers. It establishes the Post-9/11 Veterans Educational Assistance program, under which veterans and servicemembers who have served on active duty in the armed forces on or after September 11, 2001, may receive assistance towards the cost of tuition and fees, a monthly housing allowance, and a stipend for books and supplies. The Act grants authority for servicemembers who meet certain criteria to be permitted to transfer unused veterans education benefits to family members. It also increases maximum monthly benefits amounts under the Montgomery GI Bill-Active Duty program and the Reserve Educational Assistance Program.

POST-9/11 VETERANS EDUCATIONAL ASSISTANCE PROGRAM

On June 30, 2008, the President signed into law P.L. 110-252, the Supplemental Appropriations Act, 2008. Title V of P.L. 110-252, the Post-9/11 Veterans Educational Assistance Act of 2008, establishes the Post-9/11 Veterans Educational Assistance program under Chapter 33 of Title 38 of the United States Code, and makes amendments to existing veterans education programs. The Post-9/11 Veterans Educational Assistance program extends educational benefits to veterans and servicemembers who have served on active duty in the armed forces (including members of a reserve component under a call or order to active duty) for at least 90 days after September 10, 2001. The effective date for the new program is August 1, 2009, and individuals have 15 years from their discharge or release from active duty to use the benefits.

Whereas servicemembers must elect to participate in the Montgomery GI Bill-Active Duty (MGIB-AD) program at the time of their enlistment and agree to have their military pay reduced by $100 per month for 12 months, no such requirements apply to the Post- 9/11 program, which requires no contribution by servicemembers.[1]

Under the Post-9/11 Veterans Educational Assistance program, individuals who have served at least 90 days on active duty after September 10, 2001, (or who have served at least 30 continuous days on active duty and were discharged with a service-connected disability) may receive educational assistance benefits for 36 months. Individuals who have served for at least 36 months on active duty, or who were discharged with a service connected disability after 30 consecutive days of service, may receive the maximum benefit amount. Individuals who serve fewer than 36 months on active duty will be eligible for benefits calculated as a percentage of the total maximum benefits. (See Table 1)

Under the program, individuals are eligible to receive educational assistance in the form of payments for tuition and fees, a housing allowance, a books and supplies stipend, tutoring, testing and certification fees, and, in some cases, certain relocation and travel expenses. In addition, the program may provide additional funds for attending private institutions, under certain conditions, through the Yellow Ribbon GI Education Enhancement Program. The program also allows for transferability of benefits from a servicemember meeting specified criteria to a spouse and/or child(ren). (See Table 2 for more information on these benefits.)

Approved educational programs include undergraduate degrees, graduate degrees, and vocational or technical training. All training programs must be offered by an institution of higher education (IHE) and approved by the Veterans Administration.[2]

Table 1. Benefits Based on Active Duty Time Served Since 9/11/2001

Aggregate Time Served on Active Duty Since 9/11/2001	Percentage of Maximum Benefit Payable
At least 36 months	100
At least 30 continuous days on active duty and discharged due to service-connected disability	100
At least 30 months, but less than 36 months	90
At least 24 months, but less than 30 months	80
At least 18 months, but less than 24 months	70
At least 12 months, but less than 18 months	60
At least 6 months, but less than 12 months	50
At least 90 days, but less than 6 months	40

Source: Table prepared by CRS based on 38 U.S.C. §3313 and data available from the U.S. Department of Veterans Affairs.

Amendments to Other Veterans' Education Programs

In addition to the newly-enacted Post-9/11 Veterans Educational Assistance program, the following educational assistance programs are currently available to veterans and servicemembers:

- MGIB-Active Duty (MGIB-AD), for individuals who are on active duty or following separation from active duty;
- MGIB-Selected Reserves (MGIB-SR), for members of the selected reserves; and
- Reserve Educational Assistance Program (REAP), for members of reserve components who are called or ordered to active duty in response to a war or national emergency as declared by the President or Congress.

Table 2. Post-9/11 Veterans Educational Program Benefit Amounts

Benefit	Amount
Tuition and fees[a]	An individual is entitled to 36 months of tuition and fees (limited to the amount of undergraduate tuition charged at the most expensive public institution in the state in which the servicemember or veteran is enrolled).
Housing Allowance[b]	An individual is entitled to a monthly housing stipend amount equal to the monthly basic allowance for housing (BAH) for a member with dependents in pay grade E-5 in the military housing area in which the institution of higher education (IHE) is located.
Books and Supplies[c]	An individual is entitled to a $1,000 annual stipend for books and required educational expenses.
Tutoring	An individual is entitled to payment, not to exceed $100 per month and up to a maximum of $1,200, for tutorial assistance, provided it is certified the individual needs tutoring to pass a course required for the approved program of education.
Testing and Certification	An individual is entitled to payment, not to exceed the lesser of the test fee or $2,000, for one licensing or certification test.
Relocation or Travel Assistance	An individual who resides in a rural county and who has to relocate a distance of at least 500 miles, or must travel by air to attend an IHE, is entitled to a single payment of up to $500.
Yellow Ribbon	In cases where an IHE's tuition and fees are not covered by the tuition and fees payment benefit, the government may provide up to 50% of the remaining tuition and fees costs if the IHE voluntarily enters into an agreement to match an equal percentage.
Transferability	The program allows the Secretary of Defense to authorize the branches to permit servicemembers who have served at least six years and who agree to serve at least four more years to transfer between 18 and 36 months of educational benefits to a spouse and/or child(ren).

Source: Table prepared by CRS based on 38 U.S.C. Chapter 33 and data available from the U.S. Department of Veterans Affairs.

a. There may be great variation from state to state in tuition and fees amounts. For example, in 2006, undergraduate in-state tuition and fees at the most expensive public IHE ranged from $2,160 at the University of the District of Columbia in Washington, D.C. to $12,750 at the Benjamin Franklin Institute of Technology in Massachusetts. Figures obtained from the Integrated Postsecondary Education Data System (IPEDS) at the National Center for Education Statistics (NCES) at [http://nces.ed.gov/ipeds/].

b. There may be great variation from state to state and within states for BAH stipends. For example, in 2008, the BAH for pay grade E-5 with dependents ranged from $667 per month to $2,512 per month [http://141 .1 16.74.201/bah/acrobat/2008/!FINAL%202008%20'With' %20BAH% 20Rates.pdf]. Individuals on active duty or pursuing an education on a less-than-half-time basis are not eligible for the housing allowance.

c. Individuals on active duty are not eligible for the books and supplies stipend.

Maximum monthly benefit amounts for full-time enrollment in eligible programs, as of October 1, 2007, are $1,101.00 for active duty members (MGIB-AD) who enlist for three years or more; $880.80 for individuals in the selected reserves (REAP) who are called to active duty and who serve more than two consecutive years on active duty; and $317.00 for members of the selected reserves (MGIB-SR) who are not serving on active duty. P.L. 110-252 increases the maximum rate for MGIB-AD to $1,321 for the period August 1, 2008, through September 30, 2009. The maximum reimbursement rate for REAP increases to $1,056.80 as of August 1, 2008.[3]

Previously, under the MGIB-AD program, the different service branches were authorized to operate limited transferability programs, but only the Army offered such a program. P.L. 110-252 provides for transferability of educational benefits for MGIB-AD, MGIB-SR, and REAP, effective the date of enactment.

Individuals eligible for the MGIB-AD, MGIB-SR, or REAP programs on August 1, 2009, may elect to receive benefits under the Post-9/11 Veterans Educational Assistance Act. Individuals may be able to receive benefits under multiple veterans educational assistance programs (to a maximum of 48 months), but may not receive benefits under more than one program at a time.

Additional Resources

- The *GI Bill Website* of the Department of Veterans Affairs contains information on the Post-9/11 Veterans Educational Assistance program, as well as MGIB-AD, MGIB-SR, and REAP [http://www.gibill.va.gov/].
- For more information about the different federal education benefits available to veterans and military personnel, see CRS Report RL34549, *A Brief History of Veterans' Education Benefits and Their Value*, by David P. Smole and Shannon S. Loane.

End Notes

[1] For more information about the Montgomery GI Bill, see CRS Report RL34549, *A Brief History of Veterans' Education Benefits and Their Value*, by David P. Smole and Shannon S. Loane.

[2] For more information see [http://www.gibill.va.gov/GI_Bill_Info/search_programs.htm].

[3] The benefit amounts shown for each program are for full-time institutional training. The amounts are less for individuals who attend school less than full-time and who served less than the aforementioned number of years. Links to the latest education benefits payment rate schedules for each of the three programs are available at [http://www.gibill.va.gov/ GI_Bill_Info/rates.htm].

In: Veterans' Benefits and Care
Editor: Mathew H. Bradley

ISBN: 978-1-60692-500-3

Chapter 15

VETERANS' HEALTH CARE ISSUES

Sidath Viranga Panangala

SUMMARY

The Department of Veterans Affairs (VA) provides services and benefits to veterans who meet certain eligibility criteria. VA carries out its programs nationwide through three administrations and the Board of Veterans Appeals (BVA). The Veterans Health Administration (VHA) is responsible for veterans' health care programs. The Veterans Benefits Administration (VBA) is responsible for providing compensation, pensions, and education assistance, among other things. The National Cemetery Administration's (NCA) responsibilities include maintaining national veterans cemeteries.

VHA operates the nation's largest integrated health care system. Unlike most other federal health programs, VHA is a direct service provider rather than a health insurer or payer for health care. VA health care services are generally available to all honorably discharged veterans of the U.S. Armed Forces who are enrolled in VA's health care system. VA has a priority enrollment system that places veterans in priority groups based on various criteria. Under the priority system, VA decides each year whether its appropriations are adequate to serve all enrolled veterans. If not, VA could stop enrolling those in the lowest-priority groups.

Since the terrorist attacks of September 11, 2001, U.S. Armed Forces have been deployed in two major theaters of operation. Operation Enduring Freedom (OEF) in Afghanistan and Operation Iraqi Freedom (OIF) constitute the largest sustained ground combat mission undertaken by the United States since the Vietnam War. Veterans from these conflicts and from previous wars are exerting tremendous stress on the VA health care system. With increased patient workload and rising health care costs, the 110th Congress is focused on such issues as how to contain costs and at the same time maintain high-quality health care services to veterans who need them. Among other things, Congress may address the best method of funding for veterans' health care, while continuing to focus on ensuring a "seamless transition" process for servicemembers moving from the military health system into the VA health care system, improving mental health care services for veterans with Post Traumatic

Stress Disorder (PT SD), and improving rehabilitation and mental health services for those with Traumatic Brain Injuries (TBI).

In recent years, VA has made an effort to realign its capital assets, primarily its buildings, to better serve veterans' needs. VA established the Capital Asset Realignment for Enhanced Services (CARES) initiative to identify how well the geographic distribution of VA health care resources matches the projected needs of veterans. Given the tremendous interest in the implementation of the CARES initiative in the previous Congress, the 110th Congress will likely continue to monitor the CARES implementation. H.R. 327 was enacted into law (P.L. 110-110) on November 5. The House has passed several measures to improve and expand health care services to veterans: H.R. 327, H.R. 612, H.R. 1315, H.R. 1470, H.R. 2199, H.R. 2623, and H.R. 2874. The Senate VA Committee has reported the following measures: S. 1233, S. 2004, S. 2142, S. 2160, and S. 2162.

INTRODUCTION

Overview

This chapter provides an overview of major issues facing veterans' health care during the 110th Congress. The report's primary focus is on *veterans* and not *military retirees*. While any person who has served in the armed forces of the United States is regarded as a veteran, a military retiree is someone who has generally completed a full active duty military career (almost always at least 20 years of service), or who is disabled in the line of military duty and meets certain length of service and extent of disability criteria, and who is eligible for retired pay and a broad range of nonmonetary benefits from the Department of Defense (DOD) after retirement. A veteran is someone who has served in the armed forces (in most, but not all, cases for a few years in early adulthood), but may not have either sufficient service or disability to be entitled to post-service retired pay and nonmonetary benefits from DOD.[1] *Generally, all military retirees are veterans, but not all veterans are military retirees.* For the purposes of veterans' benefits, a veteran is defined as a person who served in the active military, naval, or air service, and who was discharged or released under conditions other than dishonorable.[2]

Currently, there are two health care systems that care for servicemembers and veterans. The Defense Health Program (DHP) in the DOD provides for worldwide medical and dental services to active duty military personnel, and other eligible beneficiaries.[3] Once they are discharged from their respective service branches, servicemembers become eligible for care and treatment provided by the Department of Veterans Affairs (VA). Prior to discussing major health care issues, this chapter provides a brief overview of the VA, the Veterans Health Administration (VHA) within the VA which oversees the largest integrated health care system in the country, and the veteran population it serves.[4] To provide context to the issues discussed in the second part of this chapter, a basic overview of eligibility for health care under the veterans health care system is presented.

Historical Background

Beginning with the early colonial settlements of America, the nation has provided benefits in varying degrees to those who have worn the uniform and suffered physical disabilities in service to the nation. For instance, in 1718, the colony of Rhode Island enacted legislation that provided benefits not only to every officer, soldier or sailor who served in the colony's armed services, but also to the wives, children, parents, and other relations who had been dependent upon a slain servicemember. "The physically disabled were to have their wound carefully tended and healed at the colony's expense, while at the same time an annual pension was provided to him out of the general treasury sufficient for the maintenance of himself and family, or other dependent relatives."[5]

While pension and disability benefits provided to veterans were gradually increased and in some cases decreased since the early colonial period, hospital and medical care for veterans on a level similar to the care provided today was not available until World War I. The VA health care system has evolved and expanded since World War I. Congress has enlarged the scope of the VA's health care mission, and has enacted legislation requiring the establishment of new programs and services. Through numerous laws, some narrowly focused, and others more comprehensive, Congress has also extended to additional categories of veterans eligibility for the many levels of care the VA now provides. No longer a health care system focused only on service-connected veterans, the VA has become a "safety net" for the many lower-income veterans who have come to depend upon it.[6] Furthermore, with the fragmented private-sector health care system, the lack of universal access to health care services, and the growing number of people joining the ranks of the uninsured, many veterans — even some with private health insurance — have chosen to receive care through the VA.[7]

Department of Veterans Affairs (VA)

The history of the present-day VA can be traced back to July 21, 1930, when President Hoover issued Executive Order 5398, creating an independent federal agency known as the Veterans Administration by consolidating many separate veterans' programs.[8] On October 25, 1988, President Reagan signed legislation (P.L. 100-527) creating a new federal cabinet-level Department of Veterans Affairs to replace the Veterans Administration, effective March 15, 1989. VA carries out its veterans' programs nationwide through three administrations and the Board of Veterans Appeals (BVA). The Veterans Health Administration (VHA) is responsible for veterans' health care programs. The Veterans Benefits Administration (VBA) is responsible for compensation, pension, vocational rehabilitation, education assistance, home loan guaranty and insurance among other things. The National Cemetery Administration's (NCA) responsibilities include maintaining 120 national cemeteries in 39 states and Puerto Rico. The Board of Veterans Appeals (BVA) renders final decisions on appeals on veteran benefits claims.[9]

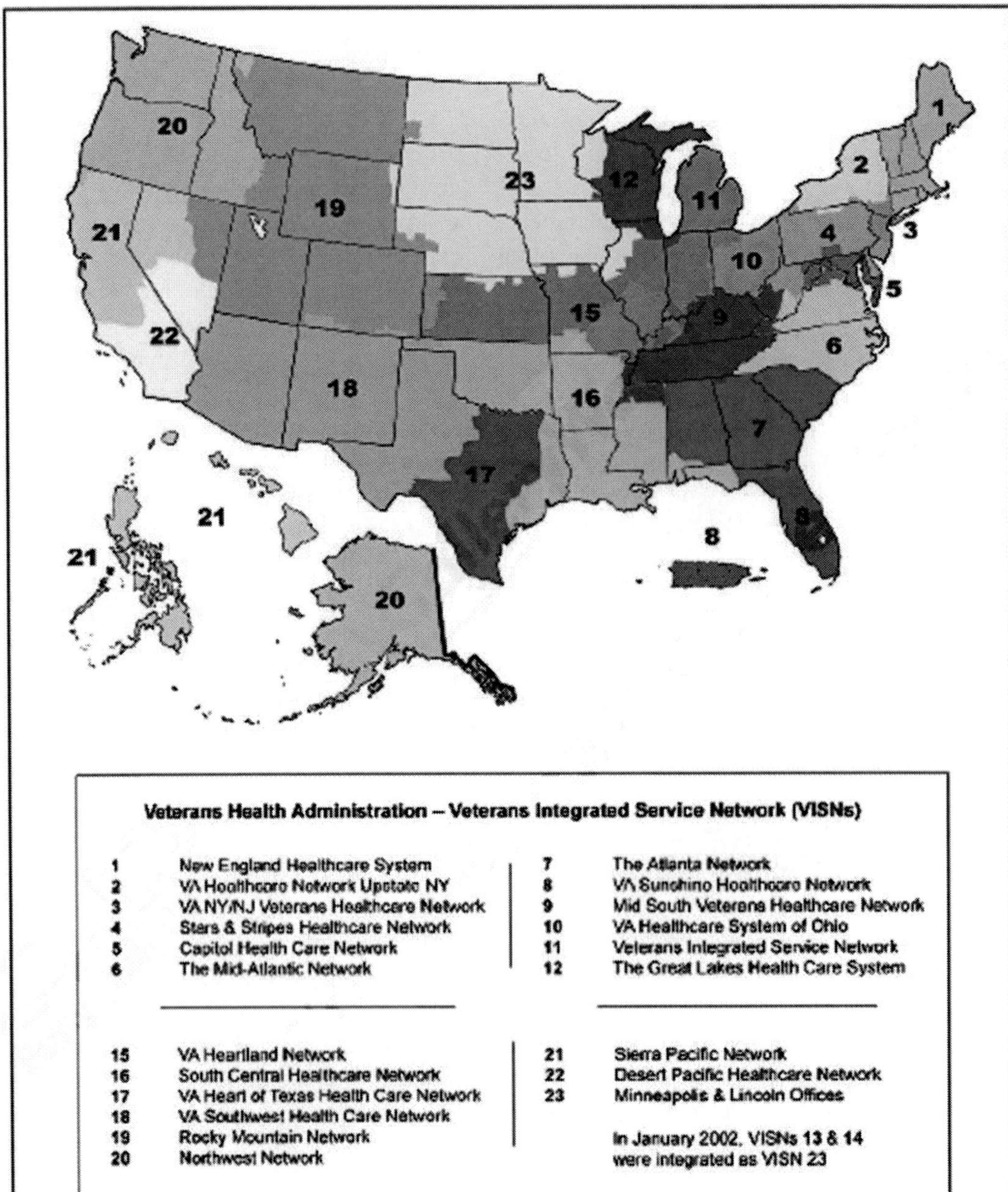

Note: VISN 21, the Sierra Pacific Network, includes northern and central California, northern Nevada, Hawaii, the Philippines, and several Pacific islands including Guam and American Samoa.

Figure 1. Veterans Integrated Services Networks (VISNs)

Veterans' Health Care System

VHA operates the nation's largest integrated direct health care delivery system.[10] VA's health care system is organized into 21 geographically defined Veterans Integrated Service Networks (VISNs) (see **Figure 1**). While policies and guidelines are developed at VA headquarters and applied throughout the VA health care system, management authority for basic decision making and budgetary responsibilities are delegated to the VISNs.[11] Congressionally appropriated medical care funds are allocated to the VISNs based on the Veterans Equitable Resource Allocation (VERA) system, which generally bases funding on patient workload.[12] Prior to the implementation of the VERA system, resources were allocated to facilities primarily on the basis of their historical expenditures. Unlike Medicare, which administers medical care through the private sector, the VA provides care directly to veterans.

In FY2007, VHA operated 155 medical centers, 135 nursing homes, 717 ambulatory care and community-based outpatient clinics (CBOCs),[13] 45 residential rehabilitation treatment programs, and 209 Vet Centers (generally these are community-based, non-medical facilities that offer counseling services).[14] VHA also pays for care provided to veterans by independent providers and practitioners on a fee basis under certain circumstances. Inpatient and outpatient care is provided in the private sector to eligible dependents of veterans under the Civilian Health and Medical Program of the Department of Veterans Affairs (CHAMPVA).[15] In addition, VHA provides grants for construction of state-owned nursing homes and domiciliary facilities, and collaborates with the Department of Defense (DOD) in sharing health care resources and services. Today, VHA has been commended by peer reviewed journals and independent studies as an outstanding health care system whose "performance now surpasses that of other health systems on standardized quality measures."[16] The journal *Neurology* in its November 2006 issue noted that "The VA has achieved remarkable improvements in patient care and health outcomes, and is a cost-effective and efficient organization. Its enrollees are provided comprehensive coverage ... and the system is especially suited to manage chronic disease."[17] In 2005, *Health Care Papers* dedicated a complete issue to examining the transformation of VHA, and the lessons that could be learned by other countries struggling to use their healthcare resources appropriately.[18] Furthermore, VA has led private-sector health care in the American Customer Satisfaction Index for both inpatient and outpatient services.[19]

Veterans Health Information Systems and Technology Architecture (VistA)

The previously discussed achievements are related in part to the VHA's development and use of electronic health records. Since 1985, VHA has had an automated information system with extensive clinical and administrative capabilities which supports ambulatory, inpatient, and long-term care. VistA is the single, integrated health information system used throughout VA in all health care settings. VistA applications are comprised of three types of packages: the clinical package, the administration and financial package, and the infrastructure package. The clinical package includes applications such as the Computerized Patient Record System (CPRS). In addition to CPRS, VistA includes VistA Imaging and Bar-Code Medication Administration.

The CPRS is a single integrated system for VA health care providers. All aspects of a patient's medical record are integrated, including active problems, allergies, current medications, laboratory results, vital signs, hospitalizations and outpatient clinic history, alerts of abnormal results, among other things. It is used in about 1,300 VHA facilities around the country. CPRS also incorporates data from scheduling, laboratory, radiology, consults and clinic notes into a single integrated patient record.[20] Remote data view allows clinicians to see health data from any other VA facility where the veteran has received care. Also as a complement to CPRS, VistA includes VistA Imaging. This application provides a multimedia, online patient record that integrates traditional medical chart information with medical images including X-rays, pathology slides, video views, scanned documents, and cardiology exam results, among other images.

The Bar Code Medication Administration (BCMA) is an application that validates the administration of medications, including intravenous medications, in real time for inpatients in all VA medical centers. This ensures that the patient receives the correct medication, at the correct dosage and at the right time. BCMA also provides visual alerts. For instance, if the software detects a potential medical error, it alerts the nurse administering the medication. These alerts require the nurse to review and correct the reason for the alert before actually administering the drug to the patient. The overall cost of maintaining the VistA system is $87 per patient annually.[21]

In 2006, Harvard University's Kennedy School of Government awarded the VA the Innovations in American Government Award for its electronic health records system. In presenting this award the Kennedy School stated that

> VistA saves lives and ensures continuity of care even under the most extreme circumstances. Many of the thousands of residents who fled the Gulf Coast because of Hurricane Katrina left behind vital health records. Records for the 40,000 veterans in the area were almost immediately available to clinicians across the country, even though the VA Medical Center in Gulfport, Mississippi, was destroyed and New Orleans VA Medical Center was closed and evacuated. Veterans were able to resume their treatments, refill their prescriptions, and get the care they needed because their medical records were immediately accessible to providers at other VA facilities.[22]

VETERAN POPULATION

At the end of FY2006 the veterans population in the United States was approximately 24 million, and of these 17.8 million were war veterans. According to the VA, the total veteran population is expected to decline to 21.7 million by 2011, and 18.1 million by 2020. VA attributes this decline to the number of veteran deaths exceeding the number of new separations from the military.[23] The largest population of veterans are living in California, followed by Florida and Texas (**Figure 2**). In FY2005 there were approximately 7.7 million veterans enrolled in the VA health care system (**Figure 3**). Most VISNs showed enrollments between 26%-30% of the total eligible veteran population in those VISNs; two VISNs (VISN 5 and VISN 11) showed enrollments below 25%. The total number of veterans enrolled in VA's health care system is estimated to increase to almost 8.0 million veterans in FY2008. It should be noted that in any given year not all veterans seek care from VA, either because they are not ill or because they have other sources of care such as private health insurance.

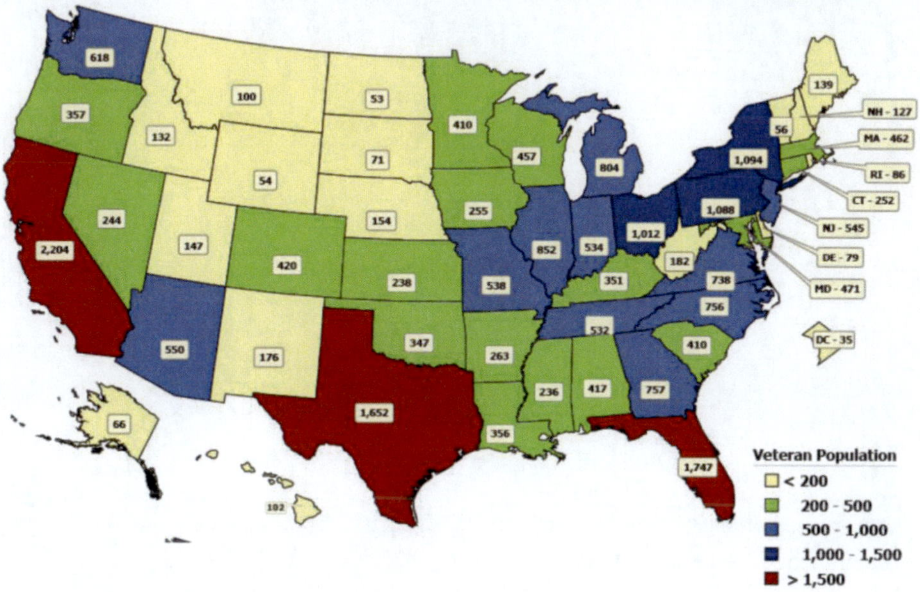

Source: Department of Veterans Affairs.

Figure 2. Veteran Population by State as of September 30, 2006 (in thousands)

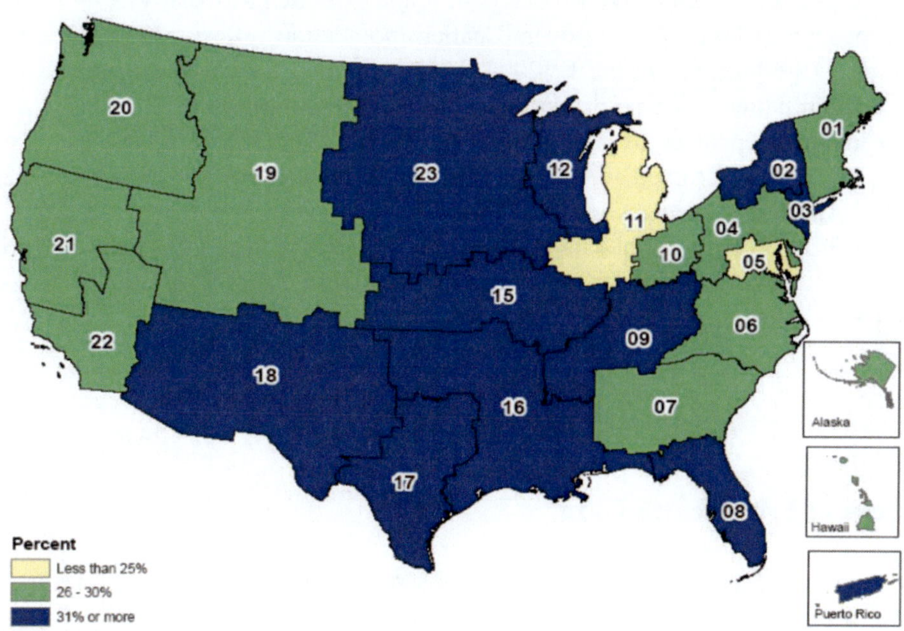

Source: Department of Veterans Affairs.

Figure 3. Percent of Veterans Enrolled in the VA Health Care System by VISN, FY2005

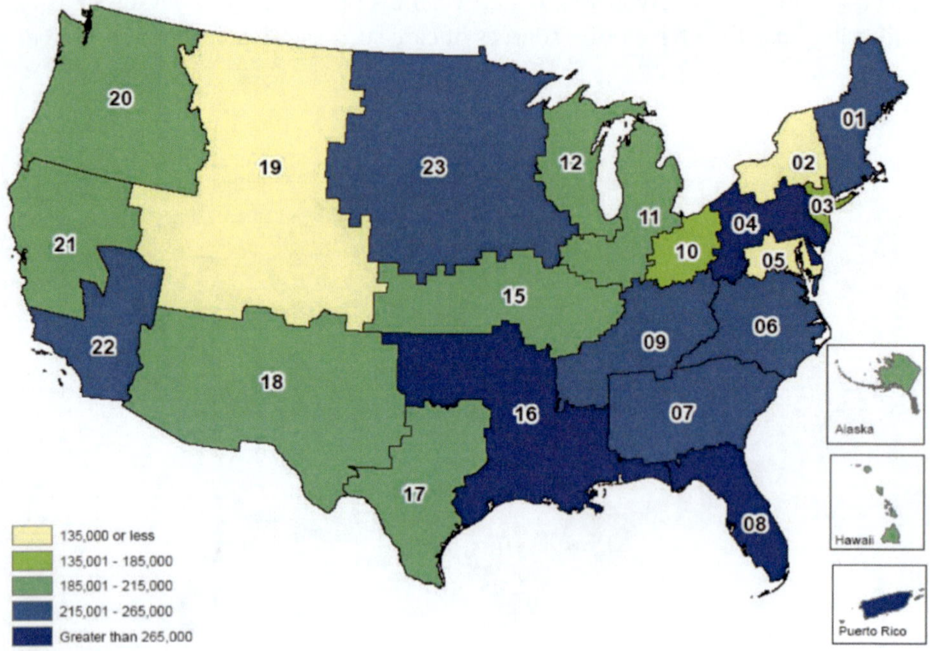

Source: Department of Veterans Affairs.

Figure 4. Number of Patients by VISN, FY2005

In FY2005, VHA provided care to approximately 4.9 million unique patients. The greatest number of patients were in VISNs 4, 8 and 16. Each of these VISNs had more than 265,000 patients (**Figure 4**). The overall patient population reflects where the total veteran population is the largest. During FY2007, VHA provided health care to about 5.2 million unique veteran patients. These patients generated 64.4 million outpatients visits and almost 800,000 inpatient episodes of care.[24] According to VHA estimates, the number of unique veteran patients is estimated to increase by approximately 109,000 between FY2007 and FY2008.[25] And VA is expected to treat about 5.3 million veteran patients in FY2008. Patients in Priority Groups 1-6 (described below) — those veterans with service-connected conditions, lower incomes, special health care needs, and service in Iraq or Afghanistan — will comprise 75% of the total veteran patient population in FY2008.

ELIGIBILITY FOR VETERANS' HEALTH CARE

"Promise of Free Health Care"

To understand some of the issues discussed later in this chapter, it is important to understand eligibility for VA health care, VA's enrollment process, and its enrollment priority groups. Unlike Medicare or Medicaid, VA health care is not an entitlement program. Contrary to numerous claims made concerning "promises" to military personnel and veterans with regard to "free health care for life," not every veteran is automatically entitled to medical care from VA.[26] Prior to eligibility reform in 1996, all veterans were technically eligible for some care, however, the actual provision of care was based on available resources.[27]

The Veterans' Health Care Eligibility Reform Act of 1996, P.L. 104-262, established two eligibility categories and required VHA to manage the provision of hospital care and medical services through an enrollment system based on a system of priorities.[28] P.L 104-262 authorized VA to provide all needed hospital care and medical services to veterans with service-connected disabilities, former prisoners of war, veterans exposed to toxic substances and environmental hazards such as Agent Orange, veterans whose attributable income and net worth are not greater than an established "means test," and veterans of World War I. These veterans are generally known as "higher priority" or "core" veterans.[29] The other category of veterans are those with no service-connected disabilities and with attributable incomes above an established "means test."

Table 1. Health Enrollment Process

Step 1	The veteran may apply for enrollment in person at a VA health care facility, by mail, or by completing an on-line application. VHA uses the military service, demographic and, as applicable, financial information collected on the application form as the basis for determining whether the veteran qualifies for VA health care benefits.
Step 2	The local VA health care facility receives the application for enrollment and intake staff enter the data into the Veterans Health Information Systems and Technology Architecture (VistA). VistA automatically queries the Master Patient Index (MPI) to determine if a record has already been established, if not it uniquely identifies the veteran record. At this time, the intake staff may also query VBA for compensation and pension and/or known military status information. Typically, the veteran is provided a preliminary eligibility determination at the conclusion of an in-person application for enrollment.
Step 3	VistA transmits the veteran data to the Eligibility and Enrollment System (national system).
Step 4	The Eligibility and Enrollment System establishes the veteran's record and queries the Social Security Administration (SSA) to verify the veteran's Social Security Number (SSN). Note: SSN verification does not occur in real time and is not on the critical path.
Step 5	The Enrollment System queries VBA to reconfirm the compensation and pension and/or military status. Currently, this is done in a batch mode; however, when VHA deploys Enrollment System Redesign (ESR), the Enrollment System will immediately trigger a query to VBA; as a result the cycle time, for the enrollment process noted above will be reduced by another day.
Step 6	The Enrollment System verifies the veteran's enrollment eligibility and shares this data with VistA (at the local level). Note: If the Enrollment System is unable to verify eligibility, then the system sends the local VA Medical Center a bulletin to alert them to take further action (i.e., confirm whether the veteran has qualifying military service). The Enrollment System establishes an enrollment record upon transmission of verifying data by the local station.
Step 7	The Enrollment System produces the letter to the veteran with the official enrollment determination.
Step 8	The veteran receives the letter from VA telling him or her about their eligibility and enrollment determination.

Source: Appendix C. *Task Force on Returning Global War on Terror Heroes* report, Department of Veterans Affairs.

P.L. 104-262 also authorized VA to establish a patient enrollment system to manage access to VA health care. As stated in the report language accompanying P.L. 104-262,

> [t]he Act would direct the Secretary, in providing for the care of 'core' veterans, to establish and operate a system of annual patient enrollment and require that veterans be enrolled in a manner giving relative degrees of preference in accordance with specified priorities. At the same time, it would vest discretion in the Secretary to determine the manner in which such enrollment system would operate.[30]

Furthermore, P.L. 104-262 was clear in its intent that the provision of health care to veterans was dependent upon the available resources. The Committee report accompanying P.L. 104-262 states that the provision of hospital care and medical services would be provided to "the extent and in the amount provided in advance in appropriations Acts for these purposes. Such language is intended to clarify that these services would continue to depend upon discretionary appropriations."[31]

VHA Health Care Enrollment

As stated previously, P.L. 104-262 required the establishment of a national enrollment system to manage the delivery of inpatient and outpatient medical care. The new eligibility standard was created by Congress to "ensure that medical judgment rather than legal criteria will determine when care will be provided and the level at which care will be furnished."[32]

For most veterans, entry into the veterans' health care system begins by completing the application for enrollment. Some veterans are exempt from the enrollment requirement if they meet special eligibility requirements.[33] A veteran may apply for enrollment by completing the Application for Health Benefits (VA Form 10-1 0EZ) at any time during the year and submitting the form online or in person at any VA medical center or clinic, or mailing or faxing the completed form to the medical center or clinic of the veteran's choosing.[34] See **Table 1** for steps in the enrollment process.

Once a veteran is enrolled in the VA health care system the veteran remains in the system and does not have to re-apply for enrollment annually. However, those veterans who have been enrolled in Priority Group 5 based on income must submit a new VA Form 10-1 0EZ annually with updated financial information demonstrating inability to defray the expenses of necessary care.[35]

Veteran's Status

Eligibility for VA health care is primarily based on "veteran's status" resulting from military service. Veteran's status is established by active-duty status in the military, naval, or air service and an honorable discharge or release from active military service. Generally, persons enlisting in one of the armed forces after September 7, 1980, and officers commissioned after October 16, 1981, must have completed two years of active duty or the full period of their initial service obligation to be eligible for VA health care benefits. Servicemembers discharged at any time because of service-connected disabilities are not held to this requirement. Also, reservists that were called to active duty and who completed the term for which they were called, and who were granted an other than dishonorable discharge are exempt from the 24 continuous months of active duty requirement. National Guard members who were called to active duty by federal executive order are also exempt from this two year requirement if: 1) they completed the term for which they were called, and 2) were granted an other than dishonorable discharge.

When not activated to full-time federal service, members of the reserve components and National Guard have limited eligibility for VA health care services. Members of the reserve components may be granted service-connection for any injury they incurred or aggravated in the line of duty while attending inactive duty training assemblies, annual training, active duty for training, or while going directly to or returning directly from such duty. Additionally, reserve component servicemembers may be granted service-connection for a heart attack or stoke if such an event occurs during these same periods. The granting of service-connection makes them eligible to receive care from VA for those conditions. National Guard members are not granted service-connection for any injury, heart attack, or stroke that occurs while performing duty ordered by a governor for state emergencies or activities. [36]

Priority Groups

After veteran's status has been established, VA next places applicants into one of two categories. The first group is composed of veterans with service-connected disabilities or with incomes below an established means test. These veterans are regarded by VA as "high priority" veterans, and they are enrolled in Priority Groups 1-6 (see **Appendix 1**). Veterans enrolled in Priority Groups 1-6 include:

- veterans in need of care for a service-connected disability;[37]
    - veterans who have a compensable service-connected condition;
    - veterans whose discharge or release from active military, naval or air service was for a compensable disability that was incurred or aggravated in the line of duty;
    - veterans who are former prisoners of war (POWs);
    - veterans awarded the purple heart;
    - veterans who have been determined by VA to be catastrophically disabled (these are veterans who have a permanent severely disabling injury, disorder, or disease that compromises the ability to carry out the activities of daily living);
    - veterans of World War I;
    - veterans who were exposed to hazardous agents (such as Agent Orange in Vietnam) while on active duty; and
    - veterans who have an annual income and net worth below a VA-established means test threshold.

VA also looks at applicants' income and net worth to determine their specific priority category and whether they have to pay copayments for nonservice-connected care. In addition, veterans are asked to provide VA with information on any health insurance coverage they have, including coverage through employment or through a spouse. VA may bill these payers for treatment of conditions that are not a result of injuries or illnesses incurred or aggravated during military service.

The second group is composed of veterans who do not fall into one of the first six priority groups. These veterans are primarily those with nonservice-connected medical conditions and with incomes and net worth above the VA established means test threshold. These veterans are enrolled in Priority Group 7 or 8 (see **Appendix 1**).[38]

Health Services

VHA provides a standard benefits package to all enrolled veterans. Broadly, this includes preventive care services (e.g., immunizations, physical examinations, health care assessments, screening tests); inpatient and outpatient medical care, surgery, and mental health care, including care for substance abuse; prescription drugs, including over-the-counter drugs and medical and surgical supplies; and durable medical equipment and prosthetic and orthotic devices, including eyeglasses and hearing aids.

Medical Care for Returning Injured Servicemembers

Overview

The *National Strategy for Combating Terrorism* issued in September 2006, stated that the "War on Terror will be a long war."[39] Along with all other facets of the U.S. government, it is likely that the U.S. military will continue to play a leading role in this "long war." Since the terrorist attacks of September 11, 2001, U.S. Armed Forces have been deployed in two major theaters of operation. Operation Enduring Freedom (OEF) in Afghanistan and Operation Iraqi Freedom (OIF) constitute the largest sustained ground combat mission undertaken by the United States since the Vietnam War. Veterans from these conflicts and from previous wars are exerting tremendous stress on the VA health care system. With increased patient workload and rising health care costs, the 110th Congress is focused on ensuring a "seamless transition" process for veterans moving from active duty into the VA health care system.

Compared with previous wars that the nation has fought, because of the advancement in battle field medicine, a larger proportion of soldiers are surviving their injuries. In World War II, 30% of the U.S. servicemembers injured in combat died. In Vietnam, the proportion dropped to 24%. In OEF and OEF operations about 10% of those injured have died.[40] In November 2007, DOD reported that over 30,000 servicemembers have been wounded in action since the beginning of OEF and OEF.[41] With increasing numbers of soldiers returning from Iraq and Afghanistan — both injured and non-injured — Congress and veterans' advocates are very concerned that returning servicemembers may not have a smooth transition from DOD health care to VA health care. The final report of the President's Commission on Care for America's Returning Wounded Warriors acknowledged that handoffs between inpatient and outpatient care and between the two separate DOD and VA health care and disability systems are problematic.[42] *It should be noted that injured servicemembers receiving care in VA health care facilities are not considered veterans until they are formally discharged from active duty service.*[43]

OEF and OIF Veterans

Since the onset of OEF and OIF, more than 1.6 million servicemembers have served in these two theaters of operation, making them potentially eligible for veterans benefits.[44] Since FY2002, 751,273 OEF and OIF veterans have separated (discharged) from active duty.[45] Of this amount, 362,237, or 48%, were active duty troops, while 389,036, or 52%, were separated National Guard and Reserve component members. Approximately 35%, or 263,909, of all separated OEF and OIF veterans since FY2002 have sought care from VA. About 96% of the veterans who sought care have received outpatient care, while 4%, or a little more than 10,000, have been hospitalized at least once in a VHA facility. **Figure 5** provides a breakdown of the five major diagnoses among returning OIF and OEF veterans. While diseases of the musculoskeletal system have the highest frequency of diagnosis, mental disorders ranks second among major diagnoses. Mental disorders may include, among other conditions, nondependent abuse of drugs, alcohol dependent syndrome, and PTSD.

Figure 6 below provides data on the number of OEF and OIF discharges per fiscal year. The number of new discharges was highest in FY2004, followed by FY2003, whereas FY2006 had the lowest number of discharges. However, note that the numbers in the graph are from FY2002-FY2006 and do not reflect the most recent data presented above, which includes FY2007 3rd quarter data.

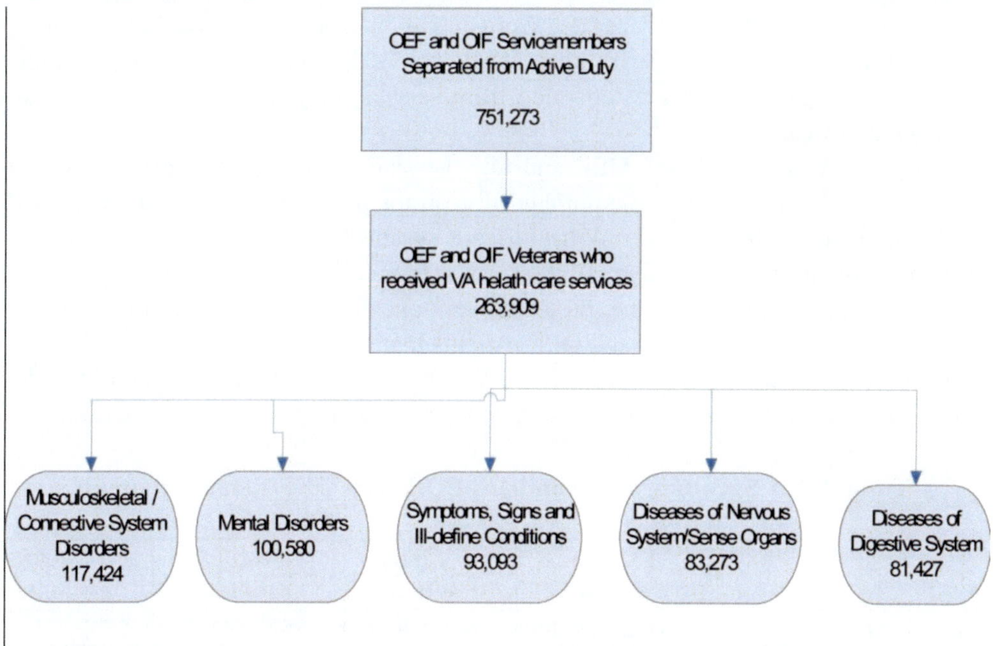

Source: CRS Analysis of VA Data.

Notes: These diagnoses are based on broad International Classification of Diseases 9th Revision (ICD-9) categories. These data are cumulative data since FY2002, with data on hospitalizations and outpatient visits as of June 30, 2007. A veteran is counted only once in any single diagnostic category but can be counted in multiple categories. Therefore, above numbers add up to greater than 263,909.

Figure 5. Frequency of Major Diagnoses among OEF and OIF Veterans

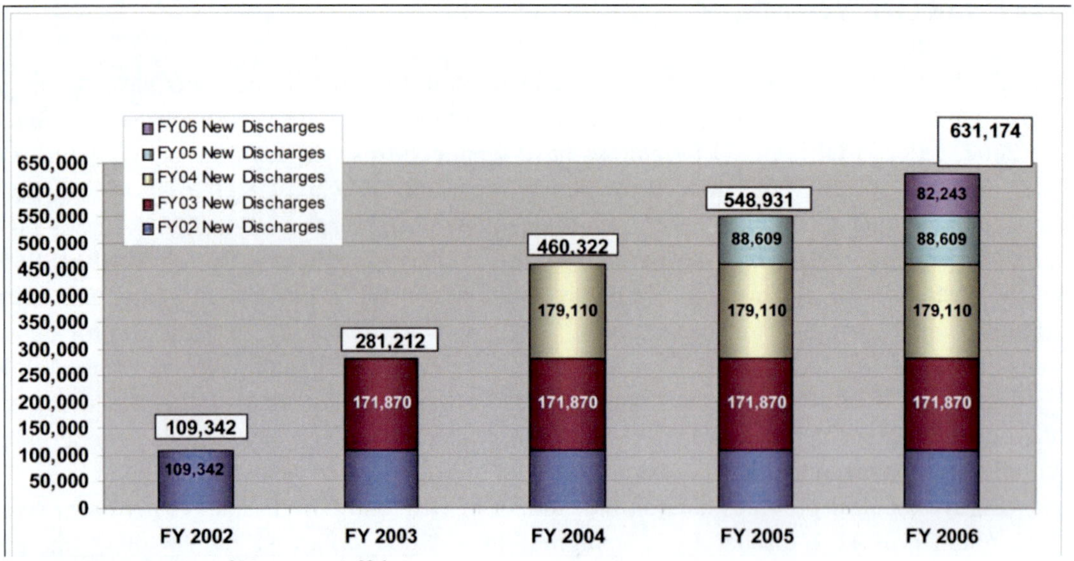

Source: Department of Veterans Affairs.

Figure 6. Cumulative Number of OIF and OIF Veterans Discharged from FY2002-FY2006

Although National Guard and Reserve component members make up 52% of OIF and OEF servicemembers who have separated from active duty, they compose 34% of those who have sought VA health care since FY2002. While active duty OIF and OEF servicemembers make up 48% of those who have separated from service, they make up 36% of those who have received VA care.

VA expects to treat 263,345 OEF and OIF veterans in FY2008 (**Table 2**). This is an increase of 54,037, or 26%, over the number of veterans from these two theaters of operation that VA anticipates will enter the VA health care system in FY2007, and 108,073, or 70%, more than the number VA treated in FY2006. As seen in **Table 2,** there is a 223% increase in funding between FY2005 and the projected amount for FY2008. **Figure 7** shows the cumulative number of unique OIF and OEF patients that the VA treated between FY2002 and FY2006, with projections for FY2007 and FY2008. In FY2005 and FY2006, VA treated more OIF and OEF veterans than it had budgeted for at the beginning of the fiscal year.

Table 2. VA Spending and Number of OIF and OEF Veteran Patients

	FY2005 actual	FY2006 actual	FY2007 estimate	FY2008 estimate
Obligations[a]	$232,500,000	$404,840,000	$572,562,000	$752,438,000
Number of OEF/OIF patients	100,808	155,272	209,308	263,345
Average Annual Cost Per OIF/OEF Patient	$2,306	$2,607	$2,736	$2,857

Source: U.S. Department of Veterans Affairs, *FY2008 Congressional Budget Submissions, Medical Programs,* vol. 1 of 4, pp. 9-14.

a. Total VA spending on OEF and OIF veteran patients.

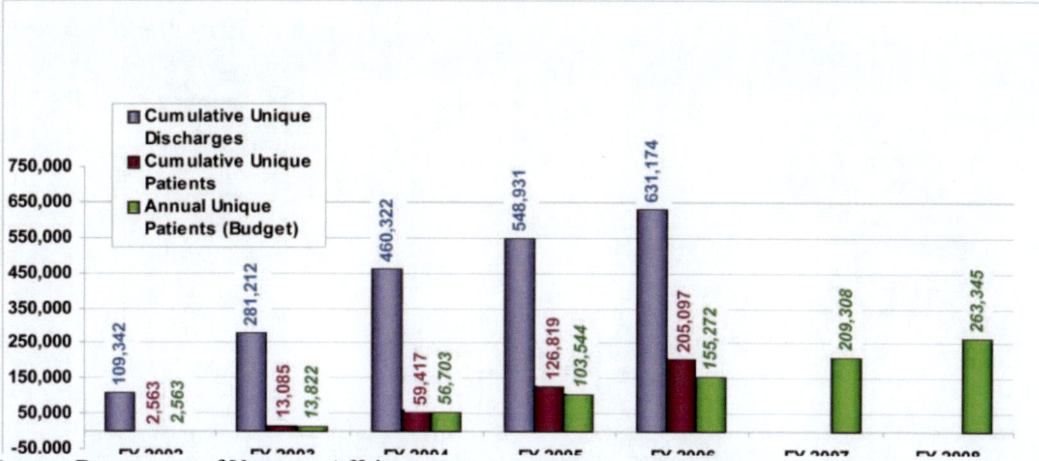

Source: Department of Veterans Affairs.

Figure 7. Cumulative Unique OIF and OEF Veteran Patients and OIF and OEF Discharges from FY2002 thru FY2006 Compared with Annual Number of Unique Patients

In March, VA testified that the number of severely injured or ill active duty servicemembers and veterans that have transitioned from DOD to VHA facilities is over 6,800;[46] of these 342 have been polytrauma patients.[47] VHA defines polytrauma as "injury to the brain in addition to other body parts or systems resulting in physical, cognitive, psychological, or psychosocial impairments and functional disability."[48]

As of April 1, there were 571 amputees reported by DOD. Since FY2002,VA's Prosthetic and Sensory Aids Service (PSAS) has provided services and products to over 22,000 OEF and OIF unique veterans. PSAS has served a total of 187 major amputees (those with upper or lower limb amputations) from OEF and OIF, including veterans and active duty servicemembers.[49]

Transition Issues

In 2003, several injured servicemembers or their parents testified on the obstacles faced during the transition from DOD's health care system to VHA.[50] However, since that time there have been significant improvements in that area as described later in this chapter. Aside from this day-to-day handoff, coordination and sharing of health information between VA and DOD has been problematic.[51] In 2003, the President's Task Force to Improve Health Care Delivery for Our Nation's Veterans identified several issues with regard to sharing of information between DOD and VA. It stated that "the VA/DOD processes for sharing information about eligible service members do not facilitate quick and accurate enrollment into VA programs."[52]

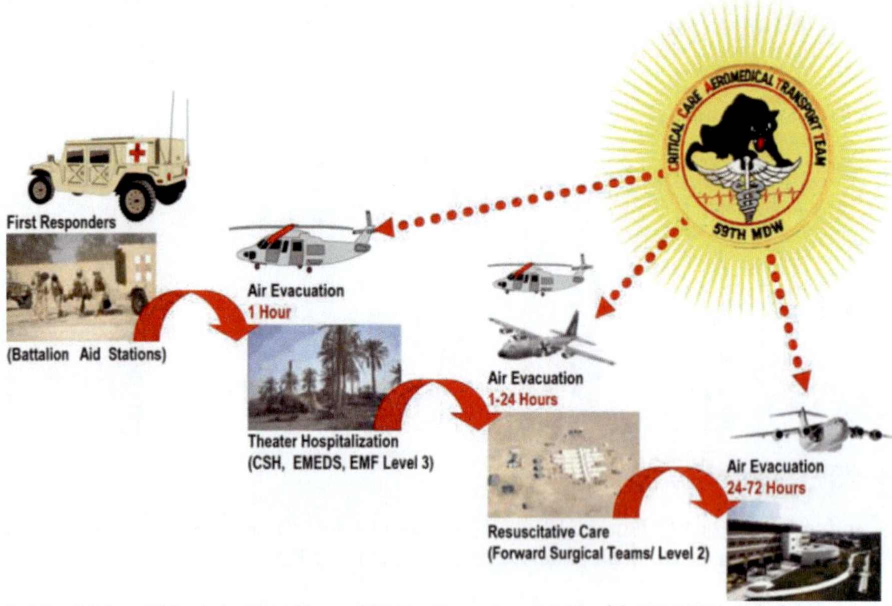

Source: DOD, Major Alfred A. Hamilton, PH.D, Government Health IT 2007 Conference, Adapted by CRS Graphics.

Figure 8. Current Level of Care from Injury to Definitive Care

In March 2005, the Government Accountability Office (GAO) testified that VA still does not have systematic access to DOD data about returning servicemembers who may need its services.[53] Again in September 2005, GAO testified that while VA has developed policies and procedures to provide OEF and OIF servicemembers and veterans with timely access to care, the sharing of health information between DOD and VA is limited.[54] In March 2007, GAO testified that despite coordination efforts by DOD and VA, these two Departments were still having problems sharing medical records.[55] Among other things, the recently appointed Task Force on Returning Global War on Terror Heroes identified that "currently, there are no formal interagency agreements between DOD and VA to transfer case management responsibilities across the military services and VA"[56] In its July 2007 report, the President's Commission on Care for America's Returning Wounded Warriors acknowledged that handoffs between the two separate DOD and VA health care and disability systems have been problematic, and recommended the integration of medical and rehabilitation programming across the two Departments.[57]

Initial Medical Care in DOD Facilities

In general, as shown in Figure 8, when a solider is injured on the battlefield he or she is stabilized in theater by a combat medic/lifesaver and then moved to a battalion aid station. If the servicemember has serious injuries he or she is transferred to a forward surgical team to be stabilized and then moved to a combat support hospital and further stabilized for a period of about two days. If the servicemember needs more specialized care he or she is evacuated from OEF and OIF conflict theaters and brought to Landstuhl Regional Medical Center (LRMC) in Germany for treatment. Most patients arrive at LRMC 24 to 72 hours after injury. In general, servicemembers remain in Germany for a period of about 4 to five days.[58] Length of stay at in-theater medical facilities is determined by the stability of the patient and the availability of medical evacuation aircraft. After further stabilization at LRMC they are evacuated to the United States and arrive at an echelon V Military Treatment Facility (MTF) such as Walter Reed Army Medical Center (WRAMC) in Washington, DC, or the National Naval Medical Center in Bethesda, Maryland. All catastrophic burn patients are flown to the Brooke Army Medical Center (BAMC) at Fort Sam Houston, Texas. BAMC has also established a specialized amputee rehabilitation center.[59]

Table 3. VHA's Polytrauma System of Care

Level I. Comprehensive Polytrauma Rehabilitation Centers (PRCs)
• provide acute comprehensive medical, surgical, and rehabilitation care for complex and severe polytraumatic injuries • serve as a resource to other facilities in the system via the development of tele-rehabilitation for consultation, best practices in polytrauma care, educational programs, and evaluation of new technology • provide all clinical services and serve concurrently as Level II sites within their respective Veterans Integrated Service Networks (VISNs)
Level II. Polytrauma Network Sites (PNSs)
• there are 21 PNSs, one in each of VHA's 21 VISNs • these sites manage veterans with complex injuries requiring specialized expertise as they return to their VISNs • these sites provide a high level of expert care, with a full range of clinical and ancillary resources • these sites provide specialized outpatient care to polytrauma patients not requiring inpatient services • these sites develop a referral network within their VISN, and identify VISN resources for TBI/polytrauma services
Level III. Polytrauma Facility Teams (PFTs)
• these facilities have more limited resources than Level I and Level II centers • Level III PFTs include a core polytrauma clinic team that could deliver a continuum of follow-up services in consultation with Level I and II centers • these facilities are more likely to be closer to a veterans home and to provide day-to-day care, contact and support
Level IV. Polytrauma Care Coordination Points of Contact (POCs)
• these sites are smaller facilities with limited resources • these sites serve as coordinators of referrals and consultations of polytrauma patients to Level I, II, or III facilities • Level IV coordinators are knowledgeable about the services available within the system of care and about the avenues for access to care

Source: Department of Veterans Affairs, Office of Inspector General, *Health Status of and Services for Operation Enduring Freedom/Operation Iraqi Freedom Veterans after Traumatic Brain Injury Rehabilitation*, (Report No. 05-01818-165), July 12, 2006.

Transfer and Care in VA Facilities

Once a seriously injured servicemember enters a major MTF, DOD can elect to send those with traumatic brain injuries (TBI) and other complex polytrauma cases to one of the four VA Polytrauma Rehabilitation Centers (PRCs) at the following locations: James A. Haley Veterans Affairs Medical Center (VAMC), Tampa, Florida; Minneapolis VAMC, Minneapolis, Minnesota; Veterans Affairs Palo Alto Health Care System, Palo Alto, California; and Hunter Holmes McGuire VAMC, Richmond, Virginia.[60] VA recently announced the decision to locate a fifth Polytrauma Center in San Antonio, Texas. As previously noted, injured servicemembers receiving care in VA health care facilities are not considered veterans until they are formally discharged from active duty service.

The PRCs have resources and clinical expertise to provide care for complex patterns of injuries, including TBI, traumatic or partial limb amputation, nerve damage, burns, wounds, fractures, vision and hearing loss, pain, mental health, and readjustment problems. In total there are currently 76 polytrauma clinic teams in the VA. These local teams of providers deliver follow up services in consultation with regional and network specialists. They also assist in management of stable patients through direct care, consultation and the use of tele-rehabilitation technologies, when needed. These PRCs have social work case managers at a ratio of one for every six patients. These case managers help assess the psychosocial needs of each patient and family, match treatment and support services to meet identified needs, coordinate services, and oversee the discharge planning process.[61] **Table 3** provides an brief summary of VHA's polytrauma system of care.

VA has stationed employees at Army and Navy hospitals to act as VHA/DOD liaisons.[62] These VA/DOD liaisons assist with the transfer of patients as they move from MTFs to VHA hospitals and clinics. In general, once the MTF decides to transfer a patient to a PRC, it refers the patient to a VA/DOD liaison. The VA/DOD liaison then contacts the liaison at the PRC. The PRC completes a medical screening and initiates the transfer process. Medical records are obtained through direct access to WRAMC and Bethesda National Naval Medical Center. However, not all medical records are available electronically. In such cases Nursing Admissions Coordinators in PRCs obtain specific paper records through the VA/DOD liaison personnel stationed at both WRAMC and Bethesda. Video teleconferencing between the MTFs and PRCs provides an opportunity for families to meet the VA interdisciplinary team and facilitate the transition-of-care process.

Upon admission to a PRC, members of the rehabilitation team individually evaluate the servicemember within 24 hours.[63] According to the VA, the rehabilitation team generally meets three times weekly to discuss each patient and to continually adjust the therapeutic plan of care. "Each patient undergoes three to six hours of therapy each day based on their individual functional and cognitive needs."[64] By July 2007, VA plans to develop 4 Residential Transitional Rehabilitation Programs co-located with the Level I PRCs. The stated goal of these programs is to improve the veterans' physical, cognitive, communicative, behavioral, psychological and social functioning under necessary supervision, and to return these patients to active duty, work, school or independent living in the community.

In July 2007, the Dole-Shalala Commission proposed the appointment of recovery coordinators to manage individualized recovery plans that would be used to guide the servicemembers' care. The Dole-Shalala Commission further recommended that these recovery coordinators possibly come from the U.S. Public Health Service, and be highly skilled and have considerable authority to be able to access resources necessary to implement the recovery plans.[65] As reported recently by GAO, the Army and the Senior Oversight Committee's[66] workgroup on case management "have initiated efforts to develop case management approaches that are intended to improve the management of servicemembers' recovery process."[67] As of October 2007, VA, DOD, and the Department of Health and Human Services (HHS) have signed a memorandum of understanding to define the role of the Public Health Service in the Recovery Coordinator program. In addition, two members of the Public Health Service Commissioned Corps have been detailed from HHS to VA and are presently working with VA and DOD to establish the Recovery Coordinator (RC) program.[68]

The RC would be designated by DOD and VA as the individual with delegated authority for oversight/coordination of the clinical and non-clinical care identified in the Individualized Recovery Plan (IRP) for every eligible severely injured/ill servicemember/veteran from initial admission to the MTF. The RC would (1) ensure the development, implementation, and oversight of the IRP and (2) ensure that the servicemembers/veterans and their families have access to all clinical and non-clinical case management services, including medical care, rehabilitation, education- and employment-related programs, and disability benefits.

According to the VA, the RC positions would be located at the following locations: Walter Reed Army Medical Center in Washington, DC; Bethesda Naval Medical Center in Bethesda, MD; Brooke Army Medical Center in San Antonio, TX; and Balboa Naval Medical Center in San Diego, CA.

VA Activities to Assist OEF and OIF Servicemembers

VA has stated that it has taken numerous steps to ease the transition of seriously injured servicemembers between DOD and VA medical facilities. VA has conducted several thousand briefings to servicemembers and their families about VA benefits and services, and about where to obtain VA health care services. VA also sends "thank-you" letters together with information brochures to each OEF and OIF veteran identified by DOD as having separated from active duty. These letters provide information on health care and other VA benefits, toll-free numbers for obtaining information, and appropriate VA websites for accessing additional information Letters and educational "tool kits"explaining VA services and benefits are also sent to each of the National Guard Adjutants General and the Reserve Chiefs. VA has stated that it has developed an outreach, education, and awareness program for the National Guard and Reserve. To ensure coordinated transition services and benefits, a Memorandum of Agreement (MOA) was signed with the National Guard in May 2005. VA is also in the process of developing MOAs with both the United States Army Reserve and the United States Marine Corps. According to VA these new partnerships will increase awareness of, and access to, VA services and benefits during the demobilization process and as service personnel return to their local communities.[69]

VA-DOD Joint Executive Committee

The VA- DOD Joint Executive Committee (JEC) was established by the National Defense Authorization Act for 2004 (P.L. 108-136). The JEC is required to report annually to Congress with recommendations for improving coordination and sharing between the two departments. As part of preparing the recommendations, P.L. 108-136 requires the JEC to: (1) review all polices, procedures, and practices related to the coordination and sharing of resources between the departments; (2) identify changes to the policies, procedures, and practices that would benefit the coordination and sharing of resources between the agencies with the goal of improving the delivery of benefits and services; (3) identify further opportunities for coordination and collaboration between the departments that would not affect the quality of care, range of services, or priorities for benefits; (4) review each department's plans for acquiring additional resources such as facilities, equipment, and technology to determine the effect on future opportunities for coordination and sharing of resources; and (5) review the implementation of activities designed to promote coordination and resource sharing between the departments. By statute, the JEC has at least two subordinate committees (for health and benefits), but may have other subordinate committees, or working groups, as deemed necessary by the Deputy Secretary of Veterans Affairs and the Under Secretary of Defense.[70] In April 2004, VA signed a Memorandum of Understanding (MOU) with DOD to provide health care and rehabilitation services to servicemembers who sustain spinal cord injury, TBI, or visual impairment. The MOU established referral procedures for transferring active duty inpatient servicemembers from DOD medical facilities to VA medical facilities.

Office of Seamless Transition

On January 3, 2005, VA established the National Veterans Affairs Office of Seamless Transition to ensure that there is no interruption of care as a servicemember moves from being a DOD patient to a VA patient, that whatever kinds of treatment are being delivered in the MTF are continued, and that treatment plans are shared. The office is composed of representatives from VHA, VBA, as well as an active duty Marine Corps officer from Marine4Life, a representative from the Army Wounded Warrior (AW2) program, and representatives from the National Guard and Reserve Components. The office also facilitates priority access to care by enrolling patients in the VA system before they leave an MTF. Major activities of this office undertaken in 2006, are summarized below:

- Placed additional VA/DOD Liaisons at the Naval Medical Center in San Diego, California, and Womack Army Medical Center at Ft. Bragg, North Carolina.
- Placed a VA certified Rehabilitation Registered Nurse at the WRAMC to assess and provide regular updates to the Polytrauma Rehabilitation Centers on the medical condition of the patients, educate families and prepare the active duty servicemember for transition to the rehabilitation phase of recovery.
- Established an OIF/OEF Polytrauma Call Center to assist seriously injured veterans. The Call Center is operational 24 hours a day, 7 days a week to answer and/or refer clinical, administrative, and benefit inquiries from OIF/OEF polytrauma patients and their families.
- Trained 54 National Guard Transition Assistance Advisors (TAAs). TAAs would serve as the statewide point of contact and coordinator, to provide advice to Guard members, their families and all other reserves as to VA benefits and services, and to assist in resolving problems with VA healthcare, benefits, and TRICARE.[71]

- o Implemented a seamless transition performance measure for FY2007. Under this performance measure severely injured OEF and OIF servicemembers who are transferred by VA/DOD Liaisons at the military treatment facilities must be assigned a VA medical center case manager prior to the transfer. This VA case manager must contact the service member/veteran within 7 calendar days of notification of the transfer.

Vet Centers

The Department has emphasized that it has enhanced its outreach efforts through the Vet Center program. This program was originally established by Congress in 1979 to meet the readjustment needs of veterans returning from the Vietnam War.[72] From their inception, Vet Centers were designed to be community-based, non-medical facilities that offered easy access to care for Vietnam veterans who were experiencing difficulty in resuming a normal civilian life.

Today, VHA's Vet Center program consists of 209 community-based centers located across the country, and in Puerto Rico, the Virgin Islands, and Guam. On February 7, 2007, the Department announced that it will be establishing 23 new centers in communities across the nation during 2007 and 2008.[73] The Vet Center program is primarily funded through the Medical Services appropriation (personnel costs), with additional funds provided from the Medical Facilities (leasing costs), Information Technology, and Medical Administration accounts. Vet Center funding is designated as specific purpose funding within the overall medical care appropriation. Funds are allocated at the direction of the Readjustment Counseling program office.

Each Vet Center is managed by a Team Leader who reports to one of the seven Readjustment Counseling Service (RCS) Regional Managers. The Chief Readjustment Counseling Officer at the VA Central Office is responsible for direct line supervision, through the seven RCS Regional Managers, of all Vet Center clinical and administrative operations. The Chief Readjustment Counseling Officer reports directly to the Under Secretary for Health.

Site selection for the new Vet Centers is based on demographic data from the U.S. Census Bureau and the DOD Defense Manpower Data Center. Initial input is provided by the seven RCS Regional Offices. Finally, recommendations and supporting data are evaluated by the Chief Readjustment Counseling Officer and the Office of the Under Secretary for Health. The final decision is made by the Under Secretary for Health. Vet Centers utilize permanently leased space and are usually staffed by one or two counselors who provide full-time services to area veterans on a regular basis. Vet Centers also remain open after normal business hours or on weekends to accommodate veterans traveling in from greater distances.

Vet Centers have hired and trained 100 new outreach workers from among the ranks of recently separated OIF and OEF veterans. In May 2007, VHA announced that it plans to recruit an additional 100 staff positions to the Vet Center program in FY2008 and another 100 staff positions for FY2009. Vet Center outreach is primarily for the purpose of providing information that will facilitate a seamless transition and the early provision of VA services to newly returning veterans and their family members upon separation from the military. These positions are being located on or near active military out-processing stations, as well as National Guard and Reserve facilities. New veteran hires are providing briefing services to transitioning servicemen and women regarding military-related readjustment needs, as well as the complete spectrum of VA services and benefits available to them and their family members. VA also has stated that it expects to add staff to 61 existing facilities to augment the services these centers provide.[74]

All combat veterans are eligible for Vet Center readjustment counseling services.[75] From FY2003 through the end of the third quarter of FY2007, the Vet Center program has provided services to 183,530 veterans and clinical services to 58,504 veterans.[76] The Vet Center program also provides bereavement counseling services to family members of those servicemembers killed while on active. From FY2003 through the end of the third quarter of FY2007, such services have been provided to more than 1,570 family members. In addition, the Vet Centers provide counseling to veterans who have experienced sexual trauma while on active duty.

Exchange of Health Information

As discussed previously, a key component of the seamless transition of patients from DOD to the VA is the exchange of medical information between the two Departments. Since the late 1 990s, VA and DOD have been working toward an interoperable medical record.[77] Before OEF and OIF, VA and DOD had been focusing on unidirectional exchange of information from DOD to VA, which would have helped VA understand the care provided to veterans while they were in the military. In June 2005, a memorandum of understanding (MOU) was signed between DOD and VA for the purposes of defining data sharing between the two departments. This MOU provides the necessary governance for the sharing of protected health information and other individually identifiable information. Later, the two Departments decided to implement a bi-directional exchange of medical information (Bidirectional Health Information Exchange — BHIE) to include information on patients' allergies, lab and radiology results, and pharmacy data. Both Departments have deployed the BHIE interface. This new interface allows VA providers to access information from all DOD health care facilities, and allows providers at all military treatment facilities to access BHIE directly from DOD's electronic medical record system. To facilitate the transfer of servicemembers from DOD treatment facilities to VA Polytrauma Rehabilitation Centers, scans of patients' radiology and medical records are now being transferred to the VA's integrated imaging system.

At present, the Clinical Health Data Repository interface is being tested in several DOD and VA locations. This interface would support the exchange of data elements in real time rather than transmitting batches of data at regular intervals. **Figure 9** shows the current and planned health information exchanges between the two Departments.

The full timeline and critical milestones supporting the exchange of medical information between the VA and the DOD are depicted in **Figure 10**.

Veterans Tracking Application (VTA)

The VTA was activated on Monday, April 23, 2007.[78] VTA would provide access to medical records in real time on wounded soldiers evacuated from Afghanistan and Iraq. Prior to this only VA's four polytrauma centers were able to access this information. The VA liaisons at the DOD MTFs and the point of contacts at the VA medical centers would now be able to use VTA to track the referral of patients from the DOD MTFs such as Walter Reed Army Medical Center to VA medical centers. According to VA, clinicians would continue to access clinical data on OEF and OIF servicemembers being treated in their facilities through DOD's Joint Patient Tracking Application (JPTA)[79] or through VTA.

The VA has stated that by the end of 2007, it expects that data in VTA will be available to providers through VistA. This VistA interface would assure that VA providers get VTA data in a format with which they are familiar and would reduce the training burden on the providers in the field.

Two-Year Eligibility for Veterans Returning from Iraq and Afghanistan

Veterans who have served or are now serving in Iraq and Afghanistan may, following separation from active duty, enroll in the VA health care system and, for a two-year period following the date of their separation, receive VA health care without copayment requirements for conditions that are or may be related to their combat service. Following this initial two-year period, they may continue their enrollment in the VA health care system but may become subject to any applicable copayment requirements.[80] For information on legislation to expand eligibility, see section on veterans health care legislation below.

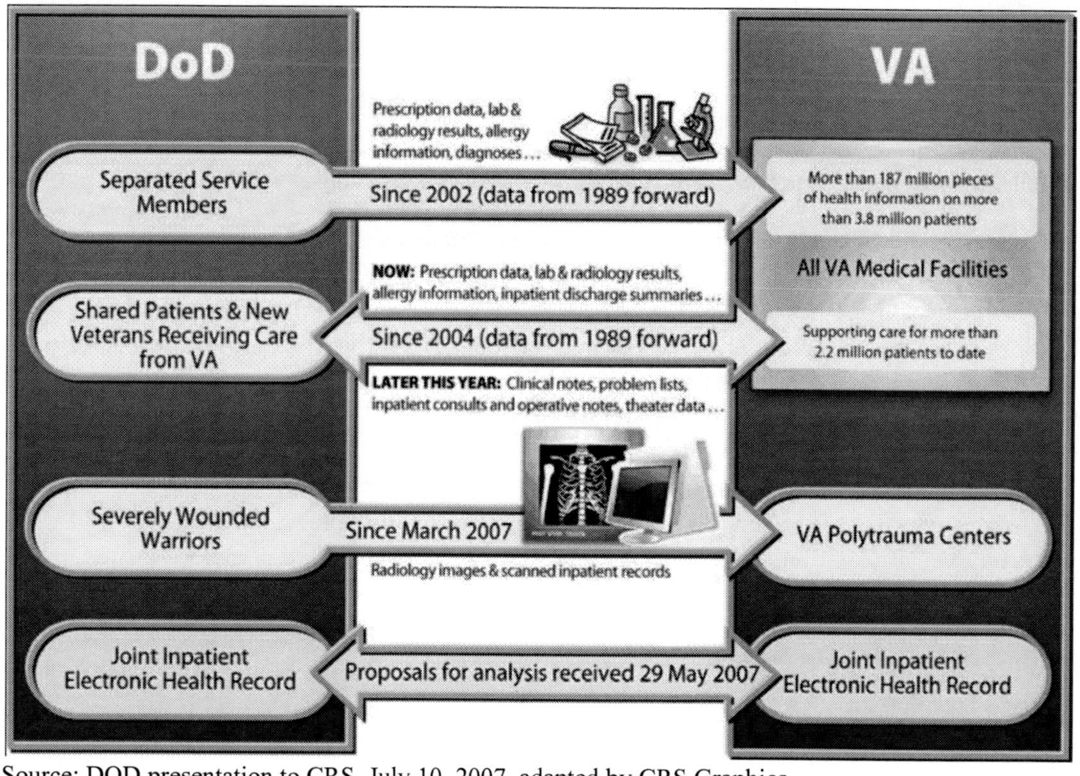

Source: DOD presentation to CRS, July 10, 2007, adapted by CRS Graphics.

Figure 9. DOD and VA Electronic Information Sharing Focus Areas

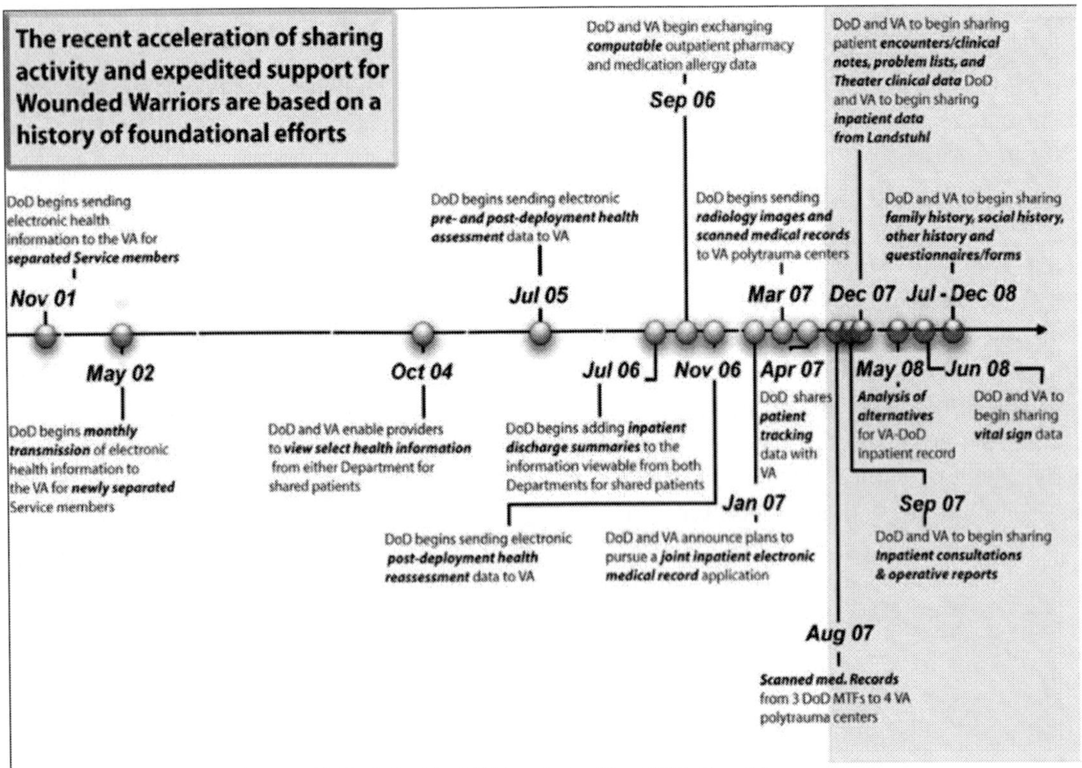

Source: DOD presentation to CRS, July 10, 2007, adapted by CRS Graphics

Figure 10. Milestones and Plans for Exchange of Medical Information

Task Force on Returning Global War on Terror Heroes

On February 18, 2007, the Washington Post reported the first in a series of articles describing problems with outpatient medical care and other services provided at the Walter Reed Army Medical Center (a DOD facility in Washington, DC) to injured servicemembers returning from combat theaters in support of OEF and OIF.[81] In response to these the President appointed several task forces and study panels to report on ways to improve services to returning servicemembers and reduce bureaucratic delays. On April 19, 2007, the interagency task force chaired by VA Secretary Nicholson issued a report providing 25 recommendations to improve delivery of federal services to returning military men and women. A summary of the health care recommendations is given below:[82]

- Develop a system of co-management and case management for returning servicemembers to facilitate ease of transfer from DOD care to VA care.
- Screen all OEF and OIF veterans seen in VA health care facilities for mild to moderate TBI.
- Assist the VA enrollment process by modifying the VA 10-10EZ form for returning servicemembers, enhance the on-line benefits package to self-identify OEF and OIF servicemembers, and expand the use of DOD military service information to establish eligibility for health care benefits.

- o Require VA to provide full support at Post-Deployment Health Reassessments for Guard and Reserve members to enroll eligible members and schedule appointments.
- o Standardize VA Liaison agreements across all military treatment facilities.
- o Expand VA access to DOD records to coordinate improved transfer of a servicemember's medical care through patient "hand-off."
- o Enhance the Computerized Patient Record System (CPRS) to more specifically track OEF and OIF servicemembers.
- o Develop a Veterans Tracking Application (VTA) and identifiers to improve monitoring of returning servicemembers (the VTA was activated in April 2007).
- o Create an "Embedded Fragment" surveillance center to monitor returning servicemembers who have possibly retained fragments of materials (shrapnel etc.) in order to provide early medical intervention.
- o Enhance capacity for OEF and OIF servicemembers to receive dental care in the private sector as VA continues to improve their capacity for dental services at their facilities.
- o Expand collaboration between VA and the Department of Health and Human Services to improve access to returning servicemembers in remote or rural areas.
- o Expand coordination on IT interoperability with the goal to adopt standardized data sharing between the VA and Indian Health Service (IHS) health care partners.

OTHER HEALTH CARE ISSUES

Post-Traumatic Stress Disorder (PTSD)

PTSD is the most prevalent mental disorder among returning OEF and OIF servicemembers and has drawn the most attention. Congress has held hearings about mental health care services provided by VA to these returning servicemembers. Demand for mental health services, including treatment for PT SD, is likely to grow not only from new soldiers returning from active combat, but also among veterans experiencing increased levels of anxiety and mental stress during wartime.[83]

OEF/OIF PTSD Data and Trends

As of June, 30 2007, VHA facilities have examined a total of 56,246 OEF and OIF veterans for potential PTSD. This includes inpatient, outpatient, and Vet Center visits. Of these veterans, 48,559 have received a possible diagnosis of PTSD.

The hallmark characteristics of PT SD include flashbacks, nightmares, intrusive recollections or re-experiencing of the traumatic event, avoidance, numbing, and hyperarousal. When such symptoms last under a month, they are typically associated with acute stress disorder, not PTSD. In order for a diagnosis of PTSD, symptoms have to persist for at least a month and cause significant impairment in important areas of daily life.

PTSD is known to have high rates of comorbidity with other anxiety disorders, major depressive disorder and substance abuse. Some studies indicate that more than 80% of people with PTSD also experience a major depressive or other psychiatric disorder.[84] Studies investigating rates of comorbidity for PTSD and lifetime prevalence of alcohol abuse have indicated rates from 68% of individuals with PTSD to as high as 82%.[85]

VA treatment programs for PTSD

Within the VA, programming for mental health is driven by the Mental Health Strategic Plan (MHSP). The goal of MHSP is to anticipate need and fill in the gaps of current mental health programs based on the CARES model (Capital Asset Realignment for Enhanced Services, discussed later in the report) and recommendations from the President's New Freedom Commission on Mental Health.

The VA delivers mental health services in a variety of clinical settings and specialized programs. Specifically, VA provides PTSD services in medical facilities, community settings, and Vet Centers. The VA medical centers include a network of more than 100 specialized programs for veterans suffering from PTSD. Outpatient PTSD programs offer three types of clinics where veterans meet with mental health professionals and PTSD specialists. PTSD Day Hospital Programs provide a "therapeutic community" offering social, recreational and vocational activities in addition to counseling throughout the week. Inpatient programs provide PTSD treatment in hospital units with 24-hour psychiatric and nursing care.

Beginning in 2005, VHA created Returning Veterans Education and Clinical Teams in medical centers to help, educate, evaluate, and treat returning veterans with mental health and psychosocial issues. These programs collaborate with other VAMC PTSD, substance abuse and mental health programs, and with polytrauma, TBI and primary care services, as well as with Vet Centers. By the close of FY2007 VA anticipates that it would have 90 of these programs operational throughout the country.

Traumatic Brain Injury (TBI)

OEF/OIF TBI Data

Among the more than 22,600 U.S. soldiers wounded in the conflicts in Iraq, Afghanistan, and other locations as of November 4, 2006, blasts from Improvised Explosive Devices (IEDs) have been by far the most common cause of injury, and 59% of blast-exposed patients at Walter Reed have been found to have a TBI.[86] On April 14, 2007, the VA began screening veterans who had seen service in Iraq or Afghanistan since the beginning of October 2001 for symptoms that may be associated with TBI.[87] Of the 61,285 veterans that VA has screened for TBI to date, 11,804 (19.26%) screened positive for TBI symptoms. At present, VA clinicians are further evaluating these 11,804 to determine whether they have actually suffered a TBI or whether the symptoms they exhibit are due to other causes, such as PTSD or other combat-related stress. A representative sample of 127 recently completed evaluations indicated that 41 veterans received a definitive diagnosis of TBI, suggesting that about one-third (32.28%) of the veterans who screen positive have actually suffered a traumatic brain injury.

TBI is the result of a severe or moderate force to the head, where physical portions of the brain are damaged and functioning is impaired. Common problems after TBI include headache, decreased memory, slow mental processing, poor attention, inability to tolerate sound, sleep disturbance, and irritability. Closely related to cognitive impairment are emotional issues such as PTSD, depression, and anxiety disorders. These psychological issues often interact with the physical injury to decrease patients' overall health status and adherence to medical regimens. Those who experience TBI may behave impulsively because of damage that removes many of the brain's checks on the regulation of behavior. Without the limits provided by these higher brain functions, these individuals may overreact to seemingly innocent or neutral stimuli.[88]

The outcome of TBI is particularly relevant for understanding PTSD because the amnesia that often occurs with TBI challenges the role of traumatic recollections in the etiology of PT SD. Studies have shown that in the absence of factual recall, individuals have delusions or reconstruct memories of trauma. These individuals may retain the delusional memories better than the factual events. Hence, traumatic recall does not have to be accurate or factual to be part of PTSD.[89]

VA Treatment of TBI

The four VA polytrauma centers in Minneapolis, Palo Alto, Richmond, and Tampa provide care to those with TBI. These facilities were designated as polytrauma centers because of their experience in medical and rehabilitative care for patients with TBI and other traumatic conditions, as well as their collaborative status with the national Defense and Veterans Brain Injury Centers (these are facilities that coordinate treatment and research for traumatic brain injuries affecting active-duty military, and veterans).[90]

Mandatory Funding for Veterans' Health Care

Veterans' advocates say that the unpredictable timing, if not uncertain funding amounts inherent in the yearly discretionary appropriations process, is a major management problem for the VA. Furthermore, veterans' groups have stated that Congress's failure to enact appropriations bills by the beginning of the fiscal year adds further strain on the VA health care system, by postponing the hiring of new medical staff, foregoing medical facility maintenance and repairs, and thereby compromising on the quality of health care provided to veterans. Therefore, national veterans' organizations have been calling for "assured funding" for veterans' health care. This has also been called "mandatory funding" by other veterans' advocates. This discussion will use mandatory funding to refer to these policy proposals.

To understand mandatory funding proposals, it is essential to understand how VA programs are funded presently. Under current law, VA programs are funded through both mandatory and discretionary spending authorities. The following programs are among mandatory spending programs: cash benefit programs, that is, compensation and pensions (and benefits for eligible survivors); readjustment benefits (education and training, special assistance for disabled veterans); home loan guarantees; and veterans' insurance and indemnities. Each of these programs is an appropriated entitlement that is funded through annual appropriations.[91] With any entitlement program, because of the underlying law, the government is required to provide eligible recipients with the benefits to which they are entitled, whatever the cost. Congress is obliged to appropriate the money necessary to fund the obligation.

If the amount Congress provides in the annual appropriations act is not enough, it is obliged to make up the difference in a supplemental appropriation. Like other entitlement programs, spending automatically increases or decreases over time as the number of recipients eligible for benefits varies. Certain of these VA entitlement benefits are indexed for inflation; the benefit amount will increase automatically based on the measured increase in the cost-of-living adjustment.

The remaining VA programs, primarily health care, medical facility construction, medical research, and VA administration, are funded through annual discretionary appropriations. Each year, Congress takes up the matter of providing budget authority for discretionary programs. As such, the amount of funds VHA can spend on discretionary programs is determined by the amount of its appropriation.

Generally, the mandatory funding proposals that have been suggested by veterans' advocates are based on a formula that takes into account the number of enrolled and nonenrolled veterans eligible for VA medical care, and the rate of medical care inflation. Proponents believe that mandatory funding will eliminate the year-to-year uncertainty about funding levels and close the gap between funding and demand for veterans' health care. Opponents believe that with these proposals spending for VHA will increase significantly as enrollment in the VA health care system soars; in most of the proposed funding formulas, automatic funding increases are primarily based on enrollment figures. Furthermore, critics believe that a static funding formula cannot adequately take into consideration the changing needs of veterans, which could affect the funding level necessary to provide a different mix of services, and that Congress is better able to evaluate the funding needs through the current annual appropriation process. For instance, not all enrolled veterans use the VA health care system in a given year. Should the number of users grow in one year and the number of enrollees remain stagnant, no additional funding would be available for the additional patients with increased utilization of health care services.

During a hearing in the 109th Congress, Chairman Buyer of the House Veterans' Affairs Committee stated that "[a]ccording to the Congressional Budget Office [CBO], mandatory funding would cost nearly half-a-trillion dollars over ten years. That would be a costly experiment. In contrast, the strong discretionary budgets of the past decade have proven responsive to change"[92] However, CBO stated that "although the bill would primarily affect funding for health care services provided by VHA, it also would result in some savings in direct spending for other government programs, primarily Medicare and Medicaid."[93]

As highlighted by some budget analysts, changing veterans' medical care into a mandatory budget authority may not solve the issue of closing the gap between funding and demand for veterans' health care. Congress can place caps on spending for mandatory programs through budget reconciliation language, which would limit spending on veterans' health programs.[94] Since Congress can act to change the formula or cap the spending amounts, the issue of uncertainty in funding amounts may not be resolved either. In recent testimony before the House Veterans Affairs Committee, Henry J. Aaron of the Brookings Institution stated that "converting the VHA to mandatory funding would not entirely insulate it from budgetary pressures. Congress could cut the per person funding amount or exclude certain groups of veterans from the formula used for computing annual funding."[95]

The Veterans Health Care Full Funding Act (H.R. 1041), Mandatory Funding for Veterans Act of 2007 (H.R. 1382), Assured Funding for Veterans Health Care Act (H.R. 2514) have been introduced in the 110th Congress. H.R. 1041 would require appropriations for VA health care to be funded based on recommendations proposed by an independent Veterans Health Care Funding Review Board. H.R. 1382 and H.R. 2514 would require the Secretary of the Treasury to make mandatory appropriations for VA health care based on a formula.

Continued Suspension of Priority Group 8 Veterans

Veterans' advocates want the suspension of Priority Group 8 veterans from enrolling in VA's health care system lifted, since they believe that all veterans must be able to receive care from VA. As discussed earlier, the Veterans Health Care Eligibility Reform Act of 1996 (P.L. 104-262) included language that stipulated that medical care to veterans will be furnished to the extent appropriations were made available by Congress on an annual basis. Based on this statutory authority, the Secretary of Veterans Affairs announced on January 17, 2003, that VA would temporarily suspend enrolling Priority Group 8 veterans.[96] Those who were in VA's health care system prior to January 17, 2003, were not to be affected by this suspension. VA claims that, despite its funding increases, it cannot provide all enrolled veterans with timely access to medical services because of the tremendous increase in the number of veterans seeking care from VA.[97]

Table 4 provides data from FY2003 through August 2006 on the number of Priority Group 8 veterans who applied for enrollment and were unable to enroll, and provides cumulative estimates from FY2006 thru FY2008. As seen in **Table 4**, the VA estimates that if the suspension on enrollment were to be lifted in FY2008, almost 1.6 million Priority Group 8 veterans would be eligible to enroll in the VA health care system.

The number of Priority Group 8 veterans already enrolled in VA's health care system is expected to decline from 1.27 million in FY2005 to 1.22 million in FY2006; this is mostly due to projected death rates for these veterans and the continued suspension of new enrollments.[98] In 2004, VA estimated that resumption of enrollment for Priority Group 8 veterans would require an additional $519 million over the FY2005 requested VHA budget, and an estimated $2.3 billion in FY2012.[99] The Senate Veterans Affairs Committee estimates that $1.113 billion would be needed to restore access for Priority Group 8 veterans. According to the Committee this number is based on VA's own estimates of what it would cost to reopen the system to Priority Group 8 veterans.[100]

Congress has shown a keen interest in providing access to VHA care for Priority Group 8 veterans, and legislation has been introduced to lift the suspension (H.R. 463, and a companion measure S. 1147). Provisions from S. 1147 have been incorporated into S. 1233 (see section on "Health Care Legislation Reported in the Senate" below).

Table 4. Impact of Priority Group 8 Suspension, FY2003-FY2008

FY2003 cumulative	FY2004 cumulative	FY2005 cumulative	2006 cumulative through August 2006	FY2006 cumulative estimate	FY2007 cumulative estimate	FY2008 cumulative estimate
93,228	192,419	263,257	327,457	830,203	1,254,460	1,570,503

Source: Department of Veterans Affairs.

Filling of Privately Written Prescriptions at VA

As part of VA's comprehensive medical care benefits package, VA provides all veterans who are enrolled for VA care with appropriate prescription medications, at the nominal charge of $8 for a 30-day supply per prescription. In general, the copayments are waived if the prescription is for a service-connected condition, if the veteran is severely disabled or indigent, or if the veteran was a former Prisoner of War (POW). VA dispenses medications, however, only to those veterans who are enrolled for, and who actually receive VA-provided care. Generally, VA does not provide medications to veterans unless those medications are prescribed by a physician who is employed by or under contract with VA.

However, there are two exceptions to this general requirement. VHA is required to provide medications, upon the order of any licensed physician, to: 1) veterans receiving additional disability compensation under Chapter 11 of Title 38 of the United States Code (U. S.C.), as a result of being permanently housebound or in need of regular aid and attendance due to a service-connected condition, or veterans who were previous recipients of such compensation and in need of regular aid and attendance; and 2) veterans receiving nonservice-connected pensions under Chapter 15 of Title 38 U.S.C. as a result of being permanently and totally disabled from a nonservice-connected disability, and who are permanently housebound or in need of regular aid and attendance.[101]

To address the growing waiting lists for primary care and specialty care appointments and to reduce the waiting times for a first appointment, VA implemented a program in September 2003 to provide access to VA prescription drugs for veterans experiencing long waits for their initial primary care appointment. This temporary program was known as the Transitional Pharmacy Benefit (TPB). Under this program, VA pharmacies and VA's Consolidated Mail Outpatient Pharmacies (CMOPs) were authorized to fill prescriptions written by non-VA (private) physicians until a VA physician could examine the veteran and determine an appropriate course of treatment. The TPB included most, but not all, of the drugs listed on the VA National Formulary (VANF).[102] To be eligible for the program, veterans had to be enrolled in the VA health care system prior to July 25, 2003, and had to have requested their initial primary care appointment prior to July 25, 2003. To qualify for this program, veterans also must have been waiting more than 30 days for the initial primary care appointment as of September 22, 2003.

Although VA anticipated that around 200,000 veterans would be eligible to participate in the program, about 41,000 veterans were ultimately deemed eligible to enroll; of those veterans, about 8,300 veterans participated. VA attributes low participation to the fact that many veterans had already received VA services by the start of the program. According to the VA, the TPB program incurred administrative costs associated with contacting private physicians to suggest formulary alternatives, as many of them had prescribed medications that were not on VA's formulary. VA has discontinued this pilot program.

There was considerable interest in the 108th and 109th Congresses in providing a prescription-only health care benefit for veterans. While several bills were introduced, none of them was enacted into law.

Capital Asset Realignment for Enhanced Services (CARES)

VA holds a substantial inventory of real property and facilities throughout the country. A majority of these buildings and property support VHA's mission. Much of VA's medical infrastructure was built decades ago when its focus was inpatient care. In the past several years VA has been shifting from a hospital-based system and, today, more than 80% of the treatment VA provides is on an outpatient basis through Community Based Outpatient Clinics (CBOCs). In 1999, GAO projected that one in four medical care dollars was spent on maintaining and operating VA's buildings and land. It estimated that VA has over 5 million square feet of vacant space which can cost as much as $35 million a year to maintain.[103]

In October 2000, VA established the CARES program with the goal of evaluating the projected health care needs of veterans over the next 20 years, and of realigning VA's infrastructure to better meet those needs. In August 2003, VA's Under Secretary for Health issued a preliminary *Draft National CARES Plan* (DNCP). The DNCP, among other things, recommended that seven VA health care facilities be closed and duplicative clinical and administrative services delivered at over 30 other VHA facilities be eliminated. The sites slated to be closed were in: Canandaigua, New York; Pittsburgh, Pennsylvania (Highland Drive Division); Lexington, Kentucky (Leestown Division); Cleveland, Ohio (Brecksville Unit); Gulfport, Mississippi; Waco, Texas; and Livermore, California. Patients currently provided services at these VHA facilities would be provided care at other nearby sites. The DNCP recommended that new major medical facilities be built in Las Vegas, Nevada, and in East Central Florida. Furthermore, the DNCP recommended significant infrastructure upgrades at numerous sites, including at or near locations where VA proposed to close facilities. In addition, the draft plan called for the establishment of 48 new high-priority CBOCs.

Following the release of the DNCP, the VA Secretary appointed a 16-member independent commission to study the draft plan. The commission was composed of individuals from a wide variety of backgrounds outside of the federal government. The CARES Commission developed and applied six factors in the review of each proposal in the DNCP: (1) impact on veterans' access to health care; (2) impact on health care quality; (3) veteran and stakeholder views; (4) economic impact on the community; (5) impact on VA missions and goals; and (6) cost to the government. The commission conducted 38 public hearings and 81 site visits throughout 2003, and submitted its recommendations to the Secretary in February 2004. After reviewing the recommendations, the Secretary announced the final details of the CARES plan in May 2004 (Secretary's CARES Decision). **Table 5** provides a timeline of major activities under the CARES process.

The final plan included consolidating the following facilities: (1) Highland Drive campus in Pennsylvania with University Drive and Heinz campuses in Pennsylvania; (2) Brecksville campus in Ohio with Wade Park campus in Cleveland, Ohio; and (3) Gulfport campus with Biloxi campus in Mississippi. The following facilities were to be partially realigned: (1) Knoxville campus in Iowa; (2) Canandaigua campus in New York; (3) Dublin campus in Georgia; (4) Livermore campus in California; (5) Montrose campus in New York; (6) Butler campus in Pennsylvania; (7) Saginaw campus in Michigan; (8) Ft. Wayne campus in Indiana; and (9) Kerrville campus in Texas.[104]

Table 5. Timeline of Major CARES Activities

Date	Activity	Description
February 2002	VA announced the results of a pilot CARES study.	The pilot study assessed current and future use of health care assets in the three markets of Network 12, which includes parts of five states: Illinois, Indiana, Michigan, Minnesota, and Wisconsin. It resulted in decisions to realign health care services and renovate or dispose of several buildings consistent with VA mission and community zoning issues.
August 2003	VA's Under Secretary for Health presented the Draft National CARES Plan.	The Under Secretary's Draft National CARES Plan included recommendations about health care services and capital assets in VA's remaining 74 markets. These recommendations reflected input from managers of VA's health care networks.
February 2004	An independent CARES Commission issued recommendations.	An independent 16-member commission appointed by the Secretary of Veterans Affairs issued recommendations to the Secretary based on its review of the Draft National CARES Plan and related documents and information obtained through public hearings, site visits, public meetings, written comments from veterans and other stakeholders, and consultations with experts.
May 2004	VA's Secretary announced the CARES decisions.	The Secretary based his decisions on a review of the CARES Commission's recommendations.
January 2005	CARES follow-up studies.	VA awarded a contract for additional studies at 18 VA facilities. These studies will include evaluating outstanding health care issues, developing capital plans, as well as determining the best use for unneeded VA property consistent with VA mission and community zoning issues.

Source: Government Accountability Office, *VA Health Care: VA Should Better Monitor Implementation and Impact of Capital Asset Alignment Decisions*, GAO-07-408, March 2007.

The final plan also called for building new hospitals in Orlando and Las Vegas; adding 156 new CBOCs, four new spinal cord injury centers, and two blind rehabilitation centers; and expanding mental health outpatient services nationwide. By opening health care access to more veterans, VA expects to increase the percentage of enrolled veterans from 28% of the veterans' population today, to 30% in 2012 and 33% in 2022. This percentage increase can be attributed in part to a projected decline in the overall veteran population. Nationally, the number of veteran enrollees is projected to increase 6% by 2012 and decrease 5% by 2022 from the number of veteran enrollees reported in 2001. VA asserts that the CARES plan will reduce the cost of maintaining vacant space over the period 2006 to 2022 from an estimated $3.4 billion to $750 million and allow VA to redirect those funds to patient care.[105]

Critics of the CARES plan contend that closures are being considered without assessing what kind of facilities will be needed for long-term care and mental health care in the future. For instance, at the time of the release of the DNCP, projections for outpatient and acute psychiatric inpatient care contained data inconsistencies on future needs. VA asserted that it would improve its forecasting models to ensure that projections adequately reflect future need. Also, some believe that the CARES plan does not focus enough on future nursing home needs, and would leave VA short of beds in a few decades. In this view, VA would not have any choice but to privatize some parts of the health care system. Moreover, some veterans' groups believe that CARES is only about closing "surplus" hospitals and do not believe that CARES will result in the building of new and modern facilities. Finally, the closure of some VA medical facilities raised serious concern among some Members of Congress who felt that they had little input into the CARES process.[106]

The Veterans Health Programs Improvement Act of 2004 (P.L. 108-422), signed into law on November 30, 2004, required VA to notify Congress of the impact of actions that may result in a facility closure, consolidation, or administrative reorganization. The law also prohibits such actions from occurring until 60 days following the notification.

The Secretary's CARES Decision identified implementation issues that required further study, including additional stakeholder input at selected sites. On September 29, 2004, the Secretary of VA established an Advisory Committee for CARES Business Plan Studies. The committee and its subcommittees generally consist of representatives from veterans' service organizations, governmental agencies, health care providers, planning agencies, and community organizations with a direct interest in the CARES process. This committee is to consult with stakeholders during implementation of the Secretary's CARES Decision. The committee is to ensure that the full range of stakeholder interests and concerns are assembled, publicly articulated, accurately documented, and considered in the development of site-level business plans.

In January 2005, VA awarded a contract to PricewaterhouseCoopers to complete studies at 18 sites throughout the country during a 13-month period, as required by the Secretary's CARES Decision.[107] Local Advisory Panels (LAPs) gathered views of stakeholders regarding the range of potential options provided by the contractor and made recommendations to the Secretary. In 2006 VA announced the Secretary's decision for some of the 18 sites. For some sites decisions have not yet been announced.

VA has begun implementing some of the projects under the CARES decisions. Specifically, as of February 2007, VA was in the process of implementing 32 of more than 100 major capital projects that were identified in the CARES process.[108] Given below in **Table 6** is a summary of the final decisions announced thus far.

Beneficiary Travel Program

In general, the beneficiary travel program reimburses certain veterans for the cost of travel to VA medical facilities when seeking health care. P.L. 76-432, passed by Congress on March 14, 1940, mandated VA to pay either the actual travel expenses, or an allowance based upon the mileage traveled by any veteran traveling to and from a VA facility or other place for the purpose of examination, treatment, or care. P.L. 85-857, signed into law on September 2, 1958, authorized VA to pay necessary travel expenses to any veteran traveling to or from a VA facility or other place in connection with vocational rehabilitation counseling or for the purpose of examination, treatment, or care. However, this law changed VA's travel reimbursement into a discretionary authority by stating that VA "may pay" expenses of travel.

Table 6. CARES Decisions on the 18 Sites

Study Site	CARES Decision
Boston, MA (VISN 1)	The contractor's final report proposed closing four Boston VAMCs and creating a single medical center for the metropolitan area. The Secretary rejected this proposal and has instructed the contractor to proceed to Stage 2 and provide more detailed analysis of several other options. The additional options include shifting inpatient psychiatry and long-term care from the Bedford VAMC facility to the Brockton VAMC, while retaining outpatient care at Bedford and consolidating services currently located at West Roxbury VAMC into the Jamaica Plain VAMC, or vice versa.
Canandaigua, NY (VISN 2)	After reviewing the contractor's final report, the Secretary rejected all proposals to move services to an off-site facility. The Secretary decided to construct a new single-floor, 120-bed nursing home and a new 50-bed residential rehabilitation facility and to renovate the outpatient building. VA will also explore partnerships with the private sector to generate revenue and complementary services for veterans by leasing under-used buildings and land. As required by the Military Quality of Life, Military Construction, Veterans Affairs, and Related Agencies Appropriations Act FY2006 (P.L. 109-114, H.Rept. 109-305), VA has designated the Canandaigua VAMC as a mental health and post traumatic stress disorder (PTSD) "Center of Excellence," and has housed its National Suicide Prevention Hot Line at Canandaigua.
Montrose/Castle Point, NY (VISN 3)	Based on the contractor's final report, the VA decided to maintain the current residential treatment program and build a multi-specialty ambulatory care facility at the Montrose campus. Furthermore, VA would completely modernize the Castle Point campus.
New York City, NY (VISN 3)	Based on the contractor's final report, the Secretary has decided to retain the existing VAMCs in both Brooklyn and Manhattan.
St. Albans, NY (VISN 3)	Based on the contractor's final report, the Secretary has decided that VA would replace existing facilities at St. Albans with a new nursing home, outpatient clinics and a domiciliary consolidated on the north end of the campus.
Perry Point, MD (VISN 5)	After reviewing the contractors report and the recommendations of the Local Advisory Panel (LAP) the Secretary decided to build a new nursing home and modernize existing mental health and outpatient facilities. VA will continue the study internally to complete a capital plan for the campus. There will be no Stage 2 study.
Montgomery, AL (VISN 7)	Based on the contractor's final report, the Secretary has decided to continue inpatient services at the Montgomery facility.
Louisville, KY (VISN 9)	Based on the contractor's final report, a new medical center will replace the current facility. VA's Office of Facility Management has created a site selection board, and is in the process of selecting an architectural and engineering firm to support the analysis of site locations.
Lexington, KY (VISN 9)	After reviewing the contractor's final report, the Secretary requested the contractor to proceed to Stage 2 and provide a more detailed study of two options selected by the Secretary. The first option is to replace all facilities on the southeastern part of the Leestown facility; and the second option is to construct appropriately sized new clinical care buildings on the central portion of the Leestown facility.

Table 6. (continued)

Study Site	CARES Decision
Poplar Bluff, MO (VISN 15)	After reviewing the contractor's report and the recommendations of the Local Advisory Panel (LAP) the Secretary decided to maintain inpatient services and added cardiology services to the existing list of services. The Secretary's decision rejected the option for the closure of Poplar Bluff inpatient services, and referral of inpatient VA care to a community hospital.
Biloxi, MS (VSIN 16)	Hurricane Katrina obviated the need for this study because the facility was destroyed. Future construction requirements are being addressed through emergency appropriations in response to Hurricane Katrina.
Muskogee, OK (VISN 16)	After reviewing the contractor's recommendations the Secretary decided to maintain inpatient services at the Muskogee VAMC and to expand psychiatric services.
Waco, TX (VISN 17)	The Military Quality of Life, Military Construction, Veterans Affairs, and Related Agencies Appropriations Act FY2006 (P.L. 109-114, H.Rept. 109-305) required VA to designate Waco VAMC as a mental health and PTSD "Center of Excellence." The Secretary decided to keep the facility open.
Big Spring, TX (VISN 18)	The contractor's final report did not recommend the closure and transfer of inpatient care, stating that the Big Spring VAMC is in good condition, quality of care is excellent and change would result in no improvements to access. Therefore, the Secretary decided that inpatient services will remain at the Big Spring VAMC.
Walla Walla, WA (VISN 20)	After reviewing the contractor's final report, the Secretary rejected options to close the Walla Walla VAMC and move the services to the Tri-Cities market. VA would replace the current Walla Walla VAMC with a new multi-specialty outpatient facility and ensure that inpatient and nursing home services are available.
White City, OR (VISN 20)	After reviewing the contractor's final report, the Secretary has decided that VA will not transfer services from the White City Southern Oregon Rehabilitation Center and Clinic (SORCC). However, VA will continue to evaluate if it will renovate or replace the current facility.
Livermore, CA (VISN 21)	After reviewing the contractor's final report, the Secretary requested the contractor to proceed to Stage 2 and provide a more detailed study of three options selected by the Secretary. The first option is to construct a new nursing home on the current site, the second option is to relocate the current nursing home care unit to a new off-site stand-alone facility co-located with ambulatory care services. The third option is to renovate the current nursing home unit and consolidate all necessary logistics and support functions.
West LA, CA (VISN 22)	After reviewing the contractor's final report, the VA has decided to completely modernize the inpatient facility for outpatient services. In addition, a new VA building to place the urns containing the remains of cremated veterans, and a new facility for the Veterans Benefits Administration Regional Office, will be housed on campus. Buildings 205, 208, and 209 have been designated for homeless veterans programs.

Source: CRS analysis of VA decision announcements.

Due to rapidly increasing costs of the beneficiary travel program, on March 12, 1987, VA published final regulations that sharply curtailed eligibility for the beneficiary travel program.[109] Under these regulations beneficiary travel payments to eligible veterans were paid when specialized modes of transportation, such as ambulance or wheelchair van, were medically required. In addition, payment was authorized for travel in conjunction with compensation and pension examinations, as well as travel beyond a 100-mile radius from the nearest VA medical care facility. It also authorized the VA to provide transportation costs, when necessary, to transfer any veteran from one health care facility (either a VA or contract care facility) to another in order to continue care paid for by the VA. The following transportation costs were not authorized under these regulations:

- Cost of travel by privately owned vehicle in any amount in excess of the cost of such travel by public transportation unless public transportation was not reasonably accessible or was medically inadvisable.
- Cost of travel in excess of the actual expense incurred by any person as certified by that person in writing.
- Cost of routine travel in conjunction with admission for domiciliary care, or travel for family members of veterans receiving mental health services from the VA except for such travel performed beyond a 100-mile radius from the nearest VA medical care facility.

Travel expenses of all other veterans were not authorized unless the veterans were able to present clear and convincing evidence to show the inability to pay the cost of transportation; or except when medically-indicated ambulance transportation was claimed and an administrative determination was made regarding the veteran's ability to bear the cost of such transportation.[110]

The Veterans' Benefits and Services Act of 1988 (P.L. 100-322, section 108), in large part restored VA travel reimbursement benefits. It required that if VA provides any beneficiary travel reimbursement under Section 111 of Title 38 U.S.C. in any given fiscal year, then payments must be provided in that year in the case of travel for health care services for all the categories of beneficiaries specified in the statute. In order to limit the overall cost of this program, the law imposed a $3 one-way deductible applicable to all travel, except for veterans otherwise eligible for beneficiary travel reimbursement who are traveling by special modes of transportation such as ambulance, air ambulance, wheelchair van, or to receive a compensation and pension examination. In order to limit the overall impact on veterans whose clinical needs dictate frequent travel for VA medical care, an $18- per-calendar-month cap on the deductible was imposed for those veterans who are pre-approved as needing to travel on a frequent basis. At present, eligible veterans are reimbursed at the rate of 11 cents a mile for routine visits and 17 cents a mile for compensation and pension exams. Although the deductible rates are set in statute, the mileage rates are left to the discretion of the Secretary. **Table 7** provides details on veterans who are currently eligible to receive travel benefits.

With the rise in gasoline prices Congress has shown interest in changing the method of determining the mileage reimbursement rate and/or eliminating the current deductible amount. S. 1233, as reported in the Senate, includes a provision that would require the VA to reimburse qualifying veterans at the particular rate authorized by the Administrator of General Services, for federal government employees traveling on official business.

Table 7. Veterans Eligible for Travel Benefits

- Veterans with service-connected disabilities rated 30% or more.
- Veterans with service-connected disabilities rated less than 30% traveling for treatment of a service-connected condition.
- Veterans in receipt of a VA pension.
- Veterans traveling for a compensation or pension (C&P) exam.
- Veterans whose income does not exceed the maximum annual
- VA pension rate with an additional aid and attendance allowance.

VETERANS HEALTH CARE LEGISLATION

Health Care Legislation Enacted into Law

Joshua Omvig Veterans Suicide Prevention Act (H.R. 327, H.Rept. 110-055, P.L. 110-110)

The House passed this measure on March 21, 2007, and the Senate passed the House measure with an amendment on September 27. The bill was signed into law on November 5, 2007. P.L. 110-110, would, among other things, require the VA to establish a comprehensive program for suicide prevention among veterans. In carrying out this comprehensive program, the VA must designate a suicide prevention counselor at each VA medical facility. Each counselor is required to work with local emergency rooms, police departments, mental health organizations, and veterans service organizations to engage in outreach to veterans. The Act also requires the VA to provide for research on best practices for suicide prevention among veterans. P.L. 110-110 requires the Secretary to provide for outreach and education for veterans and the families of veterans, with special emphasis on providing information to veterans of OIF and OEF and the families of such veterans. The Act requires VA to provide for the availability of 24-hour mental health care for veterans and to establish a 24-hour hotline for veterans to call if needed. (In July 2007, the VA established a national suicide prevention hotline for veterans. The toll-free number, 1-800-273-TALK [8255], is staffed by mental health professionals 24 hours a day, 7 days a week).

Health Care Legislation Passed by the House[111]

Returning Servicemember VA Healthcare Insurance Act of 2007(H.R. 612)

The House passed this bill on May 23, 2007. H.R. 612 as amended, would extend the eligibility period from two years to five years following discharge or release for veterans who served in combat during or after the Persian Gulf War, to receive hospital care, medical services, or nursing home care provided by the VA, without having to prove that their condition is attributable to such service. H.R. 612 also provides for an additional three years of eligibility for veterans discharged more than five years before the enactment of this Act who have not enrolled.

Chiropractic Care Available to All Veterans Act (H.R. 1470)

The House passed H.R. 1470 on May 23, 2007. The measure would require that chiropractic services be made available in not fewer than 75 VAMCs by the end of December 2009, and at all health care centers by the end of 2011.

Traumatic Brain Injury Health Enhancement and Long-Term Support Act of 2007 (H.R. 2199, H.Rept. 110-166)

The House passed this measure on May 23, 2007. H.R. 2199, as amended, would require mandatory screening of veterans for traumatic brain injury (TBI). It would also require the VA to establish a comprehensive program of care for post-acute traumatic brain injury rehabilitation. H.R. 2199, as amended, would require the VA to establish TBI transition offices at each Department polytrauma network site to coordinate health care and services to veterans who suffer from moderate to severe traumatic brain injuries. Furthermore, the measure, as passed by the House, would require the VA to establish a registry of those who served in Operation Enduring Freedom or Operation Iraqi Freedom (OEF or OIF) who exhibit symptoms associated with TBI. H.R. 2199 also includes two provisions to improve the quality of care provided to rural veterans. It would create an advisory committee on rural veterans and establish a pilot program to provide readjustment counseling, related mental health services, and benefits outreach, through mobile Vet Centers.

Veterans Benefit Improvement Act of 2007 (H.R. 1315, H.Rept. 110-266)

This measure was passed by the House on July 30, 2007. Among other things, this bill contains a provision that would require the VA to establish a Vision Education Scholarship Program under the Health Professional Education Assistance Program. Those who receive a scholarship award would be required to work for three years in a VA health care facility. H.R. 1315 also mandates the Secretary to provide financial assistance to students enrolled in a program of study leading to a degree or certificate in blind rehabilitation in a U.S. state or territory, provided they agree with applicable requirements. The purpose of this scholarship is to increase the supply of qualified blind rehabilitation specialists for the VA.

Veterans Health Care Improvement Act of 2007 (H.R. 2874, H.Rept. 110-268)

This bill was passed on July 30, 2007. Among other things, H.R. 2874 would allow VA to establish a grant program for nonprofit entities to conduct workshops to assist in the therapeutic readjustment and rehabilitation of OEF and OIF veterans. The amount of the grants would be limited to $100,000 for each calendar year, and there would be $2 million authorized each fiscal year to carry out the program. The grant program would terminate on September 30, 2011. It would also require the VA to establish a grant program for rural veterans service organizations, state veterans' service agencies, and nonprofits to provide innovative transportation options to veterans in remote rural areas to travel to VA medical facilities. Grant amounts would be limited to $50,000, and the bill authorizes $3 million for each fiscal year from 2008 to 2012 to carry out the program.

H.R. 2874 would permanently authorize VA's authority to provide higher priority health care to veterans who participated in Project Shipboard Hazard and Defense (SHAD), Project 112, or related land-based tests. Under current law, VA is authorized to provide higher priority health care to these veterans with any illness, without those veterans needing an adjudicated service-connected disability to establish their priority for care. This special treatment authority will expire on December 31, 2007. This measure would also extend through September 30, 2009, VA's authority to require certain nonservice-connected veterans to pay a $10 per diem copayment when they receive VA hospital care, and extend through October 1, 2009, VA's authority to bill a service-connected patient's third-party insurance carrier for the cost of care VA provides the veteran for any nonservice-connected condition.

H.R. 2874 would also require VA to provide readjustment counseling and mental health services for OEF and OIF veterans. Such services would include contracting with community mental health centers in areas not adequately served by VA and contracting with nonprofit mental health organizations to train OEF and OIF veterans in outreach and peer support. It also directs VA to conduct training programs for clinicians that have contracts with VA to provide such services. It would also require the VA to ensure that VA domiciliary programs are adequate in capacity and safety to meet the needs of women veterans.

Furthermore, H.R. 2874 would reduce the time that a homeless veteran would have to wait to receive dental treatment from 60 days to 30 days. Under current law, VA can provide dental services to eligible homeless veterans as long as they have been receiving care for a period of 60 consecutive days in a domiciliary, therapeutic residence, community residential care coordinated by VA, or a setting for which the VA provides funds for a grant and per diem provider.

Prohibit the collection of copayments for all hospice care provided by the VA (H.R. 2623, H.Rept. 110-267)

H.R. 2623 was passed by the House on July 30. This bill would exempt all hospice care provided through VA from copayment requirements. Under current law, a veteran receiving hospice care in a nursing home is exempt from any applicable copayments. However, if the hospice care is provided in any other setting, such as in an acute-care hospital or at home, the veteran may be subject to an inpatient or outpatient primary care copayment. By exempting all hospice care provided by the VA regardless of the setting, H.R. 2623 would align the VA health care system with the Medicare program, which does not impose copayments for hospice care regardless of the setting.

Health Care Legislation Reported in the Senate

Veterans Traumatic Brain Injury and Health Programs Improvement Act of 2007 (S. 1233, S.Rept. 110-147)

S. 1233, as amended, was ordered to be reported by the Senate Veterans' Affairs Committee on June 27, 2007.[112] This bill includes several provisions related to enhancing veterans health care. As reported, S. 1233 would require VA to develop individual rehabilitation and community reintegration plans for veterans and servicemembers with TBI who are being treated in the VA health care system. The plan would identify a case manager to oversee its long-term implementation and would specify dates for review of the plan. The bill would also authorize the VA to use non-VA facilities for the implementation of rehabilitation and community reintegration plans for traumatic brain injury under certain specified circumstances. S. 1233, as reported, would require VA to develop and implement a research, education, and clinical care program on severe TBI. It also would authorize a five-year pilot program on assisted living services for veterans with traumatic brain injury and would require the VA to provide age-appropriate nursing home care for veterans who suffer from severe TBI

The Veterans Programs Enhancement Act (P.L. 105-3 68) authorized priority eligibility for health care for a period of two years following discharge or release from active duty to any veteran who served in a combat theater of operations. S. 1233 would extend the period from two to five years. According to the committee report (S.Rept. 110-147), this extension is necessary to ensure that veterans returning from combat receive health care during their transition from military service to civilian life and to address health care issues such as PTSD, which may take years to manifest. S. 1233 would require VA to establish a Hospital Quality Report Card Initiative to inform veterans and their families of the quality and performance of VA hospitals. According to S.Rept. 110-147, "the initiative is intended to help veterans and their families to make informed health care choices."[113]

S. 1233, as reported in the Senate, would require the VA to annually — by August 1 — to publish a notice in the *Federal Register* of which categories of veterans are eligible to be enrolled in VA health care in the upcoming fiscal year. Furthermore, in any year in which the VA proposes to stop enrollment, the VA Secretary would be required to provide to the House and Senate VA Committees an estimate of the cost of enrolling all eligible veterans. After the notice is published, the VA would be required to wait 45 days before implementing any change in enrollment. According to the committee report, "this notice-and-wait requirement would provide Congress with an opportunity to oversee the enrollment of veterans in the Veterans Health Administration, and to respond to any proposed limitation on enrollment."[114] Furthermore, it is the view of the committee that when resources are provided by Congress to enable the VA to keep pace with demand for services, the VA health care system should be open to all veterans who seek care.[115]

S. 1233 would require the VA to establish a grant program to provide transportation options to veterans in rural areas. Under this grant program, VA would provide grants for rural veterans' service organizations and community-based organizations to provide transportation to veterans in remote rural areas. For each of FY2008 through FY20 12, $6 million would be authorized to be appropriated for this grant program. The grants would be awarded to state veterans' service agencies, veterans service organizations, and qualified community transportation organizations.

Among other things, S. 1233 would require VA to establish demonstration projects on alternatives for expanding care for veterans in rural areas. Under the committee-reported measure, two demonstration projects would be required to be carried out in geographically dispersed areas. It would require VA to partner with the Department of Health and Human Services (HHS) and the Indian Health Service (IHS) to expand care for Native American veterans.

Furthermore, S. 1233 would exempt veterans in Priority Group 4 (veterans who have been determined by the VA to be catastrophically disabled) from paying copayments for nonservice-connected hospital care or nursing home care. Under current law, these veterans are required to pay copayments for all nonserviceconnected care they receive from the VA.

S. 1233, as reported in the Senate, would increase reimbursement rates for travel to VA medical facilities. At present, eligible veterans are reimbursed at the rate of 11 cents a mile for routine visits and 17 cents a mile for compensation and pension exams. Under S 1233, the

VA would reimburse qualifying veterans at the particular rate authorized for government employees under section 5707(b) of Title 5 U.S.C.

On November 14, 2007, the Senate Veterans' Affairs Committee ordered the following bills reported without amendment: S. 2004 (to amend Title 38 U.S.C. to establish epilepsy centers of excellence in the Veterans Health Administration of the Department of Veterans Affairs), S. 2142 (the Veterans Emergency Care Fairness Act of 2007), S. 2160 (The Veterans Pain Care Act of 2007), and S. 2162 (Mental Health Improvements Act of 2007). The committee has not released the Committee Print versions of these bills.

APPENDIX. PRIORITY GROUPS AND THEIR ELIGIBILITY CRITERIA

Priority Group 1

Veterans with service-connected disabilities rated 50% or more disabling

Priority Group 2

Veterans with service-connected disabilities rated 30% or 40% disabling

Priority Group 3

Veterans who are former POWs

Veterans awarded the Purple Heart

Veterans whose discharge was for a disability that was incurred or aggravated in the line of duty Veterans with service-connected disabilities rated 10% or 20% disabling

Veterans awarded special eligibility classification under Title 38, U.S.C., Section 1151, "benefits for individuals disabled by treatment or vocational rehabilitation"

Priority Group 4

Veterans who are receiving aid and attendance or housebound benefits

Veterans who have been determined by VA to be catastrophically disabled

Priority Group 5

Nonservice-connected veterans and noncompensable service-connected veterans rated 0% disabled whose annual income and net worth are below the established VA means test thresholds

Veterans receiving VA pension benefits

Veterans eligible for Medicaid benefits

Priority Group 6

Compensable 0% service-connected veterans
World War I veterans
Mexican Border War veterans
Veterans solely seeking care for disorders associated with

- exposure to herbicides while serving in Vietnam; or
- ionizing radiation during atmospheric testing or during the occupation of Hiroshima and Nagasaki; or
- for disorders associated with service in the Gulf War; or
- for any illness associated with service in combat in a war after the Gulf War or during a period of hostility after November 11, 1998.

Priority Group 7

Veterans who agree to pay specified copayments with income and/or net worth *above* the VA means test threshold and income *below* the HUD geographic index

Subpriority a: Noncompensable 0% service-connected veterans who were enrolled in the VA Health Care system on a specified date and who have remained enrolled since that date

Subpriority c: Nonservice-connected veterans who were enrolled in the VA health care system on a specified date and who have remained enrolled since that date.

Subpriority e: Noncompensable 0% service-connected veterans not included in Subpriority a above

Subpriority g: Nonservice-connected veterans not included in Subpriority c above Priority Group 3

Priority Group 8

Veterans who agree to pay specified copayments with income and/or net worth *above* the VA means test threshold and the HUD geographic index

Subpriority a: Noncompensable 0% service-connected veterans enrolled as of January 16, 2003, and who have remained enrolled since that date

Subpriority c: Nonservice-connected veterans enrolled as of January 16, 2003, and who have remained enrolled since that date

Subpriority e: Noncompensable 0% service-connected veterans applying for enrollment after January 16, 2003

Source: Department of Veterans Affairs

End Notes

[1] For detailed reports on benefits available for military retirees, see CRS Current Legislative Issue "U.S. Military Personnel and Compensation" under "Defense," at [http://www.crs. gov/].

[2] 38 U.S.C. § 101; 38 CFR §3.1. Also see CRS Report RL331 13, *Veterans Affairs: Basic Eligibility for Disability Benefit Programs,* by Douglas Reid Weimer.

[3] For details on the Defense Health Program, see CRS Report RL33537, *Military Medical Care: Questions and Answers,* by Richard A. Best Jr.

[4] For detailed information on veterans' benefits issues see, CRS Report RL33985, *Veterans' Benefits: Issues in the 110th Congress*, by Carol D. Davis, Coordinator.

[5] U.S. Congress. House. Committee on Veterans' Affairs, *The Provision of Federal Benefits for Veterans*, Committee print, 84th Congress, 1st session, December 28, 1955, House Committee Print No. 171. p.2.

[6] For a detailed description of the evolution of eligibility for VA health care, see CRS Report RL32961, *Veterans' Health Care Issues in the 109th Congress*, by Sidath Viranga Panangala.

[7] Lisa Dubay, John Holahan, and Allison Cook. "The Uninsured And The Affordability Of Health Insurance Coverage," *Health Affairs - Web Exclusive*, November 30, 2006. Catherine Arnst, "The Best Medical Care in the U.S." *Business Week*, July 17, 2006 p.50.

[8] In the 1920s three federal agencies, the Veterans Bureau, the Bureau of Pension in the Department of the Interior, and the National Home for Disabled Volunteer Soldiers, administered various benefits for the nation's veterans.

[9] For details on the appeals process, see CRS Report RL33704, *Veterans Affairs: The Appeal Process for Veterans' Claims,* by Douglas Reid Weimer.

[10] Established on January 3, 1946, as the Department of Medicine and Surgery by P.L. 79- 293, succeeded in 1989 by the Veterans Health Services and Research Administration, renamed the Veterans Health Administration in 1991.

[11] Jian Gao, Ying Wang and Joseph Engelhardt, "Logistic Analysis of Veterans' Eligibility- Status Change," *Health Services Management Research*, vol. 18, (August 2005), p. 175.

[12] About 90% of the VHA appropriation is allocated through VERA. Networks also receive appropriated funds not allocated through VERA for such things as prosthetics, homeless programs, readjustment counseling, and clinical training programs. VA facilities could also retain collections from insurance reimbursements and copayments, and use these funds for the care of veterans.

[13] On June 23, 2006, VA announced plans to open 25 new CBOCs in 17 states and American Somoa. The following facilities were scheduled to become operational in CY2006:Bessemer, Alabama; Tafuna, American Samoa; Miami-Globe, Northwest Tucson and Southeast Tucson, Arizona; South Orange County, California; Dover, Delaware; Athens, Georgia; Canyon County, Idaho; Spirit Lake, Iowa; Hazard and Florence, Kentucky; Bemidji, Minnesota; Holdrege, Nebraska; Fallon, Nevada; Franklin, Hamlet, and Hickory, North Carolina; Cambridge and Newark, Ohio; Hamblen, Tennessee; Conroe, Texas; Lynchburg and Norfolk, Virginia; Rice Lake, Wisconsin.

[14] Data from the *FY2008 Congressional Budget Submissions*, vol. 4 of 4. Number of facilities include facilities damaged by Hurricane Katrina. Data on the number of CBOCs differ from source to source. Some studies count clinics located at VA hospitals while others count only freestanding CBOCs. The number represented in this chapter excludes clinics located in VA hospitals. The data are current as of September 29, 2006.

[15] For further information on CHAMPVA, see CRS Report RS22483, *Health Care for Dependents and Survivors of Veterans*, by Jacqueline Rae Roche and Sidath Viranga Panangala.

[16] Kupersmith, Joel, et al. "Advancing Evidence-Based Care For Diabetes: Lessons From The Veterans Health Administration," *Health Affairs* 26, no. 2 (2007): w156-w168 (published online January 26, 2007).

[17] Feasby, Thomas E., "Is the Canadian health care system better for neurologic care?" *Neurology,* 2006; 67: 1744-1747.

[18] Veterans Health Administration, *HealthcarePapers* vol. 5 no. 4, 2005.

[19] See [http://www.theacsi.org/], accessed January 23, 2007.

[20] Nedal Arar, Lonnie Wen, John McGrath, et al., "Communicating About Medications During Primary Care Outpatient Visits: The Role of Electronic Medical Records," *Informatics in Primary Care,* vol. 13, p. 14.

[21] Caron Golden, "VA's Model of Success," *Government Leader*, November/December, 2006, p. 27.

[22] See [http://www.excelgov.org/UserFiles/VA%20VistA%20release%20finale.pdf].

[23] U.S. Department of Veterans Affairs, Office of the Secretary, *Strategic Plan FY2006-2011*, October 2006, p.11.

[24] VHA schedules about 39 million appointments a year. According to VHA, 37 million of these are scheduled within 30 days of the request of the patient's desired date.

[25] U.S. Department of Veterans Affairs, *FY2008 Congressional Budget Submissions, Medical Programs*, vol. 1 of 4, p.2-2.

[26] For a detailed discussion of "promised benefits," see CRS Report 98-1006, *Military Health Care: The Issue of "Promised" Benefits*, by David F. Burrelli.

[27] Barbara Sydell, *Restructuring the VA Health Care System: Safety Net, Training and Other Considerations*, National Health Policy Forum, Issue Brief no. 716, March 1998. Available at [http://www.nhpf.org/pdfs_ib/IB71 6_VA_3-25-98.pdf].

[28] U.S. Congress, House Committee on Veterans Affairs, *Veterans' Health Care Eligibility Reform Act of 1996,* report to accompany H.R. 3118, 1 04th Cong. 2nd sess., H.Rept. 104-690, p. 2.

[29] Ibid. p.5.

[30] Ibid. p.6.

[31] Ibid. p.5.

[32] Ibid. p.4.

[33] Veterans do not need to apply for enrollment in VA's health care system if they fall into one of the following categories: veterans with a service-connected disability rated 50% or more (percentage ratings represent the average impairment in earning capacity resulting from diseases and injuries encountered as a result of or incident to military service; those with a rating of 50% or more are placed in Priority Group 1); less than one year has passed since the veteran was discharged from military service for a disability that the military determined was incurred or aggravated in the line of duty, but the VA has not yet rated; or the veteran is seeking care from VA for only a service-connected disability (even if the rating is only 10%).

[34] VA Form 10-1 0EZ is available at [https://www. 101 0ez.med.va.gov/sec/vha/ 101 0ez/ #Process].

[35] 38 C.F.R. § 17.36 (d)(3)(iv) (2005).

[36] 38.U.S.C. §101(24); 38 C.F.R. §3.6(c).

[37] The term "service-connected" means, with respect to disability, that such disability was incurred or aggravated in line of duty in the active military, naval, or air service. VA determines whether veterans have service-connected disabilities, and for those with such disabilities, assigns ratings from 0 to 100% based on the severity of the disability. Percentages are assigned in increments of 10%.

[38] VA considers a veteran's previous year's total household income (both earned and unearned income as well as his/her spouse's and dependent children's income). Earned income is usually wages received from working. Unearned income can be interest earned, dividends received, money from retirement funds, Social Security payments, annuities, or earnings from other assets. The number of persons in the veteran's family will be factored into the calculation to determine the applicable income threshold. 38 C.F.R. § 17.36(b)(7) (2005).

[39] National Security Council, *National Strategy for Combating Terrorism,* September 2006, p.19, available at [http://www.whitehouse.gov/nsc/nsct/2006/nsct2006.pdf].

[40] Atul Gawande, "Casualties of War - Military Care for the Wounded from Iraq and Afghanistan," *The New England Journal of Medicine*, vol.351, iss. 24, (December 2004), p. 2471.

[41] Data current as of November 24, 2007 [http://www.defenselink.mil/news/casualty.pdf].

[42] The President's Commission on Care for America's Returning Wounded Warriors, July 2007, p.2, available at [http://www.pccww.gov].

[43] Title 38 U.S.C. §§ 8111, Sharing of Department and Department of Defense Health Care Resources, provides the authority for VA and the DOD to enter into agreements and contracts for the mutual use or exchange of use of services, supplies or other resources. Title 38 U.S.C. §§ 811 1A, Furnishing of Health-care Services to Members of the Armed Forces During a War or National Emergency, authorizes VA to provide care during and immediately following a period of war, or a period of national emergency as declared by the President or Congress that involves the use of the Armed Forces in armed conflict. P.L. 97-174, Section 2(b), notes that DOD might not have adequate health care resources to care for military personnel wounded in combat and other active duty personnel. The law further notes that VA has an extensive, comprehensive health care system that could be used to assist DOD in caring for such personnel.

[44] OEF, which commenced in October 2001, conducts combat operations in Afghanistan and other locations. OIF, which began in March 2003,conducts combat operations in Iraq and other locations.

[45] Since October 2003, DOD's Defense Manpower Data Center (DMDC) has periodically (every 60 days) sent VA an updated personnel roster of troops who participated in OEF and OIF, and who have separated from active duty and become eligible for VA benefits. The roster was originally prepared based on pay records of individuals. However, in more recent months it has been based on a combination of pay records and operational records provided by each service branch. The current separation data are from FY2002 through May 31, 2007.

[46] Testimony of Acting Under Secretary for Health Department of Veterans Affairs Dr. Michael J. Kussman, in U.S. Congress, House Committee on Veterans' Affairs Subcommittee on Oversight and Investigations, hearing on *Servicemembers' Seamless Transition into Civilian Life — The Heroes Return*, 110th Cong., 1st sess., March 8, 2007.

[47] Testimony of Acting Undersecretary for Health, Department of Veterans Affairs, Michael Kussman, in U.S. Congress, House Committee on Appropriations, Subcommittee on Military Construction, Veterans Affairs and Related Agencies, hearing on *FY 2008 fundingfor the Veterans Health Administration*, 110th Cong., 1st sess., March 6, 2007.

[48] Department of Veterans Affairs, Veterans Health Administration Directive. Polytrauma Rehabilitation Centers. Washington (DC): Veterans Health Administration; Jun 8, 2005, p. 2.

[49] Data provided by the Department of Veterans Affairs.

[50] U.S. Congress, House Committee on Veterans' Affairs, Subcommittee on Health, *"Handoffs or Fumbles?" Are DOD and VA Providing Seamless Health Care Coverage to Transitioning Veterans?*, 108th Cong., 2nd sess., October 16, 2003.

[51] For detailed information on issues related to disability evaluation of returning servicemembers see, CRS Report RL33991, *Disability Evaluation of Military Servicemembers* by Christine Scott, et al.

[52] The President's Task Force to Improve Health Care Delivery for Our Nation's Veterans, Final Report, May 2003, p. 24.

[53] U.S. Government Accountability Office, *VA Disability Benefits and Health Care, Providing Certain Services to the Seriously Injured Poses Challenges*, GAO-05-444T, p. 5.

[54] U.S. Government Accountability Office, *VA and DOD Health Care: VA Has Policies and Outreach Efforts to Smooth Transition from DOD Health Care, but Sharing of Health Information Remains Limited,* GAO-05-1052T.

[55] U.S. Government Accountability Office, *DOD and VA Health Care: Challenges Encountered by Injured Servicemembers during Their Recovery Process*, GAO-07-606T, p 4.

[56] *Task Force on Returning Global War on Terror Heroes,* Executive Summary, p.2.

[57] Report of the President's Commission on Care for America's Returning Wounded Warriors, July 2007, p.2 and 13, available at [http://www.pccww.gov/].

[58] Joachim J. Tenuta, "From the Battlefields to the States: The Road to Recovery. The Role of Landstuhl Regional Medical Center in US Military Casualty Care," *Journal of the American Academy of Orthopedic Surgeons*, vol 14, (2006), S45-S47.

[59] The Center for the Intrepid, a $50 million, 60,000 sq. ft., physical rehabilitation center, and two new Fisher Houses, 21-room residences for hospitalized soldiers' families were declared open on January 29, 2007.

[60] The Veterans Health Programs Improvement Act of 2004 (P.L. 108-422) required VA to establish centers for research, education, and clinical activities related to complex trauma due to combat injuries, and the Department of Veterans Affairs, and Housing and Urban Development, and Independent Agencies Appropriations Act, 2005 (P.L. 108-447) required VA to establish a new prosthetics and integrative health care initiative. The PRCs were designated as a response to these mandates.

[61] Statement of William F. Feeley, Deputy Undersecretary for Health for Operations and Management, Department of Veterans Affairs, hearing on *Servicemembers' Seamless Transition into Civilian Life — The Heroes Return*, in U.S. Congress, House Committee on Veterans Affairs, Subcommittee on Oversight and Investigations, 110th Cong., 1st sess., March 8, 2007.

[62] There are a total of ten VA/DOD liaisons located at Walter Reed Army Medical Center, Washington, DC (two VA/DOD liaisons); National Naval Medical Center, Bethesda, Maryland; Brooke Army Medical Center, Fort Sam Houston, Texas; Eisenhower Army Medical Center, Fort Gordon, Georgia; Fort Hood Army Medical Center, Fort Hood, Texas; Madigan Army Medical Center, Tacoma, Washington (two VA/DOD liaisons); Evans Army Medical Center Fort Carson, Colorado; Camp Pendleton, San Diego, California; Womack Army Medical Center, Ft. Bragg, North Carolina.

[63] The rehabilitation team consists of a Rehabilitation Physician, Rehabilitation Nurses, Physical Therapists, Occupational Therapists, Speech and Language Pathologists, Recreation Therapists, Kinesiotherapists, Neuropsychologists, Psychologists, Dieticians, Social Worker/Case Manager, Military Liaisons, and Blind Rehabilitation Therapists.

[64] Testimony of Shane McNamee, Medical Director, Richmond Polytrauma Rehabiliation Center, Department Of Veterans Affairs, hearing on *Servicemembers ' Seamless Transition into Civilian Life — The Heroes Return*, in U.S. Congress, House Committee on Veterans Affairs, Subcommittee on Oversight and Investigations, 110th Cong., 1st sess., March 8, 2007.

[65] The President's Commission on Care for America's Returning Wounded Warriors, July 2007, pp5-6.

[66] Senior Oversight Committee is an interagency committee specifically established to address concerns about the care and services provided to returning servicemembers. The committee is co-chaired by the Deputy Secretary of VA and the Deputy Secretary of Defense.

[67] U.S., Government Accountability Office (GAO), *DOD AND VA: Preliminary Observations on Efforts to Improve Health Care and Disability Evaluations for Returning Servicemembers,* GAO-07-1 256T,p.8.

[68] Testimony of Patrick W. Dunne, Assistant Secretary for Policy and Planning, Department of Veterans Affairs, hearing on *VA and DOD Collaboration: Report of the President's Commission on Care For America's Returning Wounded Warriors; Report of the Veterans Disability Benefit Commission; and other related reports* in U.S. Congress, Senate Committee on Veterans' Affairs, October 17, 2007.

[69] Testimony of Gordon H. Mansfield, Deputy Secretary, Department of Veterans Affairs hearing on *VA/DOD Cooperation and Collaboration* in U.S. Congress, Senate Committee on Veterans' Affairs, 110th Cong., 1st sess., January 23, 2007.

[70] For more information on the JEC, see VA/DOD Joint Executive Council, *Fiscal Year 2006 Annual Report,* at [http://www.tricare.mil/DVPCO/downloads/VADoD2006.pdf].

[71] TRICARE is the health plan of the military health system. For detailed information about this program see, CRS Report RL33537, *Military Medical Care: Questions and Answers*, by Richard A. Best Jr.

[72] Established by the Veterans' Health Care Amendments of 1979 (P.L. 96-22).

[73] New Vet Centers will be located in Montgomery, Alabama; Fayetteville, Arkansas; Modesto, California; Grand Junction, Colorado; Orlando, Fort Myers, and Gainesville, Florida; Macon, Georgia; Manhattan, Kansas;

Baton Rouge, Louisiana; Cape Cod, Massachusetts; Saginaw and Iron Mountain, Michigan; Berlin, New Hampshire; Las Cruces, New Mexico; Binghamton, Middletown, Nassau County and Watertown, New York; Toledo, Ohio; Du Bois, Pennsylvania; Killeen, Texas; and Everett, Washington. During 2007, VA plans to open facilities in Grand Junction, Orlando, Cape Cod, Iron Mountain, Berlin and Watertown. The other new Vet centers are scheduled to open in 2008.

[74] Testimony of Acting Under Secretary for Health Department of Veterans Affairs Dr. Michael J. Kussman, in U.S. Congress, House Committee on Veterans' Affairs Subcommittee on Oversight and Investigations, hearing on *Servicemembers' Seamless Transition into Civilian Life — The Heroes Return*, 110th Cong., 1st sess., March 8, 2007.

[75] For a list of who is eligible for Vet Center services, see [http://www.va.gov/RCS/ Eligibility.asp].

[76] Testimony of Under Secretary for Health, Department of Veterans Affairs, Dr. Michael J. Kussman, in U.S. Congress, House Committee on Veterans' Affairs, hearing on the *Long-Term Costs of the Current Conflicts*, 110th Cong., 1st sess., October 17, 2007.

[77] In 1996, the President's Advisory Committee on Gulf War Veterans' Illnesses reported on many deficiencies in VA's and DOD's data capabilities for handling servicemembers' medical records. In November 1997, the President called for the two departments to start developing a comprehensive, lifelong medical record for each service member. In 1998 the President issued a executive order requiring VA and DOD to develop a "computer-based patient record system that will accurately and efficiently exchange information."

[78] Bob Brewin, "VA to debut new patient tracking system," *Government Executive*, April 20, 2007. Available at [http://www.govexec.com/dailyfed/0407/042007br1 .htm].

[79] The Joint Patient Tracking Application (JPTA) was created primarily as an electronic record for tracking where a patient was in the military healthcare system when moving from the battlefield to a field hospital to Landstuhl, Germany, and then on to Military Treatment facilities in the US. Although there has been some medical information inserted into the JPTA, including X-rays and scans done in theater, JPTA is not a complete medical record.

[80] The Veterans Programs Enhancement Act of 1998 (P.L. 105-368) [38 U.S.C. § 1710(e)(1)(D) and §1710(e)(3)(C)] authorized VA to provide health care for an initial two-year period after discharge from service for veterans (including National Guard and Reserve components) in combat during any period of war after the first Gulf War or during any other future period of hostilities after November 11, 1998, even if there is insufficient medical evidence to conclude that such illnesses are attributable to such service. For combat veterans who do not enroll with VA during the two-year post-discharge period, eligibility for enrollment and subsequent health care is subject to such factors as a service-connected disability rating, VA pension status, catastrophic disability determination, or financial circumstances (as described in this chapter). If their financial circumstances place them in Priority Group 8, they will be "grandfathered" into a Priority Group 8a or Priority Group 8c, and their enrollment in VA will be continued, regardless of the date of their original VA application.

[81] Dana Priest and Anne Hull, "Soldiers Face Neglect, Frustration At Army's Top Medical Facility," *Washington Post*, February 18, 2007.

[82] The Task Force on Returning Global War on Terror Heroes, Report to the President, p. 3

[83] Alan West and William Weeks, "Veterans Before, During, and After the Invasion of Iraq," *Psychiatric Services*, vol. 57. no. 2 (Febrary 2006).

[84] National Academies, Institute of Medicine, *Posttraumatic Stress Disorder: Diagnosis and Assessment*, 2006.

[85] National Academies, Institute of Medicine, *Posttraumatic Stress Disorder: Diagnosis and Assessment*, 2006, p.13.

[86] Susan Okie, "Traumatic Brain Injury in the War Zone," *New England Journal of Medicine*, Vol. 352, pp. 2043-2047 May 19, 2005; and "Reconstructing Lives — A Tale of Two Soldiers," *New England Journal of Medicine*, volume 355 pp. 2609-2615 December 21, 2006.

[87] The instrument used to screen veterans is a highly sensitive, not specific, questionnaire. The questionnaire is designed to identify everyone who may possibly have suffered a TBI. It should be noted that some of those who are identified by this questionnaire as possibly having a TBI will not, in fact, receive that diagnosis upon a subsequent in-depth evaluation.

[88] Drawn from Henry L. Lew, Guest Editorial, "Rehabilitation needs of an increasing population of patients: Traumatic brain injury, polytrauma, and blast-related injuries," *Journal of Rehabilitation Research & Development*, volume 42, no. 4 July/August 2005.

[89] Peleg T, Shalev AY, "Longitudinal Studies of PTSD: Overview of Findings and Methods," *CNS Spectrum*, vol 11, no. 8, pp. 589-602, 2006.

[90] Defense and Veterans Brain Injury Centers are located at Walter Reed Army Medical Center, Washington, DC; Wilford Hall US Air Force Medical Center, Lackland Air Force Base, TX; Brooke Army Medical Center, Fort Sam Houston, TX; Naval Medical Center-San Diego, San Diego, CA; Hunter McGuire VA Medical Center, Richmond, VA; James A Haley VA Hospital, Tampa, FL; Veterans Affairs Medical Center, Minneapolis, MN; VA Palo Alto Health Care System, Palo Alto, CA; and Lakeview Virginia NeuroCare, Charlottesville, VA (Civilian Partner Site). Further information available at [http://www.dvbic.org/index.html].

[91] For a detailed explanation on appropriated entitlements, see CRS Report RS20 129, *Entitlements and Appropriated Entitlements in the Federal Budget Process,* by Bill Heniff Jr.

[92] House Committee on Veterans' Affairs, "Committee Hears Legislative Views of Millions of Veterans," press release, September 20, 2006.

[93] U.S. Congressional Budget Office, Cost Estimate, H.R. 515 (109th Congress), Assured Funding for Veterans Health Care Act of 2005, July 25, 2005, p.1.

[94] Testimony of Richard Kogan, Center on Budget and Policy Priorities at the Alternative Processes for Funding Veterans Health Care Forum, June 3, 2004. Transcript available at [http://www.dav.org/voters

[95] U.S. Congress, House Committee on Veterans Affairs, hearing on *Funding the U.S. Department of Veterans Affairs of the Future*, 110th Congress, 1st sess.,October 3, 2007.

[96] Department of Veterans Affairs, "Enrollment — Provision of Hospital and Outpatient Care to Veterans Subpriorities of Priority Categories 7 and 8 and Annual Enrollment Level Decision; Final Rule," *68 Federal Register* 2670, January 17, 2003.

[97] For detailed information on the FY2007 veterans health care budget see, CRS Report RL33409, *Veterans' Medical Care: FY2007 Appropriations*, by Sidath Viranga Panangala.

[98] Department of Veterans Affairs, *FY2006 Budget Submission, Medical Programs*, vol. 2 of 4, pp. 2-4.

[99] U.S. Congress, Senate Committee on Appropriations, *Department Veterans Affairs, and Housing and Urban Development and Independent Agencies Appropriations for FY2005*, hearings on H.R. 5041/S. 2825, 108th Cong., 2nd sess., April 6, 2004, S.Hrg. 108-776, p. 379.

[100] Democratic and Independent Members of the Committee on Veterans' Affairs Views and Estimates on the FY2008 budget for Function 700 (Veterans' Benefits and Services), March 1, 2007.

[101] 38 U.S.C. § 17 12(d); 38 C.F.R. § 17.96.

[102] A formulary is a list of drugs approved for coverage under a drug benefit.

[103] U.S. General Accounting Office, *VA Health Care: Capital Asset Planning and Budgeting Need Improvement*, GAO/T-HEHS-99-83, March 10, 1999, pp. 1-6.

[104] The Draft National CARES Plan (DNCP) defines realignment as: moving services from one facility to another, contracting for care to ensure inpatient access to care is available when needed, and in all cases maintaining outpatient services in the community.

[105] Department of Veterans Affairs, Office of the Secretary, Secretary of Veterans Affairs, *CARES Decision*, May 2004, pp. 1-8.

[106] Honorable Bob Graham, "Statements on Introduced Bill and Joint Resolutions," remarks in the Senate, *Congressional Record*, 108th Congress, vol. 149 (June 18, 2003), p. S8135.

[107] The 18 sites are Boston, MA (VISN 1); Canandaigua, NY (VISN 2); Montrose, NY (VISN 3); New York City, NY (VISN 3); St. Albans, NY (VISN 3); Perry Point, MD (VISN 5); Montgomery, AL (VISN 7); Louisville, KY (VISN 9); Lexington, KY (VISN 9); Poplar Bluff, MO (VISN 15); Biloxi, MS (VSIN 16); Muskogee, OK (VISN 16); Waco, TX (VISN 17); Big Spring, TX (VISN 18); Walla Walla, WA (VISN 20); White City, OR (VISN 20) Livermore, CA (VISN 21); West LA, CA (VISN 22).

[108] Government Accountability Office, *VA Health Care: VA Should Better Monitor Implementation and Impact of Capital Asset Alignment Decisions,* GAO-07-408, March 2007.

[109] Veterans Administration, "Transportation of Claimants and Beneficiaries," final regulations, 52 FR 7575-01, March 12, 1987. These regulations became effective on April 13, 1987.

[110] Ibid.

[111] For benefit legislation, see CRS Report RL33985, *Veterans' Benefits: Issues in the 110th Congress,* by Carol D. Davis, Coordinator.

[112] S. 1233 contained provisions from the following bills: S. 117, S. 383, S. 472, S. 692, S. 874, S. 994, S. 1026, S. 1146, S. 1147, S. 1326, S. 1384, S. 1392, and S. 1396.

[113] U.S. Congress, Senate Committee on Veterans' Affairs, *Veterans' Traumatic Brain Injury and Other Health Programs Improvement Act of 2007*, report to accompany S. 1233, 1 10th Congress, 1st sess., S.Rept. 110-147, p. 12.

[114] Ibid, p. 13.

[115] Ibid.

CHAPTER SOURCES

The following chapters have been previously published:

Chapter 1 – This is an edited, excerpted and augmented edition of a United States Congressional Research Service publication, Report Order Code RL34598, dated July 29, 2008.

Chapter 2 – This is an edited, excerpted and augmented edition of a United States Congressional Research Service publication, Report Order Code RL33704, dated March 20, 2008.

Chapter 3 – This is an edited, excerpted and augmented edition of a United States Congressional Research Service publication, Report Order Code RL34549, dated June 25, 2008.

Chapter 4 - This is an edited, excerpted and augmented edition of a United States Congressional Research Service publication, Report Order Code RL31664, dated January 17, 2007.

Chapter 5 – This is an edited, excerpted and augmented edition of a United States Congressional Research Service publication, Report Order Code RL33323, dated May 15, 2008.

Chapter 6 – This is an edited, excerpted and augmented edition of a United States Congressional Research Service publication, Report Order Code RL33991, dated January 30, 2008.

Chapter 7 – This is an edited, excerpted and augmented edition of a United States Congressional Research Service publication, Report Order Code RL33113, dated April 24, 2008.

Chapter 8 – This is an edited, excerpted and augmented edition of a United States Congressional Research Service publication, Report Order Code RS22804, dated February 6, 2008.

Chapter 9 – This is an edited, excerpted and augmented edition of a United States Congressional Research Service publication, Report Order Code RS22483, dated June 3, 2008.

Chapter 10 – This is an edited, excerpted and augmented edition of a United States Congressional Research Service publication, Report Order Code RL34371, dated February 13, 2008.

Chapter 11 – This is an edited, excerpted and augmented edition of a United States Congressional Research Service publication, Report Order Code RL344371, dated May 5, 2008.

Chapter 12 – This is an edited, excerpted and augmented edition of a United States Congressional Research Service publication, Report Order Code RS22897, dated June 13, 2008.

Chapter 13 – This is an edited, excerpted and augmented edition of a United States Government Accountability Office (GAO), Report to Congressional Committees. Publication GAO-08-535, dated May 2007.

Chapter 14 – This is an edited, excerpted and augmented edition of a United States Congressional Research Service publication, Report Order Code RS22929, dated July 28, 2008.

Chapter 15 – This is an edited, excerpted and augmented edition of a United States Congressional Research Service publication, Report Order Code RL33993, dated November 30, 2007.

INDEX

A

B

C

F

G

H

I

J

L

M

N

T

U

V

W

X

Y

Z